New Comprehensive Biochemistry

Volume 5

General Editors

A. NEUBERGER
London

L.L.M. van DEENEN
Utrecht

ELSEVIER
AMSTERDAM · NEW YORK · OXFORD

PROSTAGLANDINS AND RELATED SUBSTANCES

Prostaglandins and related substances

Editors

C. PACE-ASCIAK and E. GRANSTRÖM
Toronto *Stockholm*

1983

ELSEVIER
AMSTERDAM · NEW YORK · OXFORD

ISBN for the series: 0444 80303 3
ISBN for the volume: 0444 80517 6

Published by:
Elsevier Science Publishers B.V.
PO Box 211
1000 AE Amsterdam
The Netherlands

Sole distributors for the U.S.A. and Canada:
Elsevier Science Publishing Co. Inc.
52 Vanderbilt Avenue
New York, NY 10017
USA

Library of Congress Cataloging in Publication Data

Main entry under title:
Prostaglandins and related substances.
(New comprehensive biochemistry; v. 5)
Includes index.
1. Prostaglandins – Metabolism – Addresses, essays, lectures. I. Pace-Asciak, C. (Cecil) II. Granström, E. (Elisabeth) III. Series. [DNLM: 1. Prostaglandins. 2. Thromboxanes. 3. Lipoxygenases. W1 NE372F v. 5/QU 90 P9672a 1983]
QD415.N48 vol. 5 [QP801.P68] 574.19'2s [612'.405] 83-11491
ISBN 0-444-80517-6

Printed in The Netherlands

PROSTAGLANDINS AND RELATED SUBSTANCES

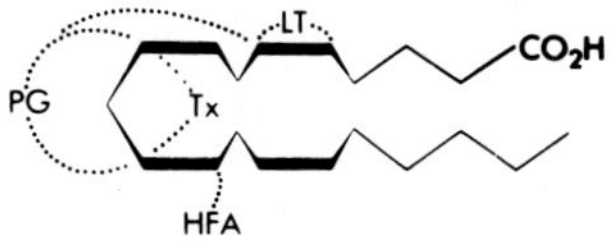

Preface

Since the chemical structures of the prostaglandins were elucidated and their biosynthesis from polyunsaturated fatty acids discovered in the early 1960's, the following two decades have seen an almost explosive development in prostaglandin research.

During the last ten years numerous discoveries were made in this field, and research was initiated in a large number of new areas. Among the mile-stones of this last decade were the isolation of the potent endoperoxide intermediates; the discovery of non-steroidal anti-inflammatory drugs as inhibitors of the fatty acid cyclooxygenase; the discovery of the mutually antagonistic endoperoxide products,

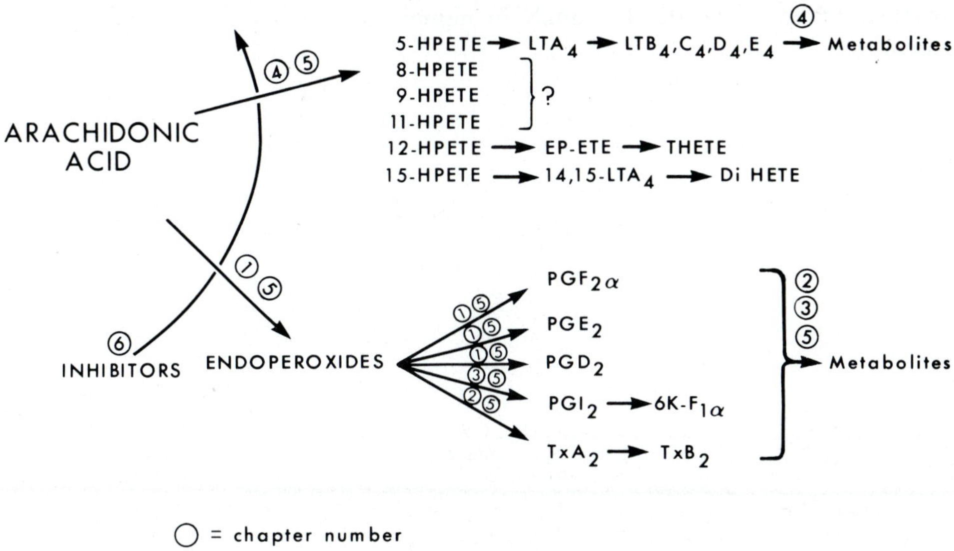

the thromboxanes and prostacyclins, whose existence had earlier gone unnoticed mostly because of their instability and the fact that they were formed only in small amounts from the precursor fatty acids; the elucidation of prostaglandin metabolism with the structure determination of a vast number of final break-down products and the identification of metabolites suitable for monitoring in various biological systems; the development of sensitive and specific quantitation methods and their application in a large number of biological studies; studies on the release of precursor fatty acids from esterified forms catalysed by various hydrolases as a key event in prostaglandin biosynthesis; the inhibition of phospholipase-catalysed fatty acid release by anti-inflammatory steroids and the elucidation of the underlying mechanism; the discovery of novel pathways in the conversion of polyunsaturated fatty acids leading to the recently discovered non-prostanoate compounds, the leukotrienes and their related products; the recognition of numerous biological roles of the members of the prostaglandin family and their involvement in the pathogenesis of a multitude of disorders and diseases; and finally, the beginning of the clinical use of certain prostaglandins in the treatment of gynecological, gastro-intestinal and circulatory conditions.

The rapid development of a greatly enhanced volume of published scientific data has increased the need for comprehensive reviews, written by scientists who are themselves active in the field, and providing the current state-of-the-science of the area.

The contributors of this volume in the New Comprehensive Biochemistry series cover the biosynthesis and metabolism of the prostaglandins, thromboxanes and leukotrienes; the analytical methods currently in use; the purification and properties of several enzymes involved in the formation and catabolism of these substances; activators and inhibitors of these enzymes; as well as the involvement of the members of the prostaglandin family in numerous physiological and pathological processes.

Bengt Samuelsson

Contents

Preface vii

Introduction. Physiological implications of products in the arachidonic acid cascade, by Marie L. Foegh and Peter W. Ramwell *xiii*

Chapter 1. The prostaglandins and essential fatty acids, by Ernst Oliw, Elisabeth Granström and Erik Änggard *1*

1. Introduction 1
2. Structure and nomenclature 2
3. Essential fatty acids 4
4. Oxygenation of essential fatty acids 8
5. Biosynthesis and metabolism of prostaglandin endoperoxides 10
6. Biological effects of prostaglandins 11
   (a) General 11
   (b) The reproductive system 13
   (c) Kidney function 14
   (d) Platelets 15
   (e) Gastrointestinal functions 15
   (f) The vascular system 16
   (g) The respiratory system 16
   (h) The nervous system 17
7. Metabolism of prostaglandins 19
8. Assay of prostaglandin production 23
9. Monooxygenase metabolism of prostaglandins and essential fatty acids 27
10. Dietary factors influencing prostaglandin production 29
11. Perspectives 33

References 34

Chapter 2. The thromboxanes, by Elisabeth Granström, Ulf Diczfalusy and Mats Hamberg *45*

1. Introduction 45
2. Discovery of thromboxanes 45
   (a) Elucidation of thromboxane structure 46
   (b) Nomenclature for thromboxanes 49
   (c) Biological effects of thromboxanes 50
3. Biosynthesis of thromboxanes 52

(a) Occurrence of thromboxane synthetase 52
(b) Purification of thromboxane synthetase 53
(c) Properties of thromboxane synthetase 54
(d) Modulation of thromboxane synthesis 55
4. Metabolism of thromboxanes 60
5. Assay methods for thromboxanes 62
(a) Assay of thromboxane A_2 62
(b) Assay of thromboxane B_2 65
(c) Pitfalls in thromboxane assay 65
(d) Assay of thromboxane metabolites 66
6. Thromboxane agonists and antagonists 67
(a) Agonists 67
(b) Antagonists 68
7. Thromboxanes and the lung 70
8. Roles of thromboxanes in platelet function 73
9. Thromboxane formation in pathological conditions 76
10. Alteration of thromboxane-prostacyclin balance in vivo: approaches in thrombosis prevention 78
References 82

Chapter 3. The prostacyclins, by Cecil Pace-Asciak and Richard Gryglewski 95

1. Introduction 95
2. Nomenclature 96
3. Biochemistry 98
(a) Biosynthesis 98
(b) Tissue distribution 99
(c) Enzyme properties 101
(d) Inhibitors 102
(e) Catabolism 102
4. Levels in biological fluids 104
(a) Plasma 104
(b) Urine 105
(c) Amniotic fluid 105
(d) Cerebrospinal fluid 107
5. Problems encountered with measurements of PGI_2 and 6-keto $PGF_{1\alpha}$ 108
6. Pharmacology 109
(a) Effects on platelets in vitro 109
(b) Antithrombotic effect in laboratory animals 110
(c) Cardiovascular effects 112
(d) Clinical trials 114
References 118

Chapter 4. The leukotrienes and other lipoxygenase products, by Göran Hansson, Curt Malmsten and Olof Rådmark 127

1. Introduction 127
2. Leukotrienes: classification and nomenclature 127
3. Biosynthesis of trienes 129
(a) Leukotrienes of types A and B 129
(b) Leukotrienes of types C, D and E (slow reacting substances SRS) 132
(c) Some characteristics of leukotriene producing systems 134

4. Other lipoxygenase products 134
(a) Lipoxygenase products 135
(b) Some properties of lipoxygenase 138
(c) Alternative preparations of lipoxygenase products 139
5. Metabolism of leukotrienes 140
(a) Metabolism of cysteinyl-containing leukotrienes 140
(b) Metabolism of LTB compounds 141
6. Biological effects of leukotrienes and other lipoxygenase products 142
(a) Effects of LTB compounds 142
(b) Effects of cysteinyl-containing leukotrienes 148
7. Assay methods for leukotrienes and other lipoxygenase products 150
(a) Assays based on biological activity 150
(b) Assays based on chromatography and UV absorption 152
(c) Gas chromatography-mass spectrometry and radioimmunoassays 154
8. Inhibitors of lipoxygenase and leukotriene synthesis, SRS antagonists 155
(a) Lipoxygenase inhibitors 155
(b) Inhibitors of other enzymes in the leukotriene pathways 157
(c) Antagonists to SRS 158
References 158

Chapter 5. Enzymes in the arachidonic acid cascade, by Shozo Yamamoto *171*

1. Introduction 171
2. Prostaglandin endoperoxide-synthesizing enzymes 171
(a) Fatty acid cyclooxygenase 172
(b) Prostaglandin hydroperoxidase 178
(c) Summary 181
3. Prostaglandin endoperoxide-metabolizing enzymes 183
(a) TXA synthase 183
(b) PGD synthase 184
(c) PGE synthase 184
(d) PGF synthase 185
(e) PGI synthase 185
(f) PGA synthase 186
(g) PGC synthase 186
(h) PGB synthase 186
4. Prostaglandin and thomboxane-catabolizing enzymes 187
(a) 15-Hydroxy-PG dehydrogenase 187
(b) 9-Hydroxy-PG dehydrogenase 190
(c) PG 9-Keto reductase 191
(d) PG Δ^{13}-reductase 192
(e) β-Oxidation 192
(f) ω-Oxidation 192
5. Lipoxygenases 193
(a) 12-Lipoxygenase 195
(b) 5-Lipoxygenase 195
(c) 15-Lipoxygenase 195
(d) Reticulocyte lipoxygenase 196
(e) PG production by soybean lipoxygenase 196
6. Cytochrome *P*-450 196
References 197

Chapter 6. Inhibitors and activators of prostaglandin biosynthesis, by William E.M. Lands and Arthur M. Hanel *203*

1. Introduction 203
2. Activators of prostaglandin biosynthesis 205
   (a) Heme 205
   (b) Peroxidase cosubstrates 205
   (c) Lipid hydroperoxides 206
3. Inhibitors of prostaglandin biosynthesis 207
   (a) General aspects 207
   (b) Mechanisms of inhibitor action 210
   (c) IC_{50} concepts and concerns 214
   (d) General data available 219
4. Summary 220

References 221

Subject index 225

INTRODUCTION

Physiological implications of products in the arachidonic acid cascade

MARIE L. FOEGH [a] and PETER W. RAMWELL [b]

Departments of Medicine [a] and Physiology and Biophysics [b], Georgetown University Medical Center, Washington, D.C. 20007, U.S.A.

Physiology is the study of function. The classical procedure used to define physiological roles is by extirpation, ablation or nerve section to reveal inadequate or inappropriate function in the absence of the postulated mechanism. This approach cannot be used to study the physiological role of arachidonate metabolites since they are not organ-localized like the adrenal steroids or concentrated in specific cells like the adrenergic transmitters. The problem is compounded also by the fact that arachidonate oxygenation is almost a universal phenomenon. Finally the metabolites are not stored like histamine or serotonin but are released immediately upon synthesis. Consequently it is always necessary to initiate synthesis to study release. Thus release is synonymous with synthesis.

The emphasis on physiology in this section also relates to the nature and quantity of the arachidonate metabolites released. For example some naive authors state that "Prostaglandins at physiological concentrations were found to be...". It is extremely difficult for such concentrations to be defined and such authors are begging the question as to what is physiological. The other 'begging' question is to assume that the cell or tissue 'sees' only one metabolite in vivo, i.e. the one in which the author is interested. This has been a particular problem in macrophage studies where the usual product measured is prostaglandin E_2 and little account has been taken of the other metabolites. In rodent and human macrophages frequently equimolar amounts of both TXB_2 and PGE_2 are released but little is known of their interaction. It is possible that the thromboxane released may completely block PGE mediated elevations in cyclic AMP, or again, because of its transient nature, TXA_2 may have little effect. Nevertheless, to avoid consideration of all the products and their interaction is simplistic.

Two other points are frequently neglected when discussing physiological roles. The first is that arachidonate metabolite receptors may be subject to regulation. Thus it is not enough to define the concentration of product formed if there are marked changes in the receptors. This appears to be the case for PGE compounds in the myometrium and liver [1]. PGE analogues clearly may down-regulate PGE receptors in the liver and estrogen down-regulates the myometrial receptors to $PGF_{2\alpha}$ and PGE_2. Other hormones may be involved; recent studies have implicated prolactin in ovarian receptor regulation and the $PGF_{2\alpha}$ receptors in the corpus luteum are known to be regulated by luteinizing hormone [2]. There is evidence from our own laboratory that estrogen and testosterone regulate prostaglandin receptors in rat aorta [3].

The second point is the role of converting and catabolising enzymes. There is now evidence for the conversion of PGI_2 to the stable product 6-keto-PGE_1 which has very similar properties [4]. There is also convincing evidence for PGE_2 to $PGF_{2\alpha}$ conversion [5] and vice versa [6]. Finally there is strong evidence that the further metabolism of PGs by prostaglandin dehydrogenase (PGDH) has a significant role as demonstrated by PGDH inhibition leading to luteolysis in rodents [7]. These therefore are points which need to be borne in mind when interpreting data as to the physiological role of arachidonate metabolites.

An approach to functional ablation has been to evaluate the effects of acute essential fatty acid (EFA) deficiency. This deficiency has been shown to cause dermatoses in both humans [8,9] and animals [10]. Van Dorp (1971) [11] reported a marked decrease in PGE_2 in skin of EFA-deficient rats and Ziboh and Hsia (1972) [12] subsequently found that topical application of PGE_2 cleared the scaly dermatoses. However, a potential difficulty is the accumulation of 5,8,11-eicosatrienoic acid (20 : 3, *n*-9) which may be responsible for some of the symptoms namely loss of skin elasticity, alopecia and scaliness. Ziboh et al. [13] showed that this trienoic acid inhibits cyclooxygenase activity. Since this fatty acid accumulates in the skin of EFA deficient rats it was tested on the skin of nude mice where at only 50 μM it significantly reduced PGE_2 and produced the scaly dermatoses. In addition it is possible that blocking the cyclooxygenase shunts arachidonate through the lipoxygenase pathway and products of this pathway are reported elevated in psoriasis [14]. Since 5,8,11-eicosatrienoic acid has proved to be a substrate for 5 lipoxygenase and thus can yield leukotrienes, it is likely that the dermatoses characteristic of EFA deficiency may not necessarily result from a PGE_2 deficiency only. Especially since lipoxygenase products are associated with psoriasis. Consequently care must be taken in interpreting data from EFA deficient animals. However it is possible to avoid the problem of redirection of synthesis by use of receptor antagonists.

Although the attempt to "ablate" or "extirpate" arachidonate metabolites by using EFA deficiency can be complex, nevertheless it is an approach to the physiological role of these metabolites which deserves further exploration since it offers so many experimental models. For example in immunology, evidence is accruing that the cyclooxygenase products which elevate cyclic AMP are immunosuppressive [15]. Feeding with essential fatty acids also produces immunosuppression [12] whilst indomethacin abrogates this effect [17]. Moreover there have been reports that cyclooxygenase inhibitors may increase anti-body response in vivo [18]. These EFA feeding experiments raises the interesting question of immune responses in Eskimos. Does the fish diet which is so rich in eicosapentaenoic acid, lead to enhanced immune response? One might anticipate this to be the case since this acid competes with arachidonate for the cyclooxygenase and thus acts as a "nutritional aspirin".

An extremely important approach to blocking all arachidonate metabolism is the use of 5,8,11,14-eicosatetraynoic acid [19]. This acetylenic analogue of arachidonate was first used to inhibit cyclooxygenase in 1970 and was replaced in 1971 by the non steroidal anti-inflammatory drugs. Later it returned to favor when it was realized that tetraynoic acid blocks the lipoxygenase pathways too. Consequently eicosatetraynoic acid treatment does not involve the complications involved in the use of either eicosapentaenoic acid or other essential fatty acids.

Eicosatetraynoic acid treatment of rats leads to the same deleterious effect on the gastro-intestinal mucosa as seen with indomethacin [20]. These effects, like the skin lesions in EFA deficiency, can be prevented by treatment with prostaglandins. The concept that prostaglandins of the E series are cytoprotective in the stomach has been suggested in several other body systems. One might also use the term cytoprotective to describe the prominent and widespread immunosuppressive effect of these types of arachidonate metabolites.

A less rigorous approach to evaluating the physiological role of the cyclooxygenase products has been to use potent cyclooxygenase inhibitors such as indomethacin. These compounds have many side effects and as discussed earlier, cyclooxygenase inhibition may lead to increased lipoxygenase product formation. Nevertheless the approach has been effective in revealing the role of the cyclooxygenase products. The most significant area has been cardiovascular homeostasis which will be discussed later in terms of renal and perinatal cardiovascular homeostasis.

The drawback to the use of cyclooxygenase inhibitors respecting arachidonate diversion to lipoxygenase products can be overcome by specific inhibition of individual pathways. This more precise approach is proving a useful method of dissecting out the roles of the individual metabolites. The importance of thromboxane synthase inhibition with the substituted imidazoles and pyrimidine was quickly appreciated. Inhibition of prostacyclin synthase with 15 hydroperoxy eicosatetraenoic acid or with tranylcypromine has been less successful. By and large the data indicate in pathophysiological models that inhibition of thromboxane synthase is protective to some degree but this may be related to an increase in prostacyclin due to divergence of the endoperoxides. An example of such divergence was seen in vitro in human peritoneal macrophages [21] as well as in vivo in baboons [22] treated with the thromboxane synthase inhibitor OKY-1581. Aiken has provided striking evidence for a physiological role for prostacyclin in the dog coronary circulation [23].

An even more precise tool is the use of receptor antagonists. In this respect the evaluation of the role of histamine is particularly instructive. Histamine was clearly recognised as a mediator of tissue injury by Sir Thomas Lewis in his classical triple response studies. This is the case now with respect to leukotrienes and thromboxane in immunological and cardiovascular pathology. But in order for histamine to be convincingly shown to have a physiological role in gastric secretion for example, it was necessary to await the development of the H_2 receptor antagonist in the early 1970s by Black [24]. In the prostaglandin area an analagous situation is particularly the case with prostacyclin. The many roles for this important metabolite have been so strongly asserted that only a specific receptor antagonist will separate the puffery from reality. The advantage of receptor antagonists is that they do not cause redirection of synthesis as is seen with thromboxane synthase inhibitors for example. It is also possible to manipulate prostaglandin receptors like other receptors with thiol reagents. The prostaglandin receptors are far more sensitive to dithiothreitol for example than acetylcholine. This approach is useful since it is reversible and moreover the receptor can be "capped" or protected with prostanoic acid [25].

Valuable clues as to the physiological roles of endogenous substances are frequently derived from glandular failure as for example in Hashimoto's disease which involves destruction of the thyroid glandular epithelium. Unfortunately no such syndrome has yet been identified with respect to arachidonate synthesis. Perhaps the nearest to such an effect is the essential fatty acid deficiency due to liver failure in cirrhosis of the liver [26]. Defects in metabolic pathways or in the absence of receptors also frequently provide valuable clues. A deficiency in platelet cyclooxygenase has been reported but this defect apparently involves only a minor bleeding tendency [27,28]. More such defects are being reported now. For example attention is being focused particularly on the relation of diabetes to decreased endothelial prostacyclin synthesis [29] and possible elevation of platelet thromboxane. Changes in the response of coronary artery preparations have also been reported in experimentally induced diabetes in the dog [31].

A number of these approaches have been applied to evaluating the role of arachidonate metabolites in perinatal physiology [32–34]. The evidence that arachidonate metabolites have a regulatory role in fetal homeostasis is becoming well established. This is because attention became directed to the key role of the ductus arteriosus. The mechanism concerning the role of arachidonic metabolites in maintaining patency is particularly interesting in that the lipoxygenase pathway does not appear to be involved and only one cyclooxygenase metabolite may be implicated namely PGE_2. However, a role for both PGD_2 and PGI_2 has been also postulated. PGD_2 increases cardiac output and reduces pulmonary and systemic resistance but is only a very weak dilator of the ductus arteriosus [35]. PGD_2 is particularly interesting as there is evidence that PGD_2 receptors appear relatively late in gestation. Thus it is possible that PGD_2 and PGE_2 may be acting synergistically. The case for PGI_2 is attractive but more conjectural. It has been suggested that if PGI_2 is the primary ductus vasodilator then the high pO_2 on delivery may destroy the notoriously susceptible prostacyclin synthase and the loss of PGI_2 permits the human ductus to be obliterated [36]. Nevertheless based upon the utility of indomethacin to close the patent ductus and the properties of the vasodilator cyclooxygenase metabolites on pulmonary vessels, as well as the ductus, there is little doubt as to the significance of their role in perinatal hemodynamics. One additional aspect is that the cyclooxygenase vasoconstrictor products $PGF_{2\alpha}$ and TXA_2 may exert a tonic constrictor effect. This is a biochemical hypothesis with little hemodynamic support. Nevertheless it would be easy to test in view of the availability of specific thromboxane synthase inhibitors, as well as receptor agonists to thromboxane and $PGF_{2\alpha}$.

A great deal of effort has been invested into determining the role of arachidonate metabolism in the kidney. As McGiff [37] points out it is useful to consider two roles for arachidonate metabolites, firstly with respect to the blood compartment and secondly with respect to tubular mechanisms. The role of the arachidonate metabolites in the regulation of the renal circulation is to protect the kidney against powerful vasoconstrictor substances such as angiotensin II [38]. The renal vascular vasodilator arachidonate metabolites such as PGE_2 are released under these circumstances and also following renal sympathetic activity [39,40]. Where the renal circulation is compromised in the diseased kidney or during dehydration then indomethacin decreases kidney function often in a reversible manner [41]. The suggestion has been offered that this deterioration may not be entirely due to lack of arachidonate vasodilator metabolites but may also be due to products with vasoconstrictor effects. The effect of leukotrienes on renin release is currently being investigated, but the vasodilator arachidonate metabolites are well known to release renin [37–39].

The renal kallikrein-kinin [40] system has been suggested as influencing renal hemodynamic as well as excretory function. This activity may also be linked to arachidonate metabolites, like PGE_2, since increased excretion of cyclooxygenase products are associated with increased kallikrein-kinin excretion. However, the physiological significance of this relationship is uncertain.

The role of arachidonate metabolites in tubular function [41,42] is more complex although the PGE compounds were shown early on to block the effect of the antidiuretic hormone (ADH) on transporting epithelia. The reason for the complexity is the effect of PGE compounds on sodium and water transport on the one hand and their effect in changing renal blood flow and intrarenal distribution on the other. It is now generally believed that the role of the vasodilator metabolites is to preserve renal homeostasis and that their effect becomes apparent when the kidney function is compromised [43]. The problem with which one is faced is to fit into this scheme the ADH-like effects of thromboxane [44] and the effects of the leukotrienes, when they are properly defined. It is possible that thromboxane and leukotrienes only become prominent in the pathological situation but this remains to be documented.

In conclusion, the oxygenation of arachidonic acid yields an extensive series of products which are universally distributed in all animal species and nearly all cells. These metabolites constitute a modulating system for maintaining homeostasis, e.g. for preserving hemostasis, hemodynamic and renal function, for signalling pain, for regulating immunological responsivity etc. One may think of them as a Claude Bernard homeostatic hormone. The role of such a universal system needs to be modulatory since so many substances involved in injury and inflammation interact with it, e.g. vasoactive amines, kallikrein and kinins, clotting factors and thrombin, complements, plasmin, platelet activating factor and oxygen derived products.

The homeostatic role of the vasodilator cyclooxygenase products in preserving hemostasis, and in pain, cytoprotection and immunosuppression can be readily appreciated and to this one can add the role of thromboxane in bleeding. It may well be that thromboxane has a very limited role probably due to its short half-life. The role of $PGF_{2\alpha}$ per se is more difficult to distinguish; an interesting view is that the conversion of PGE_2 to $PGF_{2\alpha}$ by the renal 9-ketoreductase is a method for regulating PGE_2 concentrations [45]. This idea may have general applicability since the enzyme is widely distributed. This type of conversion is especially interesting since PGI_2 is converted to its stable "mimic" 6-keto-PGE_1 by a 9-hydroxy dehydrogenase [46]. Unlike the 9 keto reductase, this latter enzyme will serve to facilitate PGI_2-like activity. Another promising interaction is the stimulation of cyclooxygenase product formation by the leukotrienes [47]. This may be a positive feedback to promote the formation of the adenylate cyclase stimulating vasodilator products.

The physiological role of thromboxane is delineated by its short half-life. The fleeting existence of this molecule serves to localize and to limit its pathogenic properties to the microvasculature during bleeding. If the synthase were to be induced, then physiology would change to pathology.

In summary, a primary homeostatic mechanism, which is present in most cells, depends upon the selective oxygenation of arachidonic acid. The role of these oxygenated products is to protect and preserve not only cells but tissues and perhaps organs. This protection is jeopardized in trauma and multiple injury. Under these circumstances, there is massive release of free arachidonate leading to formation of large amounts of oxygen-related free radicals and excessive production of deleterious arachidonate metabolites. The effect of these metabolites is mediated in part by promoting Ca^{2+} influx. Thus one can anticipate that protection can be obtained not only by interdicting arachidonate metabolites, but also by using Ca^{2+} blocking agents which are now so widely available.

References

1 Garrity, M.F. and Robertson, R.P. (1983) Adv. Prostaglandin Thromboxane Leukotriene Res. 12, 279–282.
2 Behrman, H.R. (1979) Ann. Res. Physiol. 41, 685–700.
3 Karanian, J.W., Ramey, E.R. and Ramwell, P.W. (1982) J. Androl. 3, 262–265.
4 Wong, P.Y-K., Lee, W.H., Reiss, R.F. and McGiff, J.C., (1980) Fed. Proc. 39, 392.
5 Lin, Y.M. and Jarabak, J. (1978) Biochem. Biophys. Res. Commun. 81, 1227–1234.
6 Pace-Asciak, C. (1975) J. Biol. Chem. 250, 2789–2794.
7 Lerner, L.J. and Carminati, P. (1976) Adv. Prostaglandin Thromboxane Res. 2, 645–653.
8 Hansen, A.E., Wiese, H.F., Boelsche, A.N., Haggard, M.E., Adam, D.J.D. and Davis, H. (1963) Pediatrics 31 (suppl. 1) 171–183.
9 Paulsrud, J.R., Pensler, L. Whitten, C.F., Stewart, S. and Holman, R.T. (1972) Am. J. Clin. Nutr. 25, 897–902.

10 Holman, R.T. (1971) Progr. Chem. Fats Other Lipids 9, 275–280.
11 Van Dorp, D.A. (1971) Ann. N.Y. Acad. Sci. 180, 181–199.
12 Ziboh, V.A. and Hsia, S.L. (1972) J. Lipid Res. 13, 458–467.
13 Ziboh, V.A., Nguyen, T.T., McCullough, J.L. and Weinstein, G.D. (1981) Progr. Lipid Res. 20, 857–865.
14 Hammarstrom, S., Hamberg, M., Samuelsson, B., Duell, E.A., Stawiski, M. and Voorhees, J. (1976) Adv. Prostaglandin Thromboxane Res. 2, 844.
15 Stenson, W.F. and Parker, C.W. (1982) in Lee (ed.) Prostaglandins Elsevier, New York, pp. 39–89.
16 Meade, C.J. and Mertin, J. (1976) Int. Arch. Allergy Appl. Immunol. 51, 2–24.
17 Mertin, J. and Stackpoole, A. (1978) Prostaglandins Med. 1, 283–291.
18 Goodwin, J.S., Selinger, D.S., Messner, R.P. and Reed, W.P. (1978) Infect. Immunol. 19, 430–433.
19 Ahern, D.C. and Downing, D.T. (1970) Biochim. Biophys. Acta 210, 456–461.
20 Shaw, J.E., Jessup, S.J. and Ramwell, P.W. (1972) Adv. Cyclic Nucleotide Res. 1, 479–491.
21 Foegh, M., Maddox, Y.T., Winchester, J., Rakowski, T., Schreiner, G. and Ramwell, P.W. (1983) Adv. Prostaglandin Thromboxane Leukotriene Res. 12, 45–49.
22 Casey, L.C., Fletcher, J.R., Zmudka, M.J. and Ramwell, P.W. (1982) J. Pharmacol. Exp. Ther. 222, 441–446.
23 Aiken, J.W., Shebuski, R.J., Miller, O.W. and Gorman, R.R. (1981) J. Pharm. Exp. Thep. 219, 299–308.
24 Black, J.W., Duncan, W.A., Durant, C.J., Ganellin, C.R. and Parsons, E.M. (1972) Nature 236, 385–390.
25 Johnson, M., Jessup, R. and Ramwell, P.W. (1983) Prostaglandins 4, 593–605.
26 Petit, J., Poupon, R., Chambaz, J., Bereziat, G. and Darnis, F. (1980) in Prostaglandins and Related Lipid. Prostaglandin Synthetase Inhibitors: New Clinical Applications (Ramwell, P.W., ed), Vol. 1, pp. 5–11, Alan R. Liss, New York.
27 Malmsten, C., Hamberg, M., Svensson, J. and Samuelsson, B. (1975) Proc. Natl. Acad. Sci. USA 72, 1446–1450.
28 Weiss, H.J. and Lages, B.A. (1977) Lancet i, 760–761.
29 Silberbauer, K., Schernthauer, G., Sinzinger, H., Winter, M. and Piza-Katzer H. (1979) Vasa 8, 213–216.
30 Harrison, H.E., Reece, A.H. and Johnson, M. (1978) Life Sci. 23, 351–356.
31 Sterin-Borda, L., Gimeno, M., Borda, E., del Castillo, E. and Gimeno, A.L. (1982) Prostaglandins 22, 267–278.
32 Coceani, F. and Olley, P.M. (1982) in Cardiovascular Pharmacology of the Prostaglandins, (A.G. Herman, P.M. Vanhoute, H. Denolin and A. Goossens, Eds.), pp. 303–314, Raven Press, New York.
33 Cassin, S. (1980) in Prostaglandins in the Perinatal Period (M.R. Heymann, Ed.), pp. 101–107, Grune and Stratton, New York.
34 Friedman, W.F., Printz, M.P., Skidgel, R.A., Benson, L.N. and Zednikova, M. (1982) Adv. Prostaglandin Thromboxane Leukotriene Res. 10, 277–302.
35 Sideris, E.B., Yokochi, K., Van Helder, T., Coceani, E. and Olley, P.M. (1983) Adv. Prostaglandin Thromboxane Leukotriene Res. 12, 477–482.
36 Needleman, P., Holmberg, S. and Mandelbaum, B. (1981) Prostaglandins 22, 675–682.
37 McGiff, J.C. (1981) Annu. Rev. Pharmacol. Toxicol. 21, 479–509.
38 Gerber, J.G., Olson, R.D. and Nies, A.S. (1981) Kidney Int. 19, 816–821.
39 McGiff, J.C., Spokas, E.G. and Wong, P.Y.-K. (1982) Br. J. Pharmacol. 75, 137–144.
40 Najsletti, A. and Malik, K.U. (1981) Kidney Int. 19, 860–868.
41 Gross, P.A., Schrier, R.W. and Anderson, R.J. (1981) Kidney Int. 19, 839–850.
42 Zusman, R.M. (1981) Annu. Rev. Med. 32, 359–374.
43 Kleinknecht, C., Broyer, M., Gubler, M.C. and Palcoux, J.B. (1980) N. Engl. J. Med. 302, 691.
44 Burch, R.M., Knapp, D.R. and Halushka, P.V. (1980) Am. J. Physiol. 239, F160–F166.
45 Weber, P.C., Larsson, C. and Scherer, B. (1977) Nature. 266, 65–66.
46 Wong, P.Y.-K., Lee, Wh., Chao, P.H.-W., Reiss, R.F. and McGiff, J.C. (1980) J. Biol. Chem. 255, 9021–9024.
47 Feuerstein, N., Foegh, M. and Ramwell, P.W. (1981) Br. J. Pharmacol. 72, 389–391.

Pace-Asciak / Granström (eds.) Prostaglandins and related substances

CHAPTER 1

The prostaglandins and essential fatty acids

ERNST OLIW [a], ELISABETH GRANSTRÖM [b] and ERIK ÄNGGÅRD [c]

Department of Pharmacology [a], Department of Physiological Chemistry [b], and Department of Alcohol and Drug Addiction Research [c], Karolinska Institutet, S-104 01 Stockholm, Sweden

1. Introduction

"The arachidonic acid content of active tissues is high... and it is natural to assume some important role for this highly unsaturated, long chain fatty acid". *George O. Burr and Mildred M. Burr, 1930 [1].*

Around 1930, two important but seemingly unrelated observations were made. Burr and Burr found that a deficiency state could be induced in rats on fat-free diets, which could be prevented by addition of polyunsaturated "essential" fatty acids to the diet [1,2]. At the same time two gynaecologists, Kurzrok and Lieb, discovered that human semen contained a factor that could cause either strong contraction or relaxation of human uterine smooth muscle [3]. Thirty years later, these observations could be linked together mainly through the pioneering work of von Euler, Bergström, van Dorp and their colleagues.

von Euler characterized the biological effects and the chemical nature of the factor in semen and described it as an acidic lipid, which he named prostaglandin [4,5]. von Euler also encouraged Bergström to determine the chemical structure of prostaglandin. In 1962, Bergström and coworkers announced the chemical formulae of prostaglandin (PG) E_1, E_2 and $F_{2\alpha}$ [6,7]. Two years later, Bergström and collaborators and a research group led by van Dorp showed independently that PGE_2 and $PGF_{2\alpha}$ were formed from arachidonic acid ($20:4\omega6$), one of the most abundant polyunsatured, long chain fatty acids in man and other mammals [8,9]. We know today that arachidonic acid and some other essential fatty acids are precursors of many different biologically active compounds, but it was the diverse and potent biological actions of prostaglandins on almost all organs which stimulated the interest in this research field. The literature on prostaglandins has increased almost exponentially over the last 20 years. Consequently, only a few important topics will be covered in this chapter.

2. Structure and nomenclature

The systematic nomenclature of prostaglandins and prostaglandin metabolites is based on prostanoic acid, a monocarboxylic acid with 20 carbon atoms, arranged as two side chains with 7 and 8 carbons, respectively, linked to a central cyclopentane ring (Fig. 1). Prostaglandins have functional groups with oxygen at carbons 9, 11 and 15 of prostanoic acid and also one, two or three double bonds in the side chains.

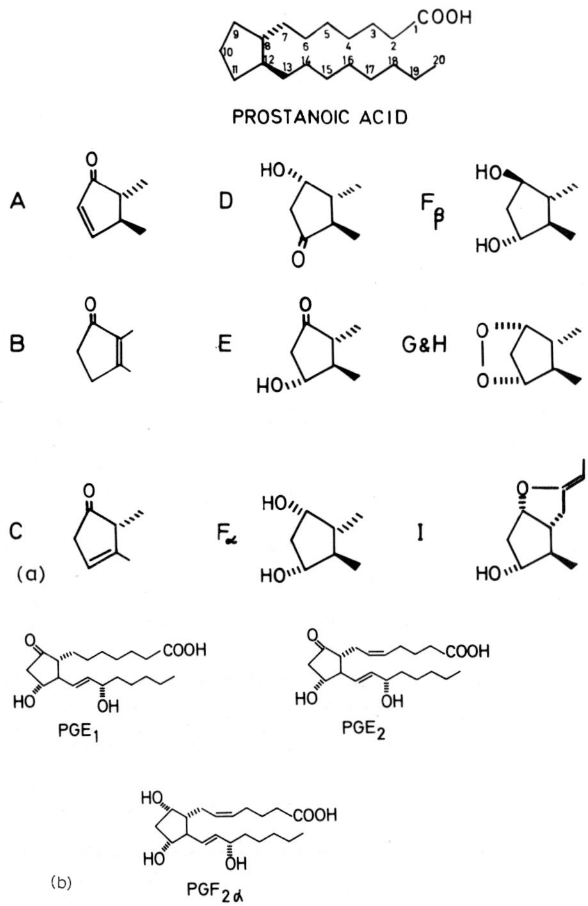

Fig. 1. (a) The structure of prostanoic acid, the carbon skeleton of the prostaglandins, and the structure and functional groups of the cyclopentane ring in prostaglandins A to I. (b) Structures of prostaglandins E_1, E_2 and $F_{2\alpha}$, the first prostaglandins to be identified (cf. refs. 6, 7).

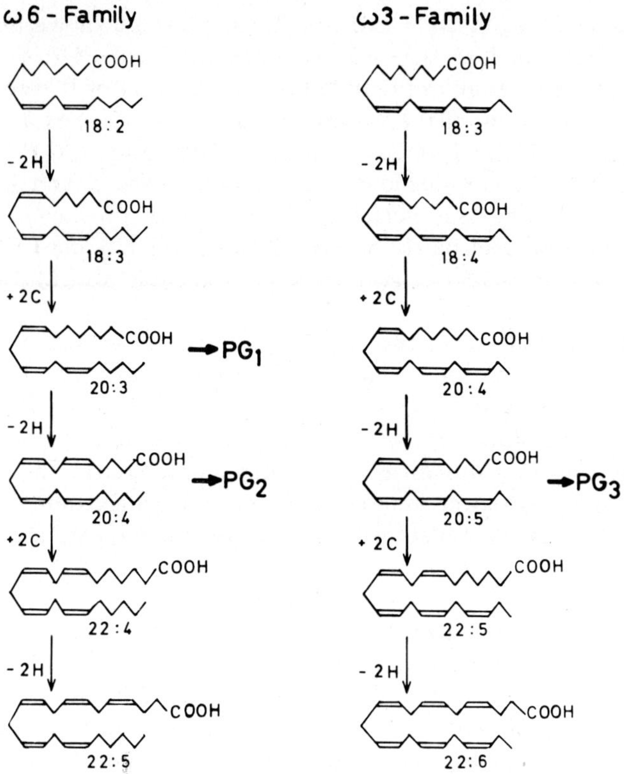

Fig. 2. Summary of the mammalian metabolism of two essential fatty acids, linoleic acid and α-linolenic acid, to other fatty acids of the ω6 and ω3 series. These fatty acids are chain-elongated and desaturated to yield the three derived essential eicosenoic acids, which are precursors of the prostaglandins of the 1-, 2- and 3-series (PG_1, PG_2 and PG_3 in this figure). Reproduced with permission from Änggård, E. and Oliw, E. (1981) Kidney Int. 19, 771–780.

Prostaglandins of the 1 series have a *trans* double bond in the Δ^{13} position and are thus derived from prost-13-*trans*-enoic acid, while prostaglandins of the 2 and 3 series have, in addition, a *cis* double bond at Δ^5 or *cis* double bonds at both Δ^5 and Δ^{17}, respectively. These prostaglandins are thus derived from prosta-5-*cis*,13-*trans*-dienoic acid and from prosta-5-*cis*,13-*trans*,17-*cis*-trienoic acid, respectively. As shown in Fig. 2, monoenoic, bisenoic and trisenoic prostaglandins are biosynthesised from the precursor acids 20 : 3ω6 (dihomo-γ-linolenic acid), 20 : 4ω6 (arachidonic acid) and 20 : 5ω3 (timnodonic acid), respectively. Furthermore, the primary prostaglandins all have a 15(S)-hydroxyl group, which seems to be important for their biological activity [10,11].

Prostaglandins are also classified by the functional groups of the cyclopentane ring. The systematic nomenclature from prostanoic acid is straightforward, but for practical reasons the non-systematic use of capital letters to denote the ring substituents has become widely accepted. The structures of the cyclopentane ring with functional groups of A, B, C, D, E, F, G, H and I prostaglandins are shown in Fig. 1. Prostaglandins of the A, B and C type can be obtained from PGE by dehydration and isomerisation of the introduced double bond. The suffix of F_α and F_β prostaglandins indicates the orientation of the 9-hydroxyl group (α or β). PGE_2 (9-keto-11α,15(S)-dihydroxyprosta-5-*cis*,13-*trans*-dienoic acid) and $PGF_{2\alpha}$ (9α,11α,15(S)-trihydroxyprosta 5-*cis*,13-*trans*-dienoic acid) as well as the E and F prostaglandins of the 1 and 3 series are often referred to as the primary prostaglandins, partly for historical reasons [6,7] and partly because they are directly derived from the endoperoxides PGG and PGH. Some authors tend to include also PGD among the primary prostaglandins.

Prostaglandins can be metabolised by one or two steps of β-oxidation (see below). These metabolites are systematically named from 2,3-dinorprostanoic acid and 2,3,4,5-tetranorprostanoic acid, respectively, but are often referred to as C_{18} and C_{16} metabolites. Carbon 20 of prostaglandins may be ω-oxidised to a carboxyl group, and this side chain may then also be β-oxidised to shorter compounds. These metabolites are often named after ω-dinorprostanoic acid or ω-tetranorprostanoic acid. Other prostaglandin metabolites are sometimes described by a combination of systematic and non-systematic nomenclature. Thus, 15-keto-13,14-dihydro-$PGF_{2\alpha}$ is often used for 9α,11α-dihydroxy-15-ketoprost-5-*cis*-enoic acid, etc.

It is conceivable that fatty acids other than the three precursor acids of prostaglandins might be substrates for the prostaglandin synthesising enzymes in some tissues. In renal papilla, 22:4ω6 (adrenic acid) is metabolised to dihomo-prostaglandins, i.e. prostaglandins elongated with two additional methylene units in the carboxyl side chain [12]. Dihomo-prostaglandins are biologically active but it is not known if they are formed in vivo. The nomenclature of thromboxanes and prostacyclin (PGI_2) is discussed in chapters 2 and 3 of this volume. The systematic nomenclature of prostaglandins has been reviewed by Nelson [13].

3. *Essential fatty acids*

A common chemical property of polyunsatured fatty acids, which are needed to maintain animals in healthy condition, seems to be *cis* double bonds at the ω6 and ω9 positions [14]. Important essential fatty acids in the diet are linoleic (18:2ω6) and α-linoleic (18:3ω3) acids, which both occur in plants. In the mammalian organism, these fatty acids can be desaturated and elongated to form the "derived" essential fatty acids, dihomo-γ-linolenic acid (20:3ω6), arachidonic acid (20:4ω6) and timnodonic acid (20:5ω3), the three precursor acids of prostaglandins (Fig. 2, see also Fig. 11). The derived essential fatty acids can also be obtained in the diet. Arachidonic and dihomo-γ-linolenic acids occur in animal tissues timnodonic acid in fish. The mammalian organism cannot introduce double bonds at the ω3 and ω6 positions of long-chain fatty acids, which partly explains why fatty acids of the ω3 and ω6 series must be provided in the diet (see refs. 15–18 for reviews). These fatty acids are also essential to man, however, deficiency states can only be induced by

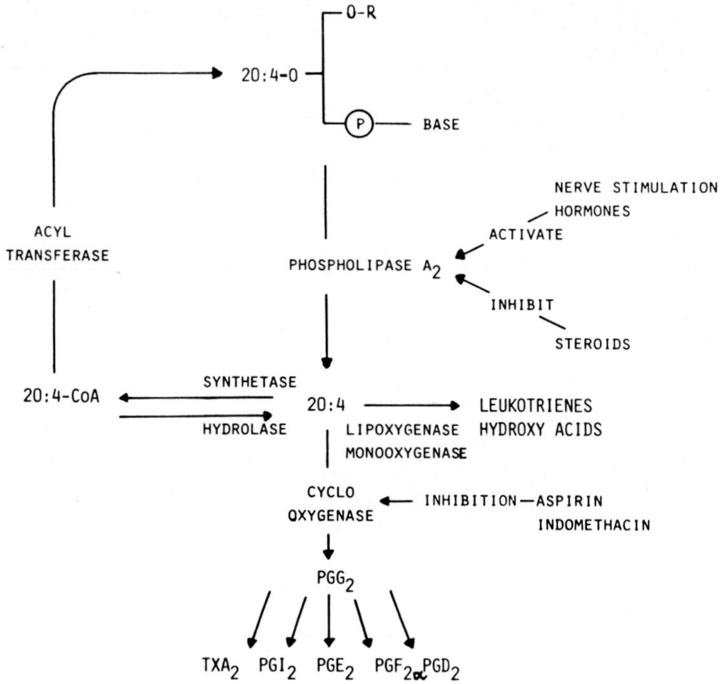

Fig. 3. Mechanism of release of arachidonic acid from glycerophospholipids for subsequent conversion to oxygenated products or for reesterification into glycerophospholipids in the 2-acyl position.

parenteral nutrition or by an extreme dietary regimen [19,20].

Polyunsaturated fatty acids are normal constituents of phospholipids in cell membranes and seem to be of importance for maintaining the fluidity of the membranes [21,22]. Polyunsaturated fatty acids are esterified to glycerophospholipids almost exclusively in the 2-acyl position [23–25]. Arachidonic acid is the most abundant of the prostaglandin precursor acids in almost all tissues. A variety of different stimuli lead to liberation of arachidonic acid from the glycerophospholipids, presumably mainly through hydrolysis by phospholipase A_2 [26]. The concentration of free arachidonic acid in unstimulated cells is normally very low, and the liberation of arachidonic acid is therefore considered to be the rate-limiting step in biosynthesis of prostaglandins and possibly other oxygenated metabolites of arachidonic acid. The mechanisms controlling arachidonic acid release are of considerable biological importance, and some of them are summarised in Figs. 3 and 4. This topic was recently reviewed by Irvine [23].

In resting tissues, arachidonic acid is presumably to a large extent rapidly esterified with CoA at the expense of ATP and then transferred into the 2-acyl position of phospholipids (e.g. lysophosphatidylcholine). Free arachidonic acid is thus in equilibrium with its arachidonoyl esters, and the formation of the latter

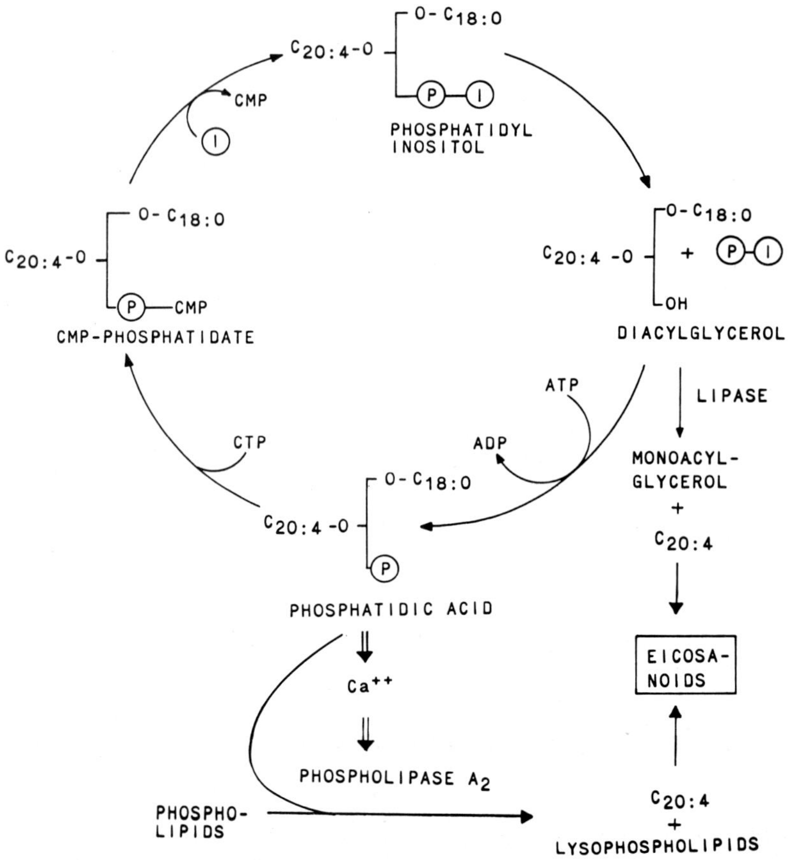

Fig. 4. The phosphatidylinositol cycle, which may yield arachidonic acid by two different mechanisms: By hydrolysis of diacylglycerol or by stimulation of phospholipase A_2 activity through release of calcium by ionophore effects of phosphatidic acid. The latter can then be recycled to phosphatidylinositol.

seems to be favoured [23,25,27,28]. It is possible that in stimulated cells a decrease in the formation of these esters may contribute to an increased level of arachidonate [23,28].

In platelets or other cells, stimulated by thrombin, bradykinin, ischaemia or by other means, there is an increased release of arachidonic acid, presumably to a large extent derived from hydrolysis of phospholipids (e.g. phosphatidylethanolamine, phosphatidylcholine and phosphatidylinositol). Phosphatidylethanolamine and phosphatidylcholine are generally believed to be hydrolysed by phospholipase A_2 [26], while phosphatidylinositol is hydrolysed by phospholipase C and then by other lipases as discussed below. It is not known whether activation of these lipases are primary or secondary events in cell activation [23]. The activity of phospholipase A_2

seems to be increased by the presence of Ca^{2+}, at least in vitro, and may also be regulated by a sequential methylation of phosphatidylethanolamine in membranes as proposed by Axelrod and coworkers [29]. The latter process, called phospholipid methylation, may increase Ca^{2+} transport over membranes and may thus stimulate Ca^{2+}-coupled cell reactions (see ref. 29 for review and refs. 30 and 31 for critical comments).

The hydrolysis of phosphatidylinositol may be of special biological interest [32,33]. This phospholipid consists largely of 1-stearoyl-2-arachidonoyl-glycero-3-phosphoinositol in many tissues (e.g. platelets, brain, liver and mouse pancreas [34,35]). Stimulation of several endocrine or exocrine glands has been found to involve an increased turnover of this phospholipid and formation of phosphatidic acid (see ref. 33 for review). This "phosphatidylinositol response" might be important for hormone induced mobilization of Ca^{2+}, at least in some tissues (see refs. 33, 36, 37 and for critical comments refs. 38 and 39).

The mechanism of an increased phosphatidylinositol metabolism has been studied in platelets stimulated with thrombin in some detail. Thrombin stimulation leads to formation of the 1,2-diacylglyceride and inositol phosphate through hydrolysis by phospholipase C (Fig. 4). According to Majerus and coworkers, the diacylglyceride is then hydrolysed by a diglyceride lipase with liberation of arachidonic acid [35,40]. In contrast, Lapetina and his colleagues [41,42] propose that the diacylglyceride is phosphorylated to phosphatidic acid, a likely calcium ionophore [43], which in turn

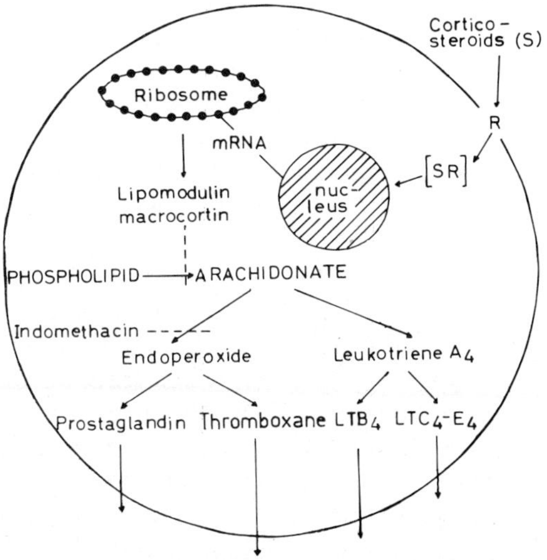

Fig. 5. Mechanism of action of corticosteroids and a non-steroidal anti-inflammatory drug (indomethacin) on cellular metabolism of arachidonic acid. Treatment with corticosteroids induces synthesis of lipomodulin or macrocortin, which inhibits the release of arachidonic acid from phospholipids. Indomethacin inhibits the enzyme fatty acid cyclo-oxygenase and thus the formation of all prostaglandins and thromboxanes.

leads to a Ca^{2+} mobilisation, stimulation of phospholipase A_2 and release of arachidonic acid from the phospholipids. Phosphatidic acid may then be converted to phosphatidylinositol by the phosphatidylinositol cycle (Fig. 4). Arachidonic acid can be released from phosphatidylinositol by these mechanisms in many other cells [44–46].

In 1975, Gryglewski and coworkers demonstrated that glucocorticoids reduced the availability of free arachidonic acid in responsive cells [47]. Similar findings were reported by Hong and Levine [48]. These observations have now been confirmed and the mechanism has been studied in detail by Flower and Blackwell [49] and by Hirata et al. [50]. Treatment with corticosteroids induces synthesis of proteins that inhibit phospholipase A activity, and these proteins have been isolated from macrophages and neutrophils. They have been named macrocortin (from macrophages) or lipomodulin (from neutrophils) but physicochemical investigations indicate that the proteins might be identical [23]. The likely sequence by which glucocorticoids induce synthesis of proteins that inhibit arachidonic acid release is summarised in Fig. 5.

In summary, arachidonic acid is rapidly liberated from and reesterified into phospholipids, but a fraction of the released arachidonic acid can also be oxygenated. The profile of oxygenated metabolites formed seems to be specific for different cell types and organs, but it is also influenced by numerous other factors.

4. Oxygenation of essential fatty acids

An obstacle in the study of the enzymatic oxygenation of polyunsaturated fatty acids is the fact that these acids can be non-enzymatically transformed to hydroperoxides and many other products [51]. Hematin and hematin-containing compounds, e.g. hemoglobin, myoglobin or cytochromes, catalyse the non-enzymatic formation of lipid hydroperoxides. Hydroperoxides may also be formed when unsaturated fatty acids are exposed to air. This autooxidation of polyunsaturated fatty acids is stimulated by light and heat and may eventually lead to complete consumption of the fatty acids.

Autooxidation of arachidonic acid leads primarily to six *cis,trans*-conjugated diene hydroperoxides as the major products [52]. The first step in their formation is the removal of a hydrogen, which is attached to carbons 7, 10, or 13 of arachidonic acid. The hydrogen is abstracted by a free radical mechanism, which leads to the formation of a radical with the W conformation [52,53]. In the next step, a hydroperoxy group is introduced at carbons 5, 8, 9, 11, 12 or 15, and a *cis,trans*-conjugated hydroperoxide is formed. The reaction mechanism is outlined in Fig. 6. 5-Hydroperoxyeicosatetraenoic acid (5-HPETE) and 9-HPETE are thus formed by hydrogen abstraction at carbon 7. An initial removal of hydrogen at carbon 10, in analogy, leads to the formation of products oxygenated at carbon 8 or 12, etc.

The *cis,trans*-conjugated hydroperoxides are the major products of autooxidation, but hydroperoxides with the *trans,trans*-configuration can also be formed. This mechanism has been studied by Porter et al. [52,53]. Oxygen addition seems to be

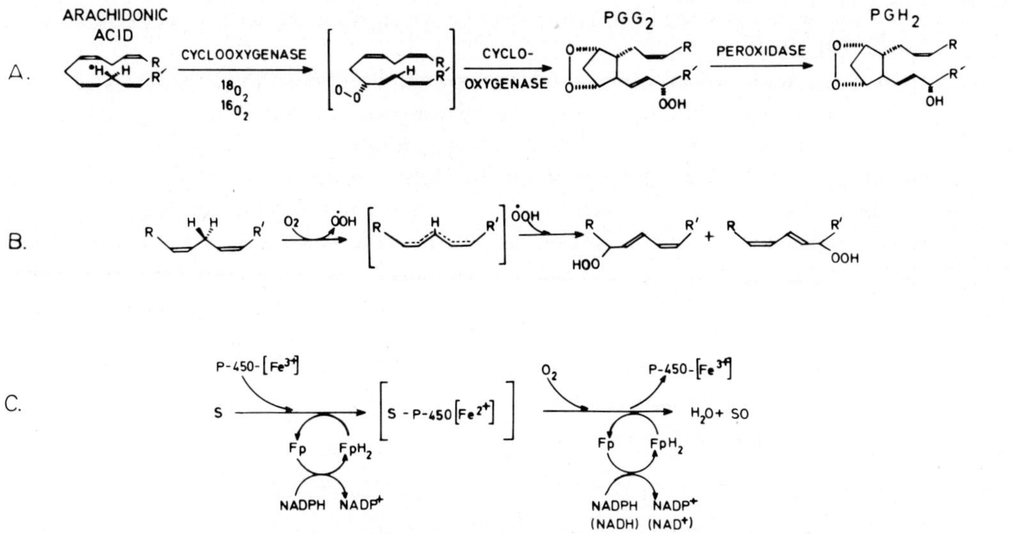

Fig. 6. Three important oxidative pathways for the metabolism of polyunsaturated fatty acids. A. The principal steps in the formation of prostaglandin endoperoxides from arachidonic acid. B. Likely mechanism for the formation of hydroperoxy *cis,trans* conjugated fatty acids by autooxidation or by lipoxygenases. In the latter case, positional as well as stereospecificity are normally found. The formed hydroperoxides may then be enzymatically transformed into leukotrienes (not shown) or to hydroxy acids. C. The enzymatic sequence in cytochrome *P*-450 mediated oxygenation. The first electron is donated from NADPH via the flavoprotein (Fp) NADPH-cytochrome-*P*-450-reductase, while the second electron comes either from NADPH or NADH. In this way the monooxygenase enzymes introduce one oxygen from air into the substrate.

reversible. 15-HPETE (*cis,trans*), for example, may lose ȮOH but the radical formed may now have two possible configurations, since the substituents at carbon 15 of 15-HPETE were free to rotate. One radical has the initial W configuration, while the other one has an isomerized configuration. The latter may be converted to the *trans,trans* hydroperoxide by addition of oxygen at carbon 11 (formation of *trans,trans* 11-HPETE). Obviously, the *trans,trans* conjugated products can be expected to be formed only in very small amounts.

Autooxidation of arachidonic acid and other polyunsaturated fatty acids may also lead to the formation of even more complex compounds. Prostaglandins, monohydroxy-epoxy-eicosatrienoic acids and other products have been described [54–57]. The formation of prostaglandins by the action of a plant lipoxygenase on arachidonic acid has also been reported [58].

Arachidonic acid is the biologically most interesting essential fatty acid of the $\omega 6$ series. Besides the normal β-oxidation, the common fate for all fatty acids in the body, arachidonic acid can be enzymatically oxygenated by three different enzyme types (Fig. 6):

(1) by lipoxygenases to form hydroperoxyeicosatetraenoic acids (e.g. 5-HPETE or 12-HPETE);
(2) by fatty acid cyclooxygenase to form prostaglandin endoperoxides; and
(3) by monooxygenases, which metabolize arachidonic acid by $\omega 1$ and $\omega 2$ hydroxylation, and by $\omega 6$, $\omega 9$, $\omega 12$ and $\omega 15$ epoxidation.

The two former routes give biologically active compounds of great biological importance, viz. the prostaglandins, thromboxanes, prostacyclin and leukotrienes.

Some tissues are particularly rich in other polyunsaturated fatty acids. Thus, $20:3\omega 6$ is abundant in ovine vesicular gland, $22:4\omega 6$ in lapine renal papilla, $22:5\omega 6$ in the testis and $22:6\omega 3$ in the brain of some species [15–18]. Interestingly, the docosatetraenoic acid ($22:4\omega 6$) can also be metabolised to biologically active compounds in the renal papilla (dihomo-prostaglandins and -thromboxanes) in vitro, however these products were less active than the corresponding prostaglandins on adenylate cyclase activity [12].

5. Biosynthesis and metabolism of prostaglandin endoperoxides

The enzyme fatty acid cyclooxygenase, that catalyses the biosynthesis of prostaglandin endoperoxides, has been demonstrated in almost all animal tissues [59]. The enzyme is particularly abundant in seminal vesicles, lungs and renal medulla. The cyclooxygenase catalyses a complex reaction, the mechanisms of which were elucidated by Samuelsson and Hamberg (see ref. 60 for review). A thorough description of the enzyme fatty acid cyclooxygenase is given in chapter 5 of this volume.

Fig. 6A shows the principal steps in the biosynthesis of prostaglandin endoperoxides. The first step is the stereospecific removal of a *pro* S hydrogen at carbon 13 and introduction of molecular oxygen at carbon 11 with a shift of the 11-*cis* double bond to the 12-*trans* position. In the next step the peroxide group, introduced at carbon 11, attacks carbon 9, leading to the formation of a peroxide between carbons 9 and 11. Simultaneously, ring closure between carbons 8 and 12 leads to the formation of the cyclopentane ring. Finally, the 14-*cis* double bond is shifted to the 13-*trans* position and a hydroperoxy group is introduced at carbon 15. This reaction sequence was elucidated in 1965–1966 (see ref. 60 for review). The existence of an intermediary prostaglandin endoperoxide was postulated by Samuelsson from experiments using $^{16}O_2/^{18}O_2$ mixture [61].

Eight years later, two groups, i.e. Hamberg and Samuelsson, and Nugteren and Hazelhof, were independently able to isolate the postulated intermediates. In fact, two endoperoxides were identified: 9α,11α-peroxido-15(S)-hydroperoxyprosta-5-*cis*,13-*trans*-dienoic acid (PGG_2) and 9α,11α-peroxido-15(S)-hydroxyprosta-5-*cis*,13-*trans*-dienoic acid (PGH_2) [62,63]. As could be expected, the endoperoxides were unstable in aqueous media and decomposed with a half-life of 4–6 min into stable prostaglandins. The endoperoxides were found to possess considerable biological activity. Among other activities, they contract certain smooth muscles and induce platelet aggregation. Furthermore, it soon became evident that the endoperoxides could also be transformed into products other than prostaglandins. Systematic studies on their biological activities and their metabolism led to the discovery of thromboxanes and prostacyclin (Chapters 2 and 3).

Fatty acid cyclooxygenase also seems to catalyse the enzymatic conversion of PGG to PGH since so far the cyclooxygenase (leading to PGG) and the hydroxyperoxidases (reduction of the hydroperoxy group at C-15) enzyme activities have not been separated [64–66]. The hydroperoxidase reaction may lead to transfer of oxygen from PGG_2 into drugs, at least in vitro (refs. 67, 68, and see ref. 69 for review). By this mechanism, toxic drug metabolites may be formed in the presence of arachidonic acid and fatty acid cyclooxygenase, and this "cooxygenation" might account for some toxic effects of paracetamol and other drugs in the kidney and the urinary tract [70].

The classical prostaglandins, E, D and F, are subsequently formed from the endoperoxides in enzymatic or non-enzymatic reactions. The endoperoxides are either isomerized to a β-hydroxy ketone (E and D type prostaglandins) or reduced to a 1,3-diol (PGF_α). Factors catalysing these conversions are described in chapter 5. Isomerisation to E prostaglandins occurs in the lung, the renal medulla and in many other tissues. Isomerases that transform endoperoxides to D prostaglandins, have, for example, been found in the cytosol of tissues from the central nervous system [71]. Formation of PGD_2 also occurs in mast cells, platelets and other cell types [72,73]. F prostaglandins are presumably to a large extent formed by non-enzymatic reduction of the endoperoxides [73].

6. Biological effects of prostaglandins

(a) General

Von Euler noted in his early studies that "prostaglandin" caused contractions of several different smooth muscle preparations and lowered the arterial blood pressure in the rabbit [4,5]. When prostaglandins became generally available for pharmacological studies, this research area expanded rapidly. It soon became apparent that prostaglandins could affect almost all body functions, at least in pharmacological doses. Indeed, the broad spectrum of prostaglandin effects has been described as "bewildering" and "awesome", and it seems today that there is hardly a single organ or function in the body that has not been shown to be influenced one way or other by prostaglandins.

If, for simplicity, we choose to focus on one single type of effect, for example smooth muscle contractility, the field unfortunately remains disturbingly complex.

First, different PGs may have opposite effects on the same organ: prostaglandins of the E type are bronchodilators whereas the F compounds are bronchoconstrictors; the cervix of the uterus is relaxed by PGEs but contracted by PGFs.

Second, the same compound may have different effects in different parts of an organ: PGE_2 may, for example, contract the corpus of the uterus and at the same time relax the cervix; prostaglandins of the E type may contract the longitudinal muscle of the gastrointestinal tract and simultaneously relax the circular muscle.

Third, an organ may respond differently during different physiological or pathological conditions. For example, the uterus is known to react differently during the various phases of the menstrual cycle and also during pregnancy.

Fourth, one compound may exert opposite actions in different species: as an illustration, $PGF_{2\alpha}$ has been found to lower the blood pressure in rabbit and cat, whereas it acts as a weak pressor in man, rat and dog.

Fifth, opposite effects can sometimes be registered with different concentrations of the same compound: low amounts of prostaglandins of the E type have proinflammatory effects, whereas high amounts are antiinflammatory.

Finally, it has even been found that two prostaglandins belonging to the same type (but differing in degree of unsaturation) may exert opposite actions: PGE_1 causes an increase in platelet cyclic AMP whereas PGE_2 lowers the cAMP levels.

The wide range of biological effects of these compounds may also be illustrated by the following, very incomplete list of activities that have been registered for one single compound, PGE_1 (ignoring species, dose, and tissue differences):

PGE_1 contracts smooth muscle in general, lowers arterial blood pressure, inhibits gastric acid secretion, exerts cytoprotection of gastric mucosa, inhibits platelet aggregation, raises cAMP levels in most cell types but lowers cAMP in bladder epithelium and adipose cells, induces vascular leakage, produces fever, dilates bronchi, stimulates pancreatic secretion, blocks resorption of sodium and water in the gastrointestinal tract, counteracts the effects of vasopressin on the distal tubules of the kidney, inhibits lipolysis, stimulates bone resorption, induces vasodilation in many vascular beds, etc. It should be noted, however, that in some cases effects are registered only by using pharmacological doses of the prostaglandin. Fig. 7 may serve as an illustration to the great complexity of this field.

In spite of this bewildering complexity of biological actions of the prostaglandins, their roles in certain organs and/or physiological processes have been relatively well

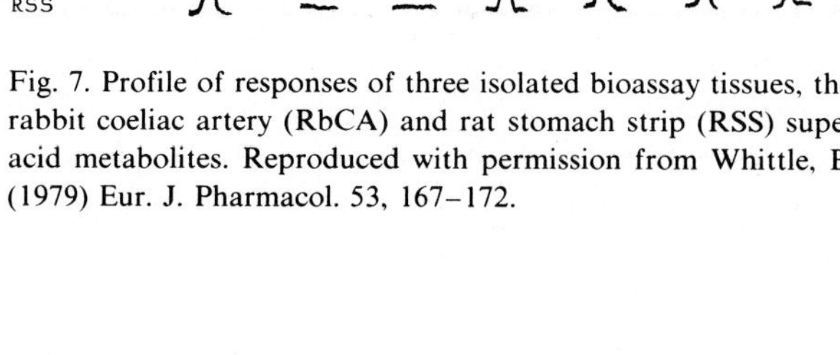

Fig. 7. Profile of responses of three isolated bioassay tissues, the rabbit transverse stomach strip (RbSS), rabbit coeliac artery (RbCA) and rat stomach strip (RSS) superfused in cascade, to several arachidonic acid metabolites. Reproduced with permission from Whittle, B.J.R., Mugridge, K.G. and Moncada, S. (1979) Eur. J. Pharmacol. 53, 167–172.

established. If we restrict our discussion to a few organ systems, the area can be more easily comprehended.

A substantial part of our knowledge stems from studies on, first, the direct effects of the prostaglandins as described above or the effects of prostaglandin precursors; second, from measurements of prostaglandin levels in body fluids or tissues; and third, from registered biological effects of inhibitors of prostaglandin biosynthesis.

In 1971, Vane and collaborators made the important discovery that aspirin, indomethacin and other non-steroidal antiinflammatory drugs (NSAIDs) were potent inhibitors of prostaglandin synthesis by a direct action on fatty acid cyclooxygenase [74–76]. NSAIDs have many other pharmacological effects in common but their effect on prostaglandin synthesis seems to correlate well with their efficiency in various inflammatory disorders. This discovery led to a renewed interest in the biological effects of NSAIDs and made studies on the physiological effects of prostaglandin synthesis inhibition possible (for reviews, see refs. 77 and 78).

NSAIDs soon found novel use in many clinical conditions. Patency of the ductus arteriosus in neonates, mastocytosis, dysmenorrhoea and other conditions are often remarkably improved by these drugs. At the same time, many adverse effects of NSAIDs can be interpreted as due to inhibition of prostaglandin synthesis. In gynaecology, for example, NSAIDs were thus found to delay parturition and cause haemorrhagic complications in the mother, and to induce premature closure of the ductus arteriosus in the infant (for reviews see refs. 79 and 80).

Prostaglandins of the 2-series, which are derived from arachidonic acid, are quantitatively dominating in most tissues. The consensus seems to be that these prostaglandins may also be of the greatest biological importance. Prostaglandins of the 1 and 3 series may be formed in many organs. The fatty acid $20:3\omega6$ is abundant in seminal vesicles, and prostaglandins, which are derived from this fatty acid (PGE_1, $PGF_{1\alpha}$) also occur in semen of several species. Let us now consider some of the most conspicuous actions of prostaglandins on various organs, keeping in mind that species variations are common.

(b) The reproductive system

It was the high concentration of prostaglandins in seminal fluid that originally led to their discovery [3–5]. Levels of certain prostaglandins in normal human seminal plasma are in the order of magnitude of several hundred $\mu g/ml$ [81–84], which is at least 10^6 fold the prostaglandin concentration in other biological fluids [cf. 85]. It is therefore surprising that the physiological roles of prostaglandins in semen are still largely unknown. Actions in the male as well as the female reproductive tract have been implicated [86]. In spite of our lack of knowledge of such roles, however, the prostaglandins have proved to be of great interest in obstetrics and gynaecology, and this area was the first one where the prostaglandins were employed as pharmacological tools [87].

Prostaglandins of the F type contract and prostaglandins of the E type relax human uterine smooth muscle in vitro [88,89]. Given intravenously, both E and F compounds elicit a prompt increase in uterine tonus with superimposed labour-like rhythmic contractions [90]. The first clinical application of prostaglandins, introduced in the late 1960s, was induction of labour at term [91,92]. Large amounts of endogenously produced prostaglandins have also been detected during normal, spontaneous labour [93–96]. That this endogenous production of prostaglandins is of considerable importance for normal labour is demonstrated by the well known prolonged duration of gestation as well as prolonged and inefficient labour that occur after intake of prostaglandin synthesis inhibitors towards the end of pregnancy [97]. Prostaglandins produced in excess by the human uterus may also be responsible for the hypercontractility of this organ found in dysmenorrhoea [98].

Of special interest is the unique effect of prostaglandins to induce abortion in the first and second trimester of pregnancy [99,100], and various prostaglandin analogues have now been developed that increase efficiency and reduce side effects when employed as abortifacients [101–104].

Prostaglandins are also of importance in animal reproduction. $PGF_{2\alpha}$ has been identified as the endogenous luteolytic hormone in many species [105,106], and administration of this prostaglandin or certain similarly acting analogues is now frequently used to synchronise estrus in domestic animals and thereby to increase the efficiency of artificial insemination [107].

For recent reviews on the roles of prostaglandins in reproduction, see e.g. refs. 108 and 109, and on prostaglandins in therapeutic use in human reproduction, e.g. refs. 79, 90, 110 and 111.

(c) Kidney function

The importance of essential fatty acids for maintaining renal function was described in one of the classical papers by Burr and Burr [1], who found the most common cause of death in essential fatty acid deficient animals to be renal failure. In spite of this early observation, more than 30 years elapsed before formation of prostaglandins in the kidney was discovered [112,113].

The renal medulla of several species has a very high capacity to form PGE_2, $PGF_{2\alpha}$, PGD_2 and PGI_2 [114–117]. The medullary prostaglandin synthesis is influenced by the sodium balance, and changes in prostaglandin biosynthesis may affect medullary blood flow and the osmotic gradient in the papilla [118–121]. Medullary prostaglandins may also counteract the tubular effects of vasopressin [122,123], while inhibition of prostaglandin synthesis by NSAIDs will augment the effects of this hormone [124]. The influence of prostaglandins on renal water excretion has recently been reviewed [125].

The renal cortex has a much lower capacity to form classical prostaglandins than the medulla [120,126,127], but the cortical vascular endothelium forms PGI_2 in relatively high amounts [120,127]. PGD_2, PGE_2 and PGI_2 are potent renal vasodilators when infused into the renal artery [116,128,129]. The arterial levels of these prostaglandins are very low, and studies with NSAIDs to inhibit prostaglandin biosynthesis indicate that prostaglandins are of little importance for maintaining renal blood flow under normal conditions [128]. Under the influence of vasoconstrictor hormones, e.g. angiotensin II, or when the blood flow is compromised by other methods, prostaglandins seem to be of greater importance, as NSAIDs may then profoundly reduce renal blood flow [128]. NSAIDs should thus be used with caution in patients with renal disease [130,131].

Cortical prostaglandins have also been implicated in the control of renin release. NSAIDs have been found to suppress renin secretion following many stimuli, while prostaglandins may augment renin release (see refs. 128, 132 and 133 for reviews). NSAIDs have also been used with success to reduce the hyperreninemia of Bartter's syndrome [134]. For general reviews on the roles of prostaglandins in the kidney, see, e.g. refs. 128, 132, 133 and 135.

(d) Platelets

The prostaglandin endoperoxides, PGG_2 and PGH_2, are both potent inducers of platelet aggregation and the release reaction [136,137]. The compounds are both efficiently converted by the platelets into the even more potent proaggregatory thromboxane A_2 [138], and the question whether the endoperoxides exert their aggregatory action per se or via TXA_2 formation has still not been conclusively settled [139,140].

The classical prostaglandins also affect platelet aggregation although they are usually inhibitory. PGE_1 and PGD_2 are potent inhibitors of platelet aggregation, presumably by increasing the concentration of cyclic AMP [141–144]. The inhibitory effect of PGE_1 persists, however, after the level of cyclic AMP has declined. The increased levels of cyclic AMP can therefore only partly explain the effects of PGE_1.

The most potent inhibitory prostaglandin is, however, PGI_2 [145]. Since platelet function is thus more influenced by the mutually antagonistic compounds, TXA_2 and PGI_2, than by other compounds in this field, this topic will be discussed more in detail in the subsequent two chapters.

(e) Gastrointestinal functions

E prostaglandins suppress gastric acid secretion in man and in experimental animals [146–148]. In lower doses, which do not inhibit gastric acid secretion, some prostaglandins also have specific protective effects on the gastric mucosa against many noxious stimuli [149]. This effect has been demonstrated in man as well as in experimental animals [150]. Gastrointestinal bleeding induced by acetylsalicylic acid or indomethacin treatment can be prevented by oral administration of prostaglandins, particularly of the E type [150,151]. This cytoprotective effect can also be used to accelerate healing of duodenal ulcer in man [152]. For reviews on the antacid and cytoprotective effects of prostaglandins, see refs. 146, 150, 153 and 154.

The prostaglandins also exert various effects on the intestines. As was mentioned above, prostaglandins of the E type may stimulate the longitudinal muscle layer but relax the circular layer. This has been found both in animals and in man [155,156].

Prostaglandins of the F and D type generally contract both types of muscle, however, both regional and species differences occur [157,158].

Gastrointestinal cramps and diarrhoea were among the first side effects to be noted when prostaglandins were employed in gynaecological practice [159,160]. Part of these actions may be attributed to such direct effects of prostaglandins on the gastrointestinal muscle layers. However, besides these effects on motility, the prostaglandins also influence water and electrolyte transport across the intestinal mucosa, thus enhancing the diarrhoea [161,162]. PGE_1, PGE_2 and $PGF_{2\alpha}$ inhibit reabsorption of water and electrolytes in the small intestine, leading to enteropooling. Other compounds, such as PGD_2 and PGI_2, exert the opposite effects [153]. It has been postulated that, e.g., the strongly diarrhoea-inducing cholera toxin and prostaglandins of the E type may act via a common mechanism, viz. increasing the cAMP content of the intestinal mucosa [163,164].

(f) The vascular system

Many autacoids have effects on the circulatory system. This is also the case with many prostaglandins. Among the first effects to be registered was the vasodilating activities of the E prostaglandins (review, ref. 165). Infusion of prostaglandins of the E type lowers the arterial blood pressure in most species [166,167]. Due to the rapid metabolic inactivation of prostaglandins in most tissues and organs (see below), it is however unlikely that these compounds are circulating hormones and thus that they affect the circulation in general. However, locally generated prostaglandins may well have effects on the microcirculation, both under normal conditions and in certain pathological processes. Many stimuli, for example ischaemia and inflammation, are known to increase prostaglandin biosynthesis, and in such situations, prostaglandins may affect the local blood flow and vascular permeability (review, ref. 133).

The potent vasodilatory effects of PGE_1 have been used with success in treatment of severe forms of Raynaud's disease as well as vascular insufficiency in systemic sclerosis and other connective tissue diseases [168]. PGE_1 and PGE_2 also relax the ductus arteriosus of newborns. Infusions of PGE_1 (50 ng/kg/min) to newborns with certain cardiac malformations, which make the persistence of the ductus essential for the systemic or pulmonary circulation, improves the clinical condition and allows surgery to be delayed to a more suitable time (see ref. 169 for a review). The tone of the ductus arteriosus seems to be balanced between the constrictor effects of oxygen, possibly also other vasoconstrictor substances, and the dilatory effects of prostaglandins formed intramurally [170]. Inhibitors of prostaglandin biosynthesis have been used to induce closure of patent ductus arteriosus of newborns, and in most cases the conventional surgical treatment could be omitted [171]. For reviews on the role of prostaglandins in the vascular system see refs. 133, 165, 172 and 173.

(g) The respiratory system

The lung has long been recognized as one of the major sites of both biosynthesis and metabolic inactivation of prostaglandins [6,174–178]. The possible physiological or pathophysiological roles of prostaglandins in the complex functions of the respiratory system, being of both respiratory, vascular and metabolic nature, have consequently been extensively studied (for reviews, see e.g. 179–182). Only one aspect will be dealt with here, viz. the possible involvement of prostaglandins in human bronchial asthma.

$PGF_{2\alpha}$ contracts and PGE_2 generally relaxes bronchial smooth muscle in vitro in many species, including man (reviews, refs. 180 and 182). Asthmatics were found to be particularly sensitive to $PGF_{2\alpha}$ [183], and a release of $PGF_{2\alpha}$ was demonstrated during allergen provoked asthma attacks [184]. Because of these findings, a role for the bronchoconstrictor $PGF_{2\alpha}$ in human asthma was postulated. Later it was found that the endoperoxides, and still later TXA_2, were considerably more potent bronchoconstrictors [185,186], and consequently these compounds were then believed to be more important in asthma than $PGF_{2\alpha}$. Thromboxane formation in human asthmatic lung has also recently been demonstrated [187]. Research in this field has however been considerably hampered by the lack of a suitable animal model. One frequently employed approximation is pulmonary anaphylaxis in the guinea pig, and numerous studies have appeared where the roles of arachidonate metabolites in this condition have been investigated (e.f. refs. 188–191). However, certain differences exist: for example, thromboxane seems to be biosynthesized much more by the guinea pig anaphylactic lung than by the human asthmatic lung [187–194]. Also, the fact that aspirin and other NSAIDs are generally ineffective in the treatment of human asthma, contradicted the postulated importance of cyclooxygenase products in this disease. Certain corticosteroids, on the other hand, are powerful tools in the treatment of this disease. This discrepancy between the effects of two types of compounds, both known to inhibit prostaglandin formation although at different levels (see above), led to the hypothesis that other, even more potent bronchoconstrictors might be formed from arachidonic acid, but via pathways separate from the cyclooxygenase catalysed step. That this was indeed the case was demonstrated when the cysteinyl containing leukotrienes were identified [195–197]; these compounds are now believed to be primarily responsible for the symptoms of human asthma [187,198–200].

The possible roles of the prostanoids in the lung are further discussed in Chapter 2.

(h) The nervous system

A number of procedures are known to cause release of prostaglandins in the brain. Electrical stimulation, trauma, hypoxia, ischaemia, hypoglycemia, convulsion, pyrogen fever all cause a rapid increase in free arachidonic acid and stimulation of prostaglandin biosynthesis. For general reviews of eicosanoids in the nervous system, see refs. 201–203.

Considerable species differences exist with respect to the pattern of prostaglandins formed in the nervous system. In mice and rats PGD_2 is by far the dominating, with lower levels of $PGF_{2\alpha}$ and PGE_2 [204–206]. $PGF_{2\alpha}$ dominates in the dog and in man [207,208], PGE_2 in the cat [209] and thromboxane B_2 in the guinea pig [210]. Some studies indicate a greater synthesis in the brain of female animals [210,211].

Higher capacity to form prostaglandins have been noted in some brain areas, notably in the hippocampus, the median eminence, pineal gland and pituitary [206,212]. In the rat and human cerebral blood vessels a high capacity for PGI_2 production was noted [208,213,214]. It is believed that high levels of 6-keto-$PGF_{1\alpha}$ in cerebrospinal fluid could originate from vascular tissue [215].

The prostaglandins in the nervous system have been implicated to have physiological roles in temperature regulation, brain circulation and possibly in neuromodulation [201]. The administration of prostaglandins of the E-series intraventricularly has been shown to have sedative effects in rodents and chickens [216]. In the mouse, a dose-dependent inhibition of picotoxin and pentahazol induced convulsion was observed [217,218]. In the cat prostaglandins inhibited penicillin induced seizures [219]. The mechanism of the anticonvulsive action of PGE compounds is not clear.

Prostaglandins of the E series have been suggested to mediate pyrogen fever (reviews, refs. 220, 221). Four lines of evidence support this hypothesis. First, a release of PGE-like activity has been observed during pyrogen fever in the cat. Second, endogenous pyrogen stimulates brain prostaglandin biosynthesis. Third, injection of small amounts of PGE_1 or PGE_2 in the anterior hypothalamus elicits fever. Fourth, inhibition of the brain cyclooxygenase by indomethacin or aspirin reduces both pyrogen fever and prostaglandin levels in the cerebrospinal fluid. However, several critical counterarguments have been raised (see refs. 203 for references). Lesions in the anterior hypothalamus reduce PGE production but not pyrogen fever. Criticism has also been raised at the unspecific methods used to measure PGE compounds in cerebrospinal fluid. Furthermore, aspirin, which inhibits prostaglandin formation in the periphery, does not appear to cross the blood brain barrier [222], and paracetamol, which is an excellent antipyretic drug, is only a weak inhibitor of fatty acid cyclooxygenase.

Vasodilating prostaglandins may play a role in maintaining cerebral blood flow. The evidence is based on the high capacity of brain blood vessels to form vasodilating eicosanoids [208,213,214] and the fact that the increase in cerebral blood flow due to hypercapnia is reduced by indomethacin treatment [223–225]. It has therefore been suggested that prostacyclin could serve as a link between cerebral metabolism and blood flow. However, the results could not be reproduced using other inhibitors of the fatty acid cyclooxygenase [226,227], and the role of prostaglandins in the maintenance of brain blood flow is not clear at present.

Eicosanoids have been suggested to play a part in the pathophysiology of several diseases of brain circulation, such as intravascular aggregation in transient ischaemic attacks (TIA) and in the severe vasospasm occurring after subarachnoid haemorrhage (for review see ref. 228).

Prostaglandins have also been suggested to have a modulating function on neuronal activity. Administration of exogenous PGE compounds has been shown to have an inhibitory effect on adrenergic neurotransmission in the peripheral nervous system [229]. This could be shown to be due to an inhibitory effect on norepinephrine release. Conversely, inhibition of prostaglandin biosynthesis led to an enhanced release of norepinephrine following nerve stimulation. Hedqvist has put forward the hypothesis that prostaglandins may be responsible for negative feedback control in sympathetic neurotransmission [229]. However, doubt has been raised as to the generality of this phenomenon, which for instance has not been shown to occur in the brain (for discussion see ref. 201).

Prostaglandins of the D type can also depress sympathetic neurotransmission [230] in the cat and increase the activity of brain adenylate cyclase [231]. The physiological relevance of these findings may, however, be limited because of the very low synthesis of PGD_2 in the cat and human nervous system [206,208,232].

Roles have been proposed for the prostaglandins in schizophrenia [233], mano-depressive psychosis [234], alcoholism [235], migraine [236] and in the mechanism of action of psychotropic drugs including cannabis [237]. It is evident that such suggestions are highly speculative at the present stage of knowledge.

7. Metabolism of prostaglandins

In view of the high biological potencies of most prostaglandins, it is not surprising that most tissues are endowed with enzymes that rapidly and extensively inactivate the compounds by metabolic degradation. The organs mainly responsible for prostaglandin uptake and metabolism are the lungs, liver and kidney. This was first demonstrated in studies employing whole body autoradiography of animals given ^{3}H-labeled prostaglandins [238,239]. These were followed by studies on each specific organ from several species (lung, refs. 240–249; liver, refs. 250–253; and kidney, refs. 254–259), as well as on numerous other organs and tissues.

Still later, a number of in vivo studies were carried out in many species, which led to the identification of a large number of final degradation products excreted into urine (e.g. the rat, 260–265; guinea pig, 266–268; rabbit, 269; monkey, 270, 271 and man, 272–278) (cf. also Fig. 8). The structures of major circulating prostaglandin metabolites were also identified [272,278,279–281].

In general, the initial metabolic attack converts the 15-hydroxyl of the prostaglandin into a keto group [240,251,282] (Fig. 9), which considerably reduces the biological activity of the compound [10, 283–287]. This reaction is followed by enzymatic reduction of the Δ^{13} double bond which further reduces the potency of the metabolites. In fact, the products of these two reactions, the 15-keto-13,14-dihydro prostaglandins (Fig. 9), are biologically essentially inactive [10, 283–287].

The first reaction is catalysed by the enzyme 15-hydroxyprostaglandin dehydrogenase (EC 1.1.1.141) (15-PGDH), which is particularly abundant in the lung, kidney, spleen and placenta [288–291], but which occurs in lower amounts also in many other cell types and tissues [288,289,292,293]. Even microorganisms have been reported to carry out this metabolic step [294]. The 15-hydroxyprostanoate dehydrogenase has been studied extensively: for a review, see e.g. ref. 293 (see also Chapter 5 of this volume).

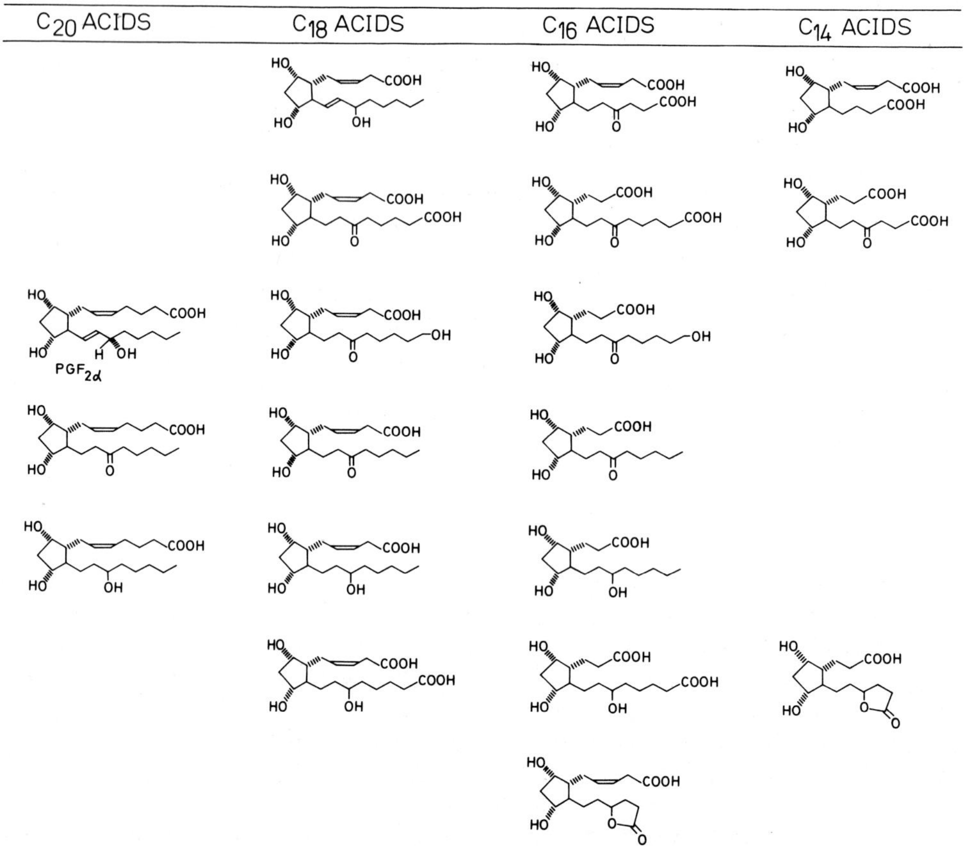

Fig. 8. Structures of urinary metabolites of prostaglandin $F_{2\alpha}$ in the human.

Dehydrogenation of the 15-hydroxyl group of a prostaglandin that has reached the blood stream is a very rapid process. Thus, a prostaglandin injected into one cubital vein of a human subject is converted almost quantitatively into 15-keto metabolites during one single passage through the pulmonary circulation, i.e. in blood samples taken from the contralateral arm vein about 1 min after the injection, less than 3% of the sample radioactivity was due to the unconverted parent prostaglandin [272,279]. The major products were identified as the corresponding 15-keto-13,14-dihydro-prostaglandins, which had considerably longer half-lives, about 10 min [272,279], and consequently accumulated to much higher levels in the circulation than the parent compounds [278]. The same findings have been reported for other species [281,295]. Such events are compatible with the efficient inactivation of biologically active prostaglandins noted in perfused organs [11,178,296,297]: as was mentioned above, 15-keto-prostaglandins have in general been found to be

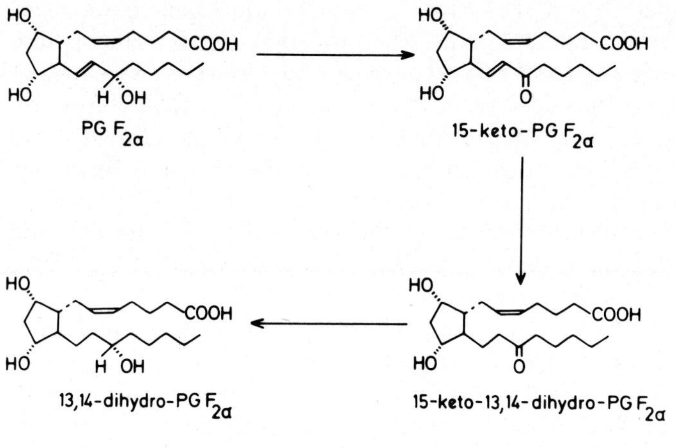

Fig. 9. Initial steps in the metabolic inactivation of prostaglandins (here $PGF_{2\alpha}$).

almost inactive. However, in certain studies considerable biological activity has been registered for this type of compounds [285,298,299]. It is, however, known that 15-ketodihydro compounds may be further metabolised into 15-hydroxy compounds (13,14-dihydroprostaglandins), either by a reversal of the dehydrogenase reaction [293] or by the action of a third enzyme in this cascade, viz. a prostaglandin 15-keto-reductase (Fig. 9). It is possible that some of the biological activity of 15-keto-prostaglandins may be attributed to this subsequently formed compound, which possesses biological potencies comparable to, or even exceeding, those of the parent prostaglandin [10,286,287].

Major final degradation products excreted into urine are generally extensively oxidised, e.g. tetranor dicarboxylic acids [262,269,272,274]. The further metabolism of the initially formed 15-keto-13,14-dihydroprostaglandins thus involves one or two steps of β-oxidation, ω1- or ω2-oxidation to ω1- or ω2-hydroxyl, ω1-aldehyde or ω2-ketone and, in the former case, also ω-carboxylic groups. Compounds with the ω-carboxylic group can be β-oxidised also from the ω-end.

β-Oxidation of prostaglandins was first studied in vitro using mitochondria from rat liver [300]. All compounds studied were found to undergo one or two steps of degradation by this mechanism. In vivo, β-oxidation is likely to follow the metabolic conversions at C-13 to C-15, since dinor and tetranor compounds were found to be poor substrates for 15-PGDH [301], whereas 15-keto prostaglandins were in general more extensively degraded than the parent compounds [300]. Later studies on β-oxidation, employing intact tissues, showed that these metabolic conversions could also take place to a considerable extent under such circumstances [252,302]. It was also demonstrated that prostaglandins were likely to utilize the common carnitine-dependent system for the β-oxidation of long-chain fatty acids [303].

ω-Oxidation of prostaglandins was first reported in 1965 [81,304] when several 19-hydroxylated prostaglandins of the A and B type were identified in human seminal plasma. It was later shown that this ω2-hydroxylation had taken place already with the primary prostaglandins [305–307], and that the conversion into corresponding A or B compounds was likely to have occurred ex vivo on storage of the seminal plasma. The site of this ω2-hydroxylation has not yet been determined.

Organs with considerable capacity for ω-oxidation (ω1- as well as ω2-hydroxylation) in several species are the liver, lung and kidney [249,308–312]; this metabolic pathway has, however, been detected also in other tissues [313].

During the last few years several studies on the mechanisms of the ω1- and ω2-hydroxylation of prostaglandins have appeared. These are discussed more in detail below (see section on Monooxygenase metabolism).

Subsequent oxidation of 20-hydroxy prostaglandins may lead to the formation of aldehyde compounds [314] and finally to ω-carboxylic metabolites [261–263,269,271,272,274,275]. After this step has taken place, one or two steps of β-oxidation can take place also from this end of the prostaglandin molecule [265,271,275–277]. Thus, several highly degraded prostaglandin metabolites have been identified in human [275–277] and rat urine [265]: C_{14} compounds which are generally tetranor, ω-dinor dicarboxylic acids but in one case a dinor, ω-tetranor dioic compound [276].

A further metabolic fate of prostaglandins is the interconversion of compounds of the E and F type. Reduction of the keto group at C-9 in PGE_2 to form F_α compounds was first noted in guinea pig liver [250] and was later found to take place also in vivo in the human [273]. The enzyme responsible for this reaction, prostaglandin 9-keto-reductase, was later found to have a widespread occurrence: it has been detected in sheep blood [315], in the kidney of several species, such as the rat [316,317], monkey [318], swine [319] and rabbit [317,320], as well as in liver and many other tissues [319,321–324]. This enzyme may well prove of great interest, since it can regulate the proportion in vivo of two prostaglandins which are often antagonistic in their actions (see above).

Interestingly, a different reduction to form an F_β compound had earlier been discovered as a major metabolic pathway of PGE in the guinea pig [226]. This reaction has also been recognised in the rat [264].

The reverse reaction has also been noted, i.e. the formation of PGE compounds from prostaglandins of the F series. This reaction is catalysed by an enzyme different from the 9-keto reductase, prostaglandin 9-hydroxy dehydrogenase [325–327]. In vivo, this reaction may take place to a considerable extent in certain species, for example the rat and the guinea pig [281], whereas it seems to be of minor importance in others, such as the human [274,280,281].

Reduction of the C-11 keto group of PGD compounds to form PGF_α metabolites has also been found, for example in sheep blood [328], in various rabbit tissues [329,330], and in an in vivo study in the monkey [271]. The enzyme, prostaglandin 11-keto-reductase, was purified to homogeneity from rabbit liver [329]. The importance of this reaction may be analogous to that of the 9-keto-reductase, viz. to regulate the balance between two prostaglandins that are agonists in certain systems but antagonists in others.

To our knowledge the opposite reaction, i.e. conversion of PGF_α compounds to PGD compounds, has not been demonstrated (yet).

8. Assay of prostaglandin production

During the past decades the prostaglandins have been postulated to be involved in a vast number of physiological processes. Also many diseases have been believed to involve derangements in arachidonate metabolism in their pathogeneses or even etiologies. One of the major obstacles in obtaining support for such hypotheses is the difficulties involved in measurements of prostaglandins in biologic material. Due to the rapid metabolic inactivation of prostaglandins after they have reached the blood stream (see above), it is feasible to assume that these compounds exert their actions close to the site of their formation. When attempts are made to measure the tissue levels of prostaglandins, it should be borne in mind that, due to their extremely high biological potencies, these compounds are not likely to be stored as such in the cells. Thus, the local in vivo concentration of prostaglandins in most tissues can be expected to be very low. Reported tissue levels of prostaglandins however span at least three orders of magnitude, i.e. from picograms to nanograms per mg tissue, even in studies of very similar design carried out on the same tissue. It is known that the prostaglandin concentration in cells and tissues with high capacity for prostaglandin biosynthesis increases rapidly with time following ischaemia or mechanical stimulation or by other means. Thus, the sampling technique is extremely important, when assay of primary prostaglandins is intended: this pertains to tissue as well as blood samples. A rapid interruption of the artifactual ex vivo biosynthesis is mandatory: deep-freezing of e.g. a tissue biopsy within seconds using liquid nitrogen may be necessary (e.g. refs. 119, 331, 332). Another technique leading to rapid inactivation of the prostaglandin synthesizing enzymes is the use of microwaves on the studied tissue in situ [333]. The addition of a prostaglandin synthesis inhibitor to the samples may however not be sufficient, since the time required for efficient inhibition may be relatively long, whereas prostaglandin biosynthesis is a very rapid process.

Because of these problems, assay of primary prostaglandins in tissues or blood may be of relatively little physiological relevance. An alternative to the measurement of true endogenous levels of prostaglandins is to assay the *capacity* for prostaglandin biosynthesis in the studied cell or tissue type instead. This approach has been used in many studies in this field (e.g. refs. 206, 334).

In many pathophysiological situations, an overproduction of certain prostaglandins or related compounds is suspected, for example in dysmenorrhoea, inflammatory diseases, asthma or thrombotic disorders. A subnormal production may however also be at hand, such as is postulated in duodenal ulcer (see above). Theoretically, it should be easier to demonstrate an overproduction of a prostaglandin than an underproduction, at least with a reasonably sensitive assay method. In reality, however, this is not necessarily the case. Many factors influence the outcome of such a study, apart from the quality of the assay. One of the most important factors is probably the variability of the prostaglandin output, which may result in irregular fluctuations in the tissue or blood levels of these compounds. This renders the timing and/or the frequency of the sample collection a crucial factor. Unless the samples are taken at exactly the right times or with very short intervals, even a comparatively long and pronounced prostaglandin release may be missed entirely [335].

When the pitfalls in prostaglandin assay became recognized, interest turned to certain prostaglandin metabolites and derivatives instead. It was discovered that the circulating levels of their initial metabolites, the 15-keto-13,14-dihydro compounds, were some 50-fold higher than those of the parent compounds [278]. Furthermore, the metabolic half-lives of these metabolites in the circulation were considerably longer, around 10 min, compared to less than 1 min for the parent prostaglandin [272,279]. These findings, taken together with the fact that 15-ketodihydro compounds are not formed as artifacts during blood sampling, rendered these metabolites far more suitable as targets for measurement.

To date a very large number of biological studies have been carried out where the endogenous $PGF_{2\alpha}$ production has been followed in various situations by monitoring 15-keto-13,14-dihydro $PGF_{2\alpha}$ in peripheral plasma instead of $PGF_{2\alpha}$ itself. The corresponding PGE_2 metabolite proved more difficult to measure because of its pronounced chemical instability: several dehydrated derivatives as well as highly polar conjugates are rapidly formed in biological material, leading to the rapid disappearance of the monitored metabolite [336,337]. This assay problem however got its solution when a stable degradation product of the metabolite was identified [336,337]. The formation of this degradation product, 11-deoxy-13,14-dihydro-15-keto-11β,16ξ-cyclo-PGE_2, can be quantitatively induced by treatment of the samples with alkali, and subsequent assay of this bicyclic prostaglandin gives a very reliable estimation of the original metabolite levels in the sample [338,339].

An alternative to blood analyses, which has been used successfully in many studies, is measurement of the prostaglandin content of urine instead [335]. Depending on the aim of the study either the primary prostaglandins (which mostly reflect the renal prostaglandin biosynthesis [128,340]) or suitable metabolites (which reflect the total body synthesis of prostaglandin [266,272]) may be monitored.

Since the major part of a prostaglandin that is released into the blood stream will eventually be excreted as degradation products into the urine, there is no risk of missing even a short surge of prostaglandin production, provided 24 h portions of urine are analysed. This approach may thus seem ideal, however, in human clinical studies it may for practical reasons be difficult to ascertain that the whole 24 h portion was actually collected, thereby reducing the reliability of this approach. Relating the prostaglandin metabolite levels to the creatinine excretion into urine may give a somewhat safer measurement [341]. However, an obvious draw-back of urine analyses is that rapid changes in prostaglandin production cannot be seen, consequently temporal endocrine relationships may thus be difficult to study with this approach.

Judging from these difficulties, the safest alternative may after all be measurement of prostaglandin levels in blood. Unfortunately, however, other problems then appear. Although it can be definitely stated that the 15-keto-13,14-dihydro metabolites are circulating compounds, in contrast to the parent primary prostaglandins, their metabolic half-life of about 10 min still implies that they are very short-lived substances. In the normal clinical situation, where it may be desirable to draw conclusions from only one or a very limited number of samples, measurements of the 15-ketodihydro compounds cannot be trusted to give a true picture of the endogenous situation.

Recent metabolic studies on the profiles of prostaglandin metabolites in the circulation have provided alternative targets for measurements: it was demonstrated both in man [280] and in several animal species [281,342,342a] that more degraded, "urinary-type" metabolites gradually accumulated in blood and in fact dominated the metabolic picture for a long time after the initial C_{20} metabolite had disappeared. That such shorter compounds are in many cases more reliable prostaglandin parameters was also demonstrated in several clinical studies [280,343,344].

Concerning the methods employed for quantitative measurements of the prostaglandins (or their metabolites), three types of methods have long dominated this area. These are bioassay, gas chromatography-mass spectrometry, and radioimmunoassay. Such assay methods have been covered in numerous review articles and volumes (see e.g. refs. 345, 346 and references in those volumes).

Bioassay is often the method of choice when biologically active compounds are monitored, and may also be the only possible method, for example when assaying compounds of unknown structure, or highly unstable substances, such as PGI_2 or TXA_2. The widely used organ bath technique has more recently been developed into the more sensitive and specific superfusion cascade type, where frequently amounts in the low nanogram range of a compound can be estimated, and where confusion with other bioactive compounds can be minimised [347]. Bioassay is, however, not possible to use for assay of prostaglandin metabolites, which are generally biologically inactive. In such cases one of the other method types may be employed.

Gas chromatography-mass spectrometry, using the reverse isotope dilution method [348], has been used mainly during the past decade. The method is based on the addition to the sample of a large amount of the compound to be measured, but labeled with a stable isotope (e.g. deuterium). This compound acts as a carrier during the subsequent purification procedure and then as an internal standard during the final GC/MS step. Selected ions, characteristic of the isotope labeled as well as the natural (e.g. protium) form of the compound, are monitored using the mass spectrometer, and the amount of the natural prostaglandin is calculated from the measured proportion between the two forms. This method is often highly specific and has generally been used as a reference method for the other assay types.

The assay method that is most widely used today is probably radioimmunoassay. This method, based on the competition between radiolabeled and "cold" molecules of a compound for antibody binding sites, is very sensitive and has a high sample capacity. The method may however be very non-specific, and a large number of highly unrealistic data have unfortunately been published, based on this methodology (for a review, see e.g. ref. 349).

During the last few years, other analytical methods have gradually come into increasing use as alternatives to the above-mentioned assay types. With the growing complexity of the prostaglandin family, analysis of biological materials is now often aimed more at obtaining total profiles of prostanoids than at measuring absolute amounts of one single compound. This has become facilitated by the improvement of chromatographic separation techniques that has occurred with the introduction of high performance liquid chromatography (HPLC) as well as the increased use of capillary columns in gas chromatography.

The problem in common for such techniques is the detection method. Methods based on conventional flame ionization detection in gas chromatography, or changes in refraction index in liquid chromatography, which should detect all compounds, are normally not sensitive enough (cf. however ref. 350). On the other hand, the more sensitive monitoring of compounds by electron capture in gas chromatography [351,352] or ultraviolet absorption in liquid chromatography [353,354] favours the few compounds that already have the desired properties, such as PGB compounds or leukotrienes. In order to assay all prostanoids in a sample, the compounds thus have to be converted into derivatives with the desired properties, i.e. easily detectable chemical groups have to be introduced. It is then customary to take advantage of the carboxyl group, which is a common feature for all naturally occurring prostanoids. This approach has recently been used in a number of analytical methods in this field. For example, prostanoid esters with fluorescent properties can be prepared by reaction with 4-bromomethyl-7-methoxycoumarin [355] or *p*-(9-anthroyloxy)phenacyl bromide [356]; in the latter case high ultraviolet absorptivity is also obtained. Such derivatives are suitable for HPLC separation and quantitation, and lower limits of detection around 20 ng [355] or 50–280 pg [356] have been reported. For analysis by gas chromatography or GC/MS, other derivatives may be preferred: electron capturing properties can be introduced into the prostanoids by converting them into pentafluorobenzoyl esters [357–359], and such derivatives are also highly suitable for analysis by the negative ion chemical ionization (NICI) type of mass spectrometry [360–362]. In the latter case the detection limit may be in the low picogram range.

The presence of a carboxyl group in all prostanoids has also been used in the "classical" assay types: this chemical group can be used to introduce labelled substituents for use as heterologous tracers in radioimmunoassay [363–365], or it may serve as a site of labeling with stable isotopes (^{18}O) for use in quantitative mass spectrometry [366].

If the analytical method is aimed only at detecting carbonyl containing compounds, various oximes may be prepared instead: methyl esters of pentafluorobenzyl oximes or p-nitrobenzyl oximes of prostaglandins of the E, D, 6-keto-E or 6-keto-F type as well as of TXB_2 have been analyzed by GC/MS methods or HPLC methods, respectively [357,367–369].

9. Monooxygenase metabolism of prostaglandins and essential fatty acids

ω-Oxidation of saturated fatty acids was originally discovered in vivo and named by Verkade et al. [370,371]. In presence of NADPH and molecular oxygen, liver microsomes were later found to catalyze ω1- and ω2-hydroxylation of saturated fatty acids [372–375]. The ω1-hydroxylating enzyme system could be solubilised and resolved into three components, which were needed for full activity, viz. the hemoprotein cytochrome *P*-450, the flavoprotein NADPH-*P*-450 reductase and a lipid factor (e.g. dilauroylphosphatidylcholine [376].). Cytochrome *P*-450 occurs in multiple forms and can oxidise a wide variety of endogenous and exogenous compounds (see ref. 377 for review). The monooxygenase reaction, which is catalyzed by these enzymes, is summarized in Fig. 10. Alkyl chains may be hydroxylated and double bonds may be epoxidized in this way [376,378,379].

ω1- and ω2-hydroxylation of saturated fatty acids has been studied in detail. In the liver these reactions may partly be catalysed by different forms of cytochrome *P*-450 [374,377,380]. Significant hydroxylation of saturated fatty acids also occurs in particulate fractions of renal cortex, lung and small intestine [381–384]. The highest activities are found in the liver and the renal cortex [377,381,385]. Hepatic monooxygenases also oxygenate many other substrates at high rates, while the renal cortical monooxygenase system seems to be rather specific for fatty acids. One form of cytochrome *P*-450 dominates in the kidneys and it catalyses formation of both ω1-

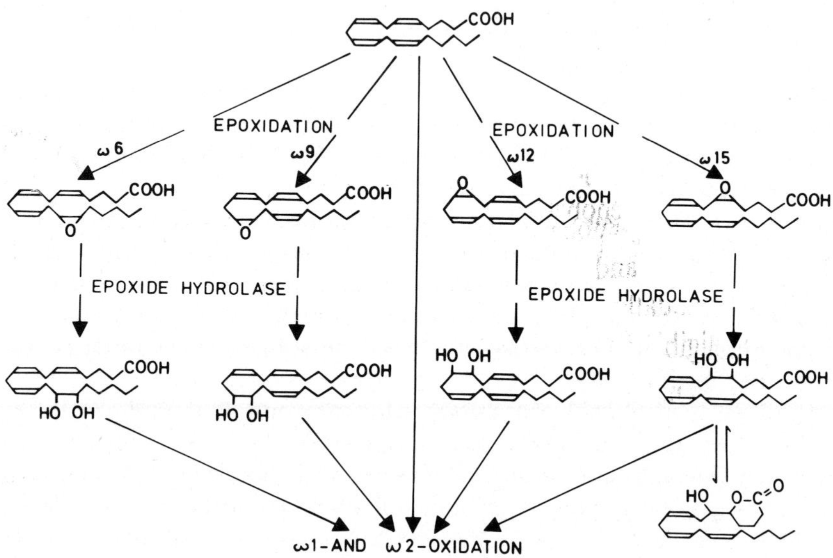

Fig. 10. Summary of the enzymatic metabolism of arachidonic acid by cytochrome *P*-450. The epoxides presumably all have the *cis* configuration although this has only been shown for the ω6 oxide. The epoxides are hydrolysed by epoxide hydrolase into the vicinal diols. Arachidonic acid and the vicinal diols may be further metabolised by ω1- and ω2-hydroxylation.

and ω2-hydroxylated products (see ref. 385 for review). Following ω1- or ω2-hydroxylation of fatty acids, soluble or microsomal enzymes may further oxidise the primary alcohol to a carboxyl group or the secondary alcohol to a ketone (e.g. ref. 386).

Quantitative studies show that only a small fraction of the fatty acids are subject to ω-oxidation in the liver under normal conditions [387]. Starvation, diabetes mellitus and ketosis apparently augment ω-oxidation of fatty acids in experimental animals and man [388–390]. In these situations, several investigators estimated that 10–40% of the fatty acids may be initially ω-oxidised [388,389,392]. The increase was probably not due to induction of the monooxygenase enzymes but could reflect a decreased rate of formation of fatty acid esters for reacylation [390]. However, monooxygenase metabolism of fatty acids is inducible. Treatment with phenobarbital increased the hepatic ω2-hydroxylation, while the ω1-hydroxylation of fatty acids was little affected [374]. Renal cortical hydroxylation of fatty acids could be induced by a high intake of fat in the diet [393].

Monooxygenase metabolism of essential fatty acids has received comparatively little attention. DiAugustine and Fouts found that in liver microsomes, linoleic acid, linolenic acid and arachidonic acid induced spectral changes of type I, which are associated with metabolism, but the products were not identified [394]. These polyunsaturated fatty acids could be expected to be ω1- and ω2-hydroxylated like their saturated counterparts and to be transformed into hydroxylated *cis,trans* conjugated products by chemical peroxidation (autooxidation) as discussed above. Recent studies show that cytochrome *P*-450 can metabolise polyunsaturated fatty acids to a large extent by epoxidation. The epoxides are rapidly hydrolysed to vicinal diols by microsomal or soluble enzymes.

The monooxygenase metabolism of arachidonic acid has been studied in greatest detail. Hepatic and renal cortical microsomes of normal rabbits were found to form two 1,2-diols as major products, viz. 11,12-dihydroxy-5,8,14-eicosatrienoic acid and 14,15-dihydroxy-5,8,11-eicosatrienoic acid [395,396].

The biosynthesis required NADPH and was inhibited by carbon monoxide. Experiments using $^{18}O_2$ strongly indicated that the 1,2-diols were formed by hydrolysis of the ω6- and ω9-epoxides of arachidonic acid, respectively [396], and these epoxides could later be isolated [397]. Other identified metabolites were formed by ω1- and ω2-oxidation [395]. Formation of several monohydroxy-eicosatetraenoic acids has also been reported [398].

Preparations of purified phenobarbital-induced cytochrome *P*-450 (*P*-450 PB-B_2 and *P*-450 LM_2 from rat and rabbit liver, respectively [377,399]), metabolised arachidonic acid by epoxidation of each of the four double bonds [397]. Using such preparations with negligible epoxide hydrolase activity, the four epoxides could be isolated [397,400]. The monooxygenase metabolism of arachidonic acid is summarised in Fig. 10. In the presence of soluble or microsomal epoxide hydrolase, the corresponding 1,2-diols are rapidly formed. Liver and renal cortical microsomes may further metabolise the 1,2-diols by ω1- and ω2-oxidation to yield a family of trihydroxy compounds and other metabolites, with polarity similar to those of many prostaglandins [396,401].

Preparations of β-naphthoflavone-induced cytochrome P-450 (P-450 BNF-B_2 and P-450 LM_4) or rabbit lung microsomes did not form significant amounts of the epoxides or vicinal diols, but ω1- and ω2-hydroxylated metabolites of arachidonic acid were formed [397,402]. Epoxidation and hydroxylation may therefore be catalysed by different enzymes in the rabbit and the rat. However, in bacillus megaterium the same cytochrome P-450 enzyme seems to catalyse both types of reactions [403].

Linoleic and linolenic acid are metabolised by hepatic microsomes of the rabbit and NADPH in an analogous way [404,405]. Linolenic acid is thus transformed into three 1,2-diols, viz. 15,16-dihydroxy-9,12-octadecadienoic acid, 12,13-dihydroxy-9,15-octadecadienoic acid and 9,10-dihydroxy-12,15-octadecadienoic acid. They were the major metabolites formed and apparently stem from hydrolysis of the ω3-, ω6- and ω9-epoxides of linolenic acid, respectively. Linoleic acid can also be ω6-ω9-epoxidised by this system [395,404,405].

Unlike ω1- and ω2-hydroxylation of fatty acids, it is not known whether epoxides of essential fatty acids are formed by monooxygenases in vivo. However, isolated renal cells and hepatocytes of the rat metabolise exogenous arachidonic acid to 11,12-dihydroxy- and 14,15-dihydroxy-eicosatrienoic acids [402]. Surprisingly, the capacity of renal cells to form these 1,2-diols was several times higher than that of the isolated hepatocytes.

Alkyl chains of many other lipids can be metabolised by ω1- or ω2-hydroxylation, and, for example, prostaglandins and leukotrienes may be transformed in this way. As discussed above, ω-oxidation of prostaglandins is one of the metabolic processes that lead to formation of the main urinary metabolites.

Monooxygenase metabolism of prostaglandins has been studied in particulate fractions of several organs. Many results are analogous to those from studies with saturated fatty acids. In the liver of several species, ω1- and ω2-hydroxylation seems to be catalysed by different monooxygenases, and ω2-hydroxylation is inducible with phenobarbital treatment [311]. In renal cortex, however, one type of monooxygenase seems to catalyse both ω1- and ω2-hydroxylation of prostaglandins [406]. Pregnancy or treatment with progesterone induces a several-fold increase in ω2-hydroxylation but not in ω1-hydroxylation in rabbit lung [249,309,310,313]. The biological significance of this observation is not known.

10. Dietary factors influencing prostaglandin production

As was mentioned above, the activity of the arachidonic acid system is dependent both on the availability of arachidonic acid at the precursor storage site in membrane phospholipids and on the release and reacylation mechanisms controlling the amount of free arachidonic acid. The formation of the prostaglandin precursor acids from the dietary linoleic (18 : 2ω6) and α-linolenic (18 : 3ω3) acids is dependent on the general nutritional state and on the presence of other dietary fatty acids, which may compete at sites of interconversion and storage. A general outline of the

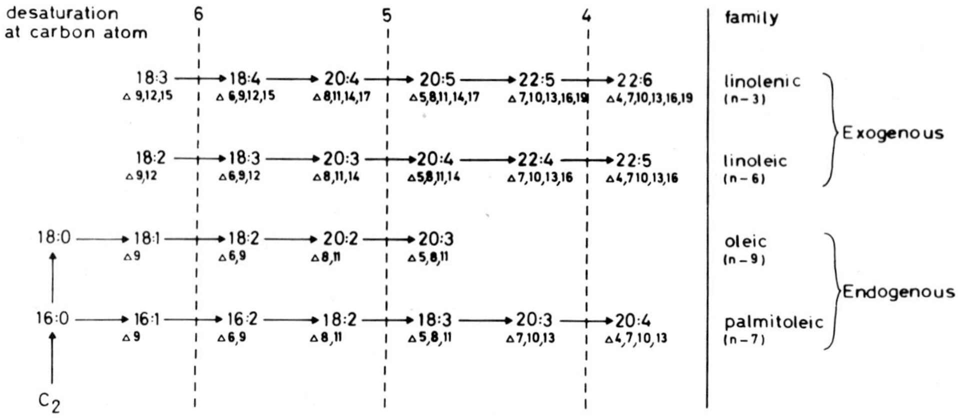

Fig. 11. Biosynthesis of polyunsaturated fatty acids from exogenous and endogenous precursors. The figures 6, 5 and 4, refer to the position of double bonds introduced by desaturases.

polyunsaturated fatty acid desaturation and chain elongation ladder is shown in Fig. 11. For reviews, see refs. 15–18 and 407–411.

Linoleic acid (18 : 2ω6) is one of the classical essential fatty acids [1,2]. It is desaturated by the Δ^6-desaturase, and then chain-elongated to form dihomo-γ-linolenic acid (20 : 3ω6), the precursor for the monoenoic prostaglandins. In most tissues it is, however, further desaturated by the Δ^5-desaturase to arachidonic acid, the precursor for the bisenoic prostaglandins. Analysis of tissue levels of these two prostaglandin precursors have revealed 3–50 fold higher concentrations of arachidonic acid [17,18]. Exceptions to this rule are the adrenal and vesicular glands, where the levels of dihomo-γ-linolenic acid are higher [18,24,412].

There is no direct evidence that α-linolenic acid (18 : 3ω3) is essential in man, and it can only cure some of the signs of essential fatty acid-deficiency in animals. Rats fed α-linolenic acid as the only source of essential fatty acids have normal reproduction except for a deficient process of parturition [408]. This is possibly due to insufficiency of the uterine prostaglandin production. It should also be noted that long chain derivatives of the ω3 series are found in high concentration in brain and retinal phospholipids, implying a specific role in brain function and in vision [413,414].

The metabolic transformation of the C_{18} essential fatty acids to their longer chain fatty acid derivatives has been studied mainly in the liver and to some extent in the brain. Animals and tissues vary greatly in their efficiency of desaturation and chain elongation [18,414,415]. Thus young rats have a particularly active system whereas cats are unable to perform this metabolic reaction. The failure of the cat family to desaturate linoleic acid has been suggested to be a possible reason behind the cats' evolution to carnivorous animals [416] (e.g. eating rats). Humans occupy an intermediate position.

The available studies indicate that a reciprocal inhibition occurs in the desaturation-chain elongation mechanisms between the fatty acids of the $\omega3$, $\omega6$ and $\omega9$ series [411] (Fig. 11). The balance between the levels of linoleic acid ($\omega6$) and linolenic acid ($\omega3$) in the diet modulates the relative rates of long chain fatty acids formed from them. Also in essential fatty acid-deficient animals oleic acid ($18:1\omega9$) can be converted to $20:3\omega9$ in appreciable quantities. This acid ("Mead acid") has thus become one of several biochemical indicators of essential fatty acid-deficiency [407–411].

Alterations in the dietary content of essential fatty acids have become one of the chief ways of providing a modulation of the prostaglandin system. Dietary regimens have ranged from frank essential fatty acid-deficiency to specific feeding programs using oils rich in $18:2\omega6$, $18:3\omega6$, $18:3\omega3$, $20:4\omega6$ and $20:5\omega3$. These studies show that essential fatty acid-deficiency decreases the in vivo prostaglandin production, whereas dietary loading with acids of the $\omega6$ series will enhance prostaglandin formation [409,410].

Essential fatty acid-deficient rats excrete less prostaglandin metabolites in urine [417], and less prostaglandins are accumulated in kidney and blood [418,419]. Only a small addition of linoleic acid (0.4–0.5% of energy) is necessary to elevate urine and tissue prostaglandins back to normal levels. Further dietary loading with $18:2\omega6$ up to 28% of dietary energy will additionally enhance the in vivo formation of prostaglandins in the rat [417]. Interestingly, dietary linoleic acid will decrease the incidence of arterial thrombosis in the rat in a dose-dependent manner and will prevent salt-induced hypertension [420].

Also in man there is evidence for a relationship between dietary linoleate and the activity of the prostaglandin system. In essential fatty acid-deficient infants Friedman and Oates noted a decreased excretion of the major urinary metabolite of PGE [421]. A quantitative relationship between dietary linoleate intake and excretion of total tetranordioic metabolites in urine has also been observed in carefully conducted feeding experiments [422]. After a 2 week diet with 0, 4 or 20% of the energy as linoleic acid given to young women, the mean excretion of metabolites convertible into tetranorprostanedioic acid was 123 ± 5.2, 175 ± 7.0 and 352 ± 10.8 μg/day, respectively. Patients given a linoleic rich diet showed a decreased platelet aggregation and a lower cardiovascular death rate [420]. Patients with recent myocardial infarction had a significantly lower proportion of linoleic acid in their erythrocyte membranes, which reflect long term dietary fat intake [423]. There is thus considerable evidence that the level of dietary intake of linoleic acid influences both prostaglandin production and the tendency for cardiovascular disease.

Since the Δ^6-desaturase is believed to be the rate limiting step in the conversion of linoleic acid to arachidonic acid, efforts have been made to utilize the relatively high content (7%) of γ-linolenic acid ($18:3\omega6$) in the evening primrose oil to influence the activity of the prostaglandin system. The essential fatty acid potency of γ-linolenic acid is 50% greater than that of linoleic acid [424]. However, there is to date no evidence on the possible relationship between dietary intake of this acid and of levels of prostaglandins and prostaglandin metabolites metabolites in vivo.

The most direct way to provide a dietary stimulation of prostaglandin production would be to feed dihomo-γ-linolenic acid or arachidonic acid, preferably in a low fat diet, to minimise competition from other unsaturated fatty acids. In feeding experiments both these approaches have been used. Hassam and Crawford gave ^{14}C-labeled dihomo-γ-linolenic acid to rats and found substantial desaturation to arachidonic acid [425]. However, 33–50% of the radioactivity was recovered as unchanged dihomo-γ-linolenic acid in plasma and liver phospholipids. Feeding this acid in larger amounts should therefore be expected to increase the precursor pools of the monoenoic prostaglandins. Indeed, feeding 1 g/kg/day of ethyl dihomo-γ-linolenate to rabbits resulted in increased incorporation in tissue phospholipids and a 20–30 fold increase in PGE_1 and a 5 fold increase in PGE_2 by a hormone responsive renal papilla preparation in vitro [426,427]. Dihomo-γ-linolenate feeding has been shown to inhibit platelet aggregation in the rat, guinea pig and baboon [18]. The production of the major urinary metabolite was increased 4.6 fold and the platelets showed less reactivity to aggregating stimuli [428]. In man dihomo-γ-linolenate feeding resulted in increased incorporation of the acid into membrane phospholipid pools [429,430]. The effects on prostaglandin production were not clear. It should be observed that dihomo-γ-linolenic acid is primarily converted to the inactive metabolite 12-hydroxy-heptadecadienoic acid by human platelets.

Intravenous administration of arachidonic acid to rabbits and dogs leads to increased formation of prostaglandins in various tissues. This technique has been widely used as an experimental tool to enhance the activity of the prostaglandin system in vivo and in vitro. If, however, the infused amounts of arachidonic acid become excessive, intravascular aggregation occurs and the animals may die. It is therefore not surprising that clinical investigators have been reluctant to administer pure arachidonate to humans. In two studies ethyl arachidonate has, however, been added to the diet of human volunteers resulting in elevated levels of phospholipid arachidonate and of urinary prostaglandin metabolites [431,432].

One of the more interesting approaches to the dietary modification of the prostaglandin system has come from observations of the protective effect of a fish diet on cardiovascular disease [433]. Since oils from fish contain large amounts of fatty acids of the ω3 series, particularly eicosapentaenoic acid (20 : 5ω3, Figs. 2 and 11), interest has been focussed on the possibility of a competition between arachidonic acid and eicosapentaenoic acid at sites of storage and prostaglandin formation. Animal experiments have shown that fish oil feeding results in decreased formation of platelet TXA_2 and vascular PGI_2 [418,434,435]. No appreciable formation of TXA_3 and PGI_3 could be shown. Eicosapentaenoic acid is thus displacing arachidonic acid from storage sites and is not converted to physiologically active eicosanoids in any significant amounts.

Clinical experiments have largely borne out these conclusions. Intake of salt water fish, providing a dietary content of up to 7–11 g of eicosapentaenoic acid per day, gave a marked increase in the ratio of 20 : 5/20 : 4 in platelet membranes [436,437]. Bleeding time, platelet aggregation and TXA_2 production was decreased upon challenge with low dose collagen. The concept of polyenoic acid competition as a dietary means of preventing thrombotic disease in man is now being tested in large scale trials. The therapeutic potential of eicosapentaenoic acid has been reviewed in ref. 438.

The incorporation of unsaturated fatty acids into membrane lipids of human and animal tissue may also be affected by other dietary factors. One of them is chronic exposure to ethanol [439–442]. Ethanol can decrease the amounts of the $\omega 6$ series of essential fatty acids in membrane lipids and can markedly lower the ratio of $C_{20:4\omega 6}/C_{18:2\omega 6}$. These changes have been attributed to a decreased absorption and/or an increased utilization of essential fatty acids and to inhibition of the Δ^6-desaturase enzyme by chronic intake of ethanol [443,444].

Like general anesthetics, ethanol appears to act by changing the fluidity of membrane lipids, leading to a perturbed function of the membrane proteins. During development of tolerance to ethanol, the membrane phospholipids acquire more saturated fatty acids, which seems to counteract the effects of ethanol on membrane function.

Another explanation for decreased levels of $C_{20:4\omega 6}$ could also be an increased metabolism, leading to prostaglandins or other compounds. In the rat, chronic ethanol exposure aggravated the biochemical indicators of essential fatty acid deficiency and increased utilization of arachidonic acid, as indicated by an increased renal excretion of prostaglandins [445]. Whether similar effects can be demonstrated in chronic alcoholism in humans must await the results of further studies.

11. Perspectives

Studies on the oxidative metabolism of arachidonic acid during the last decades have repeatedly revealed that different cells and tissues transform arachidonic acid into their own specific profile of eicosanoids. Seminal vesicles and the renal medulla form E and F prostaglandins. PGD_2 is formed by the rodent brain, by mast-cells and in small amounts by platelets. Platelets mainly transform arachidonic acid to thromboxanes and 12-hydroxy-eicosatetraenoic acid, while the vascular endothelium forms PGI_2. Yet other products are formed by monooxygenases in the liver and the renal cortex. Polymorphonuclear leukocytes and eosinophils form leukotrienes which are of paramount biological interest. It may not be too presumptuous to believe that still more routes of metabolism of arachidonic acid leading to still other biologically active principles await discovery in the future.

Acknowledgments

This study was supported in part by the Swedish Medical Research Council (proj. no. 03X-06523, 03P-5804 and 03X-05915), the Swedish Society of Medical Sciences and Jeansson's Foundation.

References

1 Burr, G.O. and Burr, M.M. (1930) J. Biol. Chem. 86, 587–621.
2 Burr, G.O. and Burr, M.M. (1929) J. Biol. Chem. 82, 345–367.
3 Kurzrok, R. and Lieb, C.C. (1930) Proc. Soc. Exp. Biol. Med. 28, 268–272.
4 von Euler, U.S. (1934) Arch. Exp. Pathol. Pharmakol. 175, 78–84.
5 von Euler, U.S. (1935) Klin. Wochenschrift 14, 1182–1183.
6 Bergström, S., Dressler, F., Krabisch, L., Ryhage, R. and Sjövall, J. (1962) Arkiv Kemi 20, 63–66.
7 Bergström, S., Dressler, F., Ryhage, R., Samuelsson, B. and Sjövall, J. (1962) Arkiv Kemi 19, 563–567.
8 Bergström, S., Danielsson, H. and Samuelsson, B. (1964) Biochim. Biophys. Acta 90, 207–210.
9 van Dorp, D.A., Beerthuis, R.K., Nugteren, D.H. and Vonkeman, H. (1964) Biochim. Biophys. Acta 90, 204–207.
10 Änggård, E. (1966) Acta Physiol. Scand. 66, 509–510.
11 Ferreira, S.H. and Vane, J.R. (1967) Nature 216, 868–873.
12 Sprecher, H., Van Rollins, M., Sun, F., Wyche, A. and Needleman, P. (1982) J. Biol. Chem. 257, 3912–3918.
13 Nelson, N.A. (1974) J. Med. Chem. 17, 911–918.
14 Thomasson, J.J. (1953) Int. Z. Vitam. Forsch. 25, 62–82.
15 Vergroesen, A.J. (1979) Ind. J. Nutr. Diet. 16, 219–230.
16 van Dorp, D.A. (1976) Acta Biol. Med. Germ. 35, 1041–1049.
17 Rivers, J.P.W. and Frankel, T.L. (1981) Br. Med. Bull. 37, 59–64.
18 Willis, A.L. (1981) Nutr. Rev. 39, 289–301.
19 Hansen, A.E., Wiese, H.F. and Boelsche, A.N. (1963) Pediatrics 31, 171–192.
20 Friedman, Z., Marks, K.H., Maisels, M.J., Thorson, R. and Naeye, R. (1978) Pediatrics 61, 694–698.
21 Berlin, E., Matusik, E.J., Jr. and Young, C., Jr. (1980) Lipids 15, 604–608.
22 Ananda Rao, G., Siler, K. and Larkin, E.C. (1979) Lipids 14, 30–38.
23 Irvine, R.F. (1982) Biochem. J. 204, 3–16.
24 Lands, W.E.M. and Samuelsson, B. (1968) Biochim. Biophys. Acta 164, 426–429.
25 Lands, W.E.M., Inoue, M., Sugiura, Y. and Okuyama, H. (1982) J. Biol. Chem. 257, 14968–14972.
26 van den Bosch, H. (1980) Biochim. Biophys. Acta 604, 191–246.
27 Lands, W.E.M. and Merkl, I. (1963) J. Biol. Chem. 238, 898–904.
28 Morita, I. and Murota, S.-I. (1980) Biochim. Biophys. Acta 619, 428–431.
29 Hirata, F. and Axelrod, J. (1980) Science 209, 1082–1090.
30 Vance, D.E. and de Kruijff, B. (1980) Nature 288, 277–279.
31 Randon, J., Lecompte, T., Chignard, M., Siess, W., Marlas, G., Dray F. and Vargaftig, B.B. (1981) Nature 293, 660–662.
32 Hokin, M.R. and Hokin, L.E. (1953) J. Biol. Chem. 203, 967–977.
33 Michell, R.H., Kirk, C.J., Jones, L.M., Downes, C.P. and Creba, J.A. (1981) Phil. Trans. R. Soc. Lond. (Biol.) 296, 123–137.
34 Marshall, P.J., Dixon, J.F. and Hokin, L.E. (1980) Proc. Natl. Acad. Sci. USA 77, 3292–3296.
35 Bell, R.L., Kennerly, D.A., Stanford, N. and Majerus, P.W. (1979) Proc. Natl. Acad. Sci. USA 76, 3238–3241.
36 Berridge, M.J. and Fain, J.N. (1979) Biochem. J. 178, 59–69.
37 Fain, J.N. and Garcia-Sáinz, J.A. (1980) Life Sci. 26, 1183–1194.
38 Hawthorne, J.N. (1982) Nature 295, 281–282.
39 Prpic, V., Blackmore, P.F. and Exton, J.H. (1982) J. Biol. Chem. 257, 11323–11331.
40 Prescott, S.M. and Majerus, P.W. (1981) J. Biol. Chem. 256, 579–582.
41 Billah, M.M., Lapetina, E.G. and Cuatrecasas, P. (1980) J. Biol. Chem. 255, 10227–10231.
42 Lapetina, E.G. (1982) Trends Pharmacol. Sci. 3, 115–118.
43 Serhan, C.N., Fridovich, J., Goetzl, E.J., Dunham, P.B. and Weissman, G. (1982) J. Biol. Chem. 257, 4746–4752.
44 Sagawa, N., Okazaki, T., MacDonald, P.C. and Johnston, J.M. (1982) J. Biol. Chem. 257, 8158–8162.

45 Benabe, J.E., Spry, L.A. and Morrison, A.R. (1982) J. Biol. Chem. 257, 7430–7434.
46 Marshall, P.J., Boatman, D.E. and Hokin, L.E. (1981) J. Biol. Chem. 256, 844–847.
47 Gryglewski, R., Panczenko, B., Korbut, R., Grodzinska, L. and Ocetkiewicz, A. (1975) Prostaglandins 10, 343–355.
48 Hong, S.-C.L. and Levine, L. (1976) Proc. Natl. Acad. Sci. USA 73, 1730–1734.
49 Flower, R.J. and Blackwell, G.J. (1979) Nature 278, 456–459.
50 Hirata, F., Schiffmann, E., Venkatasubramanian, K., Salomon, D. and Axelrod, J. (1980) Proc. Natl. Acad. Sci. USA 77, 2533–2536.
51 Gurr, M.I. and James, A.T. (1975) Lipid biochemistry. An Introduction, 2nd edn., Chapman and Hall, London. pp. 74–76.
52 Porter, N.A., Weber, B.A., Weenen, H. and Khan, J.A. (1980) J. Am. Chem. Soc. 102, 5597–5601.
53 Porter, N.A., Lehman, L.S., Weber, B.A. and Smith, K.J. (1981) J. Am. Chem. Soc. 103, 6447–6455.
54 Nugteren, D.H., Vonkeman, H. and van Dorp, D.A. (1967) Rec. Trav. Chim. 85, 1237–1245.
55 Porter, N.A., Wolf, R.A., Yarbro, E.M. and Weenen, H. (1979) Biochem. Biophys. Res. Commun. 89, 1058–1064.
56 Sevanian, A., Mead, J.F. and Stein, R.A. (1979) Lipids 14, 634–643.
57 Neff, W.E., Frankel, E.N. and Weisleder, D. (1981) Lipids 16, 439–448.
58 Bild, G.A., Bhat, S.G., Ramadoss, E.S., Axelrod, B. (1978) J. Biol. Chem. 253, 21–23.
59 Christ, E.J. and van Dorp, D.A. (1972) Biochim. Biophys. Acta 270, 537–545.
60 Samuelsson, B. (1981) The Harvey Lectures, Series 75, pp. 1–40, Academic Press, New York.
61 Samuelsson, B. (1965) J. Am. Chem. Soc. 87, 3011–3013.
62 Hamberg, M. and Samuelsson, B. (1973) Proc. Natl. Acad. Sci. USA 70, 899–903.
63 Nugteren, D.H. and Hazelhof, E. (1973) Biochim. Biophys. Acta 326, 448–461.
64 Miyamoto, T., Ogino, N., Yamamoto, S. and Hayaishi, O. (1976) J. Biol. Chem. 251, 2629–2636.
65 Van der Ouderaa, F.J., Buytenhek, M., Nugteren, D.H. and van Dorp, D.A. (1977) Biochem. Biophys. Acta 487, 315–331.
66 Ueno, R., Shimizu, T., Kondo, K. and Hayaishi, O. (1982) J. Biol. Chem. 257, 5584–5588.
67 Marnett, L.J., Wlodawer, P. and Samuelsson, B. (1975) J. Biol. Chem. 250, 8510–8517.
68 Zenser, T.V., Mattammal, M.B., Brown, W.W. and Davis, B.B. (1979) Kidney Int. 16, 688–694.
69 Marnett, L.J. (1981) Life Sci. 29, 531–546.
70 Modéus, P., Andersson, B., Rahimtula, A. and Berggren, M. (1982) Biochem. Pharmacol. 31, 1363–1368.
71 Shimizu, T., Yamamoto, S. and Hayaishi, O. (1979) J. Biol. Chem. 254, 5222–5228.
72 Roberts, L.J. II, Sweetman, B.J., Lewis, R.A., Austen, K.F. and Oates, J.A. (1980) New Engl. J. Med. 303, 1400–1404.
73 Christ-Hazelhof, E., Nugteren, D.H. and van Dorp, D.A. (1976) Biochim. Biophys. Acta 450, 450–461.
74 Vane, J.R. (1971) Nat. New Biol. 231, 232–235.
75 Smith, J.B. and Willis, A.L. (1971) Nat. New Biol. 231, 235–237.
76 Ferreira, S.H., Moncada, S. and Vane, J.R. (1971) Nat. New Biol. 231, 237–239.
77 Vane, J.R. (1978) Adv. Prostaglandin Thromboxane Res. 4, 27–44.
78 Flower, R.J. (1974) Pharmacol. Rev. 26, 33–67.
79 Novy, M.J. and Liggins, G.C. (1980) Semin. Perinatol. 4, 45–66.
80 Coceani, F. and Olley, P.M. (1980) Semin. Perinatol. 4, 109–113.
81 Hamberg, M. and Samuelsson, B. (1966) J. Biol. Chem. 241, 257–263.
82 Templeton, A.A., Cooper, J. and Kelly, R.W. (1978) J. Reprod. Fertil. 52, 147–150.
83 Tusell, J.M. and Gelpi, E. (1980) J. Chromatogr. 181, 295–310.
84 Svanborg, K., Bygdeman, M., Eneroth, E. and Bendvold, E. (1982) Prostaglandins 24, 363–375.
85 Samuelsson, B., Granström, E., Gréen, K., Hamberg, M. and Hammarström, S. (1975) Annu. Rev. Biochem. 44, 669–695.
86 Bygdeman, M. and Gillespie, A. (1981) in Prostaglandins (J.B. Lee, ed.) pp. 215–249, Elsevier, New York.
87 Bygdeman, M., Fredricsson, B., Svanborg, K. and Samuelsson, B. (1970) Fertil. Steril. 21, 622–629.

88 Goldberg, V.J. and Ramwell, P.W. (1975) Physiol. Rev. 55, 325–351.
89 Bergström, S. (1983) Nobel Lecture. in Les Prix Nobel 1982, (W. Odelberg, ed.) Almqvist and Wiksell International, Stockholm, in press.
90 Bygdeman, M. (1964) Acta Physiol. Scand. 63 (suppl. 242), 1–78.
91 Roth-Brandel, U., Bygdeman, M. and Wiqvist, N. (1970) Acta Obstet. Gynecol. Scand. 49 (suppl. 5), 1–7.
92 Karim, S.M.M., Trussell, R.R., Hillier, K. and Patel, R.C. (1969) J. Obstet. Gynaecol. Br. Commonw. 76, 769–782.
93 Bygdeman, M., Roth-Brandel, U. and Wiqvist, N. (1970) Int. J. Gynaec. Obstet. 8, 162.
94 Gréen, K., Bygdeman, M., Toppozada, M. and Wiqvist, N. (1974) Am. J. Obstet. Gynecol. 120, 25–31.
95 Granström, E. and Kindahl, H. (1976) Prostaglandins 12, 759–783.
96 Hamberg, M. (1974) Life Sci. 14, 247–252.
97 Fuchs, A.-R., Husslein, P., Sumulong, L. and Fuchs, F. (1982) Prostaglandins 24, 715–722.
98 Lewis, R.B. and Schulman, J.O. (1973) Lancet ii, 1159–1161.
99 Wiqvist, N., Widholm, O., Nillius, S.J. and Nilsson, B. (eds.) (1979) Dysmenorrhoea and Prostaglandins. Acta Obstet. Gynecol. Scand. (suppl. 87) 5–117.
100 Wiqvist, N. and Bygdeman, M. (1970) Lancet i, 889.
101 Lichtmann, A.S., Bronner, P. and Mishell, D.R. (1974) Contraception 9, 403–408.
102 Bygdeman, M., Gréen, K., Lundström, V., Ramadan, M., Fotiou, S. and Bergström, S. (1976) Prostaglandins 12 (suppl.) 27–51.
103 Karim, S.M.M., Sivasamboo, R. and Ratnam, S.S. (1974) Prostaglandins 6, 349–354.
104 Pulkkinen, M.O. (1978) Prostaglandins 15, 161–167.
105 Gréen, K., Vesterqvist, O., Bygdeman, M., Christenssen, N.J. and Bergström, S. (1982) Prostaglandins 24, 451–466.
106 Roberts, J.S., Barcikowski, B., Wilson, L., Skarnes, R.C. and McCracken, J.A. (1975) J. Steroid Biochem. 6, 1091–1097.
107 Horton, E.W. and Poyser, N.L. (1976) Physiol. Rev. 56, 595–651.
108 Edqvist, L.-E. and Kindahl, H., eds. (1981) Prostaglandins in Animal Reproduction. Acta Vet. Scand. (suppl. 88) 1–390.
109 Stabenfelt, G.H., Edqvist, L.-E., Kindahl, H., Gustafsson, B. and Bane, A. (1978) J. Am. Vet. Med. Assoc. 172, 667–675.
110 Poyser, N. (1981) Prostaglandins in Reproduction. Prostaglandin Research Studies Series, Vol. 2, pp. 1–272, John Wiley and Sons, England.
111 Gréen, K., Christenssen, N. and Bygdeman, M. (1981) J. Reprod. Fert. 62, 269–281.
112 Lee, J.B., Covino, B.G., Takman, B.H. and Smith, E.R. (1965) Circ. Res. 17, 57–77.
113 Hamberg, M. (1969) FEBS Lett. 5, 127–130.
114 Blackwell, G.J., Flower, R.J. and Vane, J.R. (1975) Biochim. Biophys. Acta 398, 178–190.
115 Schwartzman, M., Gafni, Y. and Raz, A. (1976) Eur. J. Biochem. 64, 527–534.
116 Friesinger, C.G., Oelz, O., Sweetman, B.J., Nies, A.S. and Data, J.L. (1978) Prostaglandins 15, 969–981.
117 Berlin, T., Cronestrand, R., Nowak, J., Sonnenfeldt, T. and Wennmalm, Å. (1979) Acta Physiol. Scand. 106, 441–445.
118 Tobian, L. and O'Donnell, M. (1976) Fed. Proc. 35, 2388–2392.
119 Tobian, L., O'Donnell, M. and Smith, P. (1974) Circ. Res. 34/35, suppl. I, I–83–I86.
120 Oliw, E., Lundén, I., Sjöquist, B. and Änggård, E. (1979) Acta Physiol. Scand. 105, 359–366.
121 Stahl, R.A., Attallah, A.A., Block, D.L. and Lee, J.B. (1979) Am. J. Physiol. 237, F344–F349.
122 Orloff, J., Handler, J.S. and Bergström, S. (1965) Nature 205, 397–398.
123 Grantham, J.J. and Orloff, J. (1968) J. Clin. Invest. 47, 1154–1161.
124 Andersson, R.J., Bed, T., McDonald, K.M. and Schrier, R.W. (1975) J. Clin. Invest. 56, 420–426.
125 Zusman, R.M. (1981) Annu. Rev. Med. 32, 359–374.
126 Larsson, C. and Änggård, E. (1976) J. Pharm. Pharmacol. 28, 326–328.
127 Sun, F.F., Taylor, B.M., McGuire, J.C. and Wong, P.Y.K. (1981) Kidney Int. 19, 760–770.

128 Dunn, M.J. and Hood, V.L. (1977) Am. J. Physiol. 233, F 169–184.
129 Gerber, J.G., Branch, R.A., Nies, A.S., Gerkens, J.G., Strand, D.G., Hollifield, J. and Oates, J.A. (1978) Prostaglandins 15, 81–88.
130 Kimberly, R.P., Gill, J.R., Bowden, R.E. Keiser, H.R. and Plotz, P.H. (1978) Annu. Intern. Med. 89, 336–341.
131 Kimberly, R.P. and Plotz, P.H. (1977) New Engl. J. Med. 296, 418–424.
132 Weber, P.C., Scherer, B., Seiss, W., Held, E. and Schnermann, J. (1979) Klin. Wochenschrift 57, 1021–1029.
133 McGiff, J.C. (1981) Annu. Rev. Pharmacol. Toxicol. 21, 479–509.
134 Gill, J.R. and Bartter, F.C. (1978) Am. J. Med. 65, 766–772.
135 Gerber, J.G., Anderson, R.J., Schrier, R.W. and Nies, A.S. (1982) Adv. Prostaglandin Thromboxane Leukotriene Res. 10, 227–254.
136 Hamberg, M., Svensson, J., Wakabayashi, T. and Samuelsson, B. (1974) Proc. Natl. Acad. Sci. U.S.A. 71, 345–349.
137 Malmsten, C., Hamberg, M., Svensson, J. and Samuelsson, B. (1975) Proc. Natl. Acad. Sci. USA 72, 1446–1450.
138 Hamberg, M., Svensson, J. and Samuelsson, B .(1975) Proc. Natl. Acad. Sci. USA 72, 2994–2998.
139 Needleman, O., Minkes, M. and Raz, A. (1976) Science 193, 163–165.
140 Fitzpatrick, F.A. and Gorman, R.R. (1977) Prostaglandins 14, 881–889.
141 Salzman, E.W. (1974) Stroke 5, 296.
142 McDonald, J.W.D. and Stuart, R.K. (1973) J. Lab. Clin. Med. 81, 838–849.
143 Marguis, N.R., Vigdahl, R.L. and Tavormina, P.A. (1969) Biochem. Biophys. Res. Commun. 36, 965–972.
144 Salzman, E.W. and Neri, L. (1969) Nature 224, 609–611.
145 Moncada, S. and Vane, J.R. (1979) Pharmacol. Rev. 30, 293–331.
146 Robert, A. (1976) Adv. Prostaglandin Thromboxane Res. 2, 507–520.
147 Newman, A., Prado, P., de Moraes-Filho, J., Philippakos, D. and Misiewicz, J. (1975) Gut 16, 272–276.
148 Robert, A., Nylander, B. and Andersson, S. (1974) Life Sci. 14, 533–538.
149 Robert, A., Nezamis, J.E., Lancaster, C. and Hanchar, A.J. (1979) Gastroenterology 77, 433–443.
150 Robert, A. (1981) Prostaglandins 21 (suppl.), 89–96.
151 Johansson, C., Kollberg, B., Nordemar, R., Samuelson, K. and Bergström, S. (1980) Gastroenterology 78, 479–483.
152 Kollberg, B. and Slezak, P. (1982) Prostaglandins 24, 527–536.
153 Robert, A. (1979) in The Prostaglandin System. Endoperoxides, Prostacyclin and Thromboxanes. (F. Berti and G.P. Velo, eds.) NATO Advanced Study Institutes Series, Vol. A36, pp. 393–400, Plenum Press, New York.
154 Peskar, B.M. (1980) Hepato-Gastroenterology 27, 330–336.
155 Bennett, A., Eley, K.G. and Sholez, G.B. (1968) Br. J. Pharmacol. 34, 639–647.
156 Bennett, A., Eley, K.G. and Stodeley, H.L. (1975) Br. J. Pharmacol. 54, 197–204.
157 Bennett, A., Hensby, C.N., Sanger, G.J. and Stamford, I.F. (1979) in The Prostaglandin System. Endoperoxides, Prostacyclin and Thromboxanes. (F. Berti and G.P. Velo, eds.) NATO Advanced Study Institutes Series, Vol. A36, pp. 365–375, Plenum Press, New York.
158 Sanger, G.J. and Bennett, A. (1979) Ibid, pp. 377–391.
159 Bygdeman, M., Roth-Brandel, U. and Wiqvist, N. (1970) Am. J. Obstet. Gynecol. 106, 567–572.
160 Roth-Brandel, U., Bygdeman, M., Wiqvist, N. and Bergström, S. (1970) Lancet i, 190–191.
161 Matuchansky, C. and Bernier, J.J. (1973) Gastroenterology 64, 1111–1118.
162 Cummings, J.H., Newman, A., Misiewicz, J.J., Milton-Thomson, G.J. and Billings, J.A. (1973) Nature 243, 169–171.
163 Kimberg, D.V., Field, M., Johnson, J., Henderson, A. and Gershon, E. (1971) J. Clin. Invest. 50, 1218–1230.
164 Sharp, G.W.G. and Hynie, S. (1971) Nature 229, 266–269.
165 Nakano, J. (1973) in The Prostaglandins. Pharmacological and Therapeutic Advances (M.F. Curth-

bert, ed.), pp. 23–124, William Heineman Med. Books, London.
166 Änggård, E. and Bergström, S. (1963) Acta Physiol. Scand. 58, 1–12.
167 Malik, K.M. and McGiff, J.C. (1976). in Prostaglandins: Physiological, Pharmacological and Pathological Aspects (S.M.M. Karim, ed.) pp. 103–200, MPT Press Ltd.
168 Martin, M.F.R., Dowd, P.M., Ring, E.F.J., Cooke, E.D., Dieppe, P.A. and Kirkby, J.D.T. (1981) Ann. Rheum. Dis. 40, 350–354.
169 Heymann, M.A. (1981) Am. Heart J. 101, 837–843.
170 Coceani, F. and Olley, P.M. (1973) Can. J. Physiol. Pharmacol. 51, 220–225.
171 Heymann, M.A., Rudolph, A.M. and Silverman, N.H. (1976) New Engl. J. Med. 295, 530–533.
172 Horton, R., Zipser, R. and Fishman, M. (1981) Med. Clin. North Am. 65, 789–808.
173 Mitchell, J.R. (1981) Br. Med. J. 282, 590–594.
174 Änggård, E. and Samuelsson, B. (1965) J. Biol. Chem. 240, 3518–3521.
175 Änggård, E., Gréen, K. and Samuelsson, B. (1965) J. Biol. Chem. 240, 1932–1940.
176 Bergström, S., Carlson, L.A. and Weeks, J.R. (1968) Pharmacol. Rev. 20, 1–48.
177 Änggård, E. (1966) Dissertation, Karolinska Institutet, Stockholm.
178 Piper, P.J., Vane, J.R. and Wyllie, J.H. (1970) Nature 225, 600–604.
179 Said, S.I. (1982) Annu. Rev. Physiol. 44, 257–268.
180 Mathé, A.A., Hedqvist, P., Strandberg, K. and Leslie, C.A. (1977) New Engl. J. Med. 296, 850–855 and New Engl. J. Med. 296, 910–914 (parts I and II).
181 Hyman, A.L., Spannhake, E.W. and Kadowitz, P.J. (1978) Am. Rev. Resp. Dis. 117, 111–136.
182 Cuthbert, M.F. and Gardiner, P.J. (1981) in The Prostaglandin System, Endoperoxides, Prostacyclin and Thromboxanes. (F. Berti and G.P. Velo, eds.) NATO Advanced Study Institutes Series, Vol. A36, pp. 323–342, Plenum Press, New York.
183 Mathé, A.A., Hedqvist, P., Holmgren, A. and Svanborg, N. (1973) Br. Med. J. 1, 193–199.
184 Gréen, K., Hedqvist, P. and Svanborg, N. (1974) Lancet ii, 1419–1421.
185 Hamberg, M., Hedqvist, P., Strandberg, K., Svensson, J. and Samuelsson, B. (1975) Life Sci. 16, 451–462.
186 Svensson, J., Strandberg, K., Tuvemo, T. and Hamberg, M. (1977) Prostaglandins 14, 425–436.
187 Dahlén, S.-E., Hansson, G., Hedqvist, P., Björck, T., Granström, E. and Dahlén, B. (1983) Proc. Natl. Acad. Sci. USA, 80, 1712–1716.
188 Piper, P.J. and Vane, J.R. (1969) Nature 223, 29–35.
189 Folco, G.C., Omini, C., Sautebin, L. and Berti, F. (1981) in The Prostaglandin System. Endoperoxides, Prostacyclin and Thromboxanes. (F. Berti and G.P. Velo, eds.) NATO Advanced Study Institutes Series, Vol. A36, pp. 343–364, Plenum Press, New York.
190 Boot, J.R., Cockerill, A.F., Dawson, W., Mallen, D.N.B. and Osborne, D.J. (1978) Int. Arch. Allergy Appl. Immunol. 57, 159–164.
191 Burka, J.F., Ali, M., McDonald, J.W.D. and Paterson, N.A.M. (1981) Prostaglandins 22, 683–691.
192 Hamberg, M., Svensson, J., Hedqvist, P., Strandberg, K. and Samuelsson, B. (1976) Adv. Prostaglandin Thromboxane Res. 1, 495–501.
193 Hamberg, M., Hedqvist, P. and Rådegran, K. (1980) Acta Physiol. Scand. 110, 219–221.
194 Ally, A.I., Boucher, R., Knowles, M.R. and Eling, T.E. (1982) Prostaglandins 24, 575–584.
195 Hammarström, S., Murphy, R.C., Samuelsson, B., Clark, D.A., Mioskowski, C. and Corey, E.J. (1979) Biochem. Biophys. Res. Commun. 91, 1266–1272.
196 Lewis, R.A., Austen, K.F., Drazen, J.M., Clark, D.A., Marfat, A. and Corey, E.J. (1980) Proc. Natl. Acad. Sci. USA 77, 3710–3714.
197 Morris, H.A., Taylor, G.W., Piper, P.J. and Tippins, J.R. (1980) Nature 285, 104–106.
198 Orange, R.P. and Austen, K.F. (1969) Adv. Immunol. 10, 105–144.
199 Samuelsson, B. (1982) in Advances in Pharmacology and Therapeutics II. (H. Yoshida, Y. Hagihara and S. Ebashi, eds.) Vol. 4, pp. 55–75, Pergamon Press, London.
200 Dahlén, S.-E., Björk, J., Hedqvist, P., Arfors, K.-E., Hammarström, S., Lindgren, J-Å. and Samuelsson, B. (1981) Proc. Natl. Acad. Sci. USA 78, 3887–3891.
201 Wolfe, L. (1982) J. Neurochem. 38, 1–14.
202 Coceani, F. (1974) Arch. Intern. Med. 133, 119–129.
203 Coceani, F. and Pace-Asciak, C.R. (1976) in Prostaglandins. Physiological, Pharmacological and

Pathological Aspects (S.M.M. Karim, ed.), pp. 1–36, MTP Press, Lancaster, PA.
204 Abdel-Halim, M.S., Hamberg, M., Sjöquist, B. and Änggård, E. (1977) Prostaglandins 14, 633–643.
205 Sun, F.F., Chapman, J.P. and McGuire, J.C. (1977) Prostaglandins 14, 1055–1074.
206 Abdel-Halim, M.S. and Änggård, E. (1979) Prostaglandins 17, 411–418.
207 Wolfe, L.S., Rostworowski, K. and Pappius, H.M. (1976) Can. J. Biochem. 54, 629–640.
208 Abdel-Halim, M.S., von Holst, H. Meyerson, B., Sachs, C. and Änggård, E. (1980) J. Neurochem. 34, 1331–1333.
209 Pickard, J.D. (1981) J. Cerebr. Blood Flow Metab. 1, 361–384.
210 Wolfe, L.S., Rostworowski, K. and Marion, J. (1976) Biochem. Biophys. Res. Commun. 70, 907–913.
211 Bennett, A., Charlier, E.M., Raja, B. and Stamford, I.F. (1977) Br. J. Pharmacol. 59, 448P–449P.
212 Narumiya, S., Ogorochi, T., Nakao, K. and Hayaishi, O. (1982) Life Sci. 31, 2093–2103.
213 Abdel-Halim, M.S., Lundén, I., Cseh, G. and Änggård, E. (1980) Prostaglandins 19, 249–258.
214 Gerritsen, M.E., Parks, T.P. and Printz, M.P. (1980) Biochim. Biophys. Acta 619, 196–206.
215 Abdel-Halim, M.S., Ekstedt, J. and Änggård, E. (1979) Prostaglandins 17, 405–409.
216 Horton, E.W. (1972) Monographs on Endocrinology, Vol. 7, pp. 117–149, Springer-Verlag, New York.
217 Rosenkranz, R.P. (1978) Prostaglandins 15, 925–942.
218 Rosenkranz, R.P. and Killam, K.F. (1979) J. Pharmacol. Exp. Ther. 209, 231–237.
219 Quesney, L.F., Gloor, P., Wolfe, L.S. and Joszef, S. (1975) Prostaglandins 10, 383–393.
220 Feldberg, W. and Milton, A.S. (1978) in Handbook of Experimental Pharmacology (Vane, J.R. and Ferreira, S.H., eds.) Vol. 50.1, pp. 615–656, Springer-Verlag, Berlin.
221 Milton, A.S. (1980) in Fever (J.M. Lipton, ed.) pp. 141–148, Raven Press, New York.
222 Abdel-Halim, M.S., Sjöquist, B. and Änggård, E. (1978) Acta Pharmacol. Toxicol. 43, 266–272.
223 Pickard, J.D. and MacKenzie, E.T. (1973) Nat. New Biol. 245, 187–188.
224 Dahlgren, N., Nilsson, B., Sakabe, T. and Siesjö, B.K. (1981) Acta Physiol. Scand. 111, 475–485.
225 Wennmalm, Å., Eriksson, S. and Wahren, J. (1981) Clin. Physiol. 1, 227–234.
226 Siesjö, B.K. (1982) 5th International Conference on Prostaglandins, Firenze, May 18–21, abstract book, p. 255.
227 Wennmalm, Å., Eriksson, S., Hagenfeldt, L., Law, D., Patrono, C. and Pinca, E. (1982) 5th International Conference on Prostaglandins, Firenze, May 18–21, abstract book, p. 257.
228 Boullin, D.J. (ed.) (1980) Cerebral Vasospasm. John Wiley and Sons, Chichester, NY.
229 Hedqvist, P. (1977) Annu. Rev. Pharmacol. Toxicol. 17, 259–279.
230 Hemker, D.P. and Aiken, J.W. (1980) Eur. J. Pharmacol. 67, 155–158.
231 Shimizu, T., Minzuno, N., Amano, T. and Hayaishi, O. (1979) Proc. Natl. Acad. Sci. USA 76, 6231–6234.
232 Bishai, I. and Coceani, F. (1980) Adv. Prostaglandin Thromboxane Res. 8, 1221–1223.
233 Ragheb, M. and Ban, T.A. (1982) Prog. Neuro-Psychopharmacol. Biol. Psychiat. 6, 87–93.
234 Horrobin, D.F. and Manku, M. (1980) Br. Med. J. 280, 1363–1366.
235 Änggård, E. (1983) Pharmacol. Biochem., in press.
236 Burstein, S. and Hunger, S.A. (1981) Rev. Pure Appl. Pharmacol. Sci. 2, 155–226.
237 Parantainen, J. and Vapaatalo, H. (1983) in Handbook of Prostaglandins and Related Compounds (Prior, C., ed.) Churchill Livingstone, London, in press.
238 Hansson, E. and Samuelsson, B. (1965) Biochim. Biophys. Acta 106, 379–385.
239 Gréen, K., Hansson, E. and Samuelsson, B. (1967) Progr. Biochem. Pharmacol. 3, 85–88.
240 Änggård, E. and Samuelsson, B. (1964) J. Biol. Chem. 239, 4097–4102.
241 Änggård, E. and Samuelsson, B. (1966) Arkiv Kemi 25, 293–300.
242 Granström, E. and Samuelsson, B. (1971) Eur. J. Biochem. 20, 451–458.
243 Sun, F.F. and Armour, S.B. (1974) Prostaglandins 7, 327–338.
244 Hook, R. and Gillis, C.N. (1975) Prostaglandins 9, 193–201.
245 Ryan, J.W., Niemeyer, R.S. and Ryan, U. (1975) Prostaglandins 10, 101–108.
246 Anderson, M.W. and Eling, T.E. (1976) Prostaglandins 11, 645–677.
247 Pace-Asciak, C.R. (1977) Prostaglandins 13, 649–660.
248 Pace-Asciak, C.R. and Miller, D. (1973) Prostaglandins 4, 351–362.

249 Powell, W.S. and Solomon, S. (1978) J. Biol. Chem. 253, 4609–4616.
250 Hamberg, M. and Israelsson, U. (1970) J. Biol. Chem. 245, 5107–5114.
251 Hamberg, M. and Samuelsson, B. (1971) J. Biol. Chem. 246, 1073–1077.
252 Dawson, W., Jessup, S.J., McDonald-Gibson, W., Ramwell, P.W. and Shaw, J.E. (1970) Br. J. Pharmacol. 39, 585–598.
253 Anderson, F.L., Jubiz, W. and Tsagaris, T.J. (1976) Am. J. Physiol. 231, 426–429.
254 Granström, E. (1971) Biochim. Biophys. Acta 239, 120–125.
255 Attallah, A.A., Payakkapan, W. and Lee, J.B. (1974) Life Sci. 14, 1521–1534.
256 Nakano, J. (1970) Br. J. Pharmacol. 40, 317–325.
257 Larsson, C. and Änggård, E. (1973) Eur. J. Pharmacol. 21, 30–36.
258 Pace-Asciak, C. (1975) J. Biol. Chem. 250, 2795–2800.
259 Pace-Asciak, C. (1977) Prostaglandins 13, 661–668.
260 Granström, E., Inger, U. and Samuelsson, B. (1965) J. Biol. Chem. 240, 457–461.
261 Gréen, K. (1971) Biochemistry 10, 1072–1086.
262 Gréen, K. (1971) Biochim. Biophys. Acta 231, 419–444.
263 Sun, F.F. (1974) Biochim. Biophys. Acta 348, 249–262.
264 Brash, A.R. and Baillie, T.A. (1979) Biochim. Biophys. Acta 572, 371–375.
265 Pace-Asciak, C.R. and Edwards, N.S. (1980) J. Biol. Chem. 255, 6106–6110.
266 Hamberg, M. and Samuelsson, B. (1972) J. Biol. Chem. 247, 3495–3502.
267 Granström, E. (1969) Eur. J. Biochem. 10, 411–418.
268 Kindahl, H. and Granström, E. (1972) Biochim. Biophys. Acta 280, 466–471.
269 Svanborg, K. and Bygdeman, M. (1972) Eur. J. Biochem. 28, 127–235.
270 Sun, F.F. and Stafford, J.E. (1974) Biochim. Biophys. Acta 369, 95–110.
271 Ellis, C.K., Smigel, M.D., Oates, J.A., Oelz, O. and Sweetman, B.J. (1979) J. Biol. Chem. 254, 4152–4163.
272 Hamberg, M. and Samuelsson, B. (1971) J. Biol. Chem. 246, 6713–6721.
273 Hamberg, M. and Wilson, M. (1973) Adv. Biosci. 9, 39–48.
274 Granström, E. and Samuelsson, B. (1971) J. Biol. Chem. 246, 5251–5263.
275 Granström, E. and Samuelsson, B. (1971) J. Biol. Chem. 246, 7470–7485.
276 Granström, E. and Samuelsson, B. (1972) J. Am. Chem. Soc. 94, 4380–4381.
277 Granström, E. (1972) Eur. J. Biochem. 25, 581–589.
278 Beguin, F., Bygdeman, M., Gréen, K., Samuelsson, B., Toppozada, M. and Wiqvist, N. (1972) Acta Physiol. Scand. 86, 430–432.
279 Granström, E. (1972) Eur. J. Biochem. 27, 462–469.
280 Granström, E., Kindahl, H. and Swahn, M.-L. (1982) Biochim. Biophys. Acta 713, 46–60.
281 Granström, E. and Kindahl, H. (1982) Biochim. Biophys. Acta 713, 555–569.
282 Änggård, E. and Larsson, C. (1971) Eur. J. Pharmacol. 14, 66–70.
283 Pike, J.E., Kupiecki, F.P. and Weeks, J.R. (1967) in 2nd Nobel Symposium, Prostaglandins, (Bergström, S. and Samuelsson, B., eds.) pp. 161–171, Almqvist and Wiksell, Stockholm.
284 Nakano, J. (1972) Br. J. Pharmacol. 44, 63–70.
285 Crutchley, D.J. and Piper, P.J. (1975) Br. J. Pharmacol. 54, 397–399.
286 Wasserman, M.A. (1975) Prostaglandins 9, 959–973.
287 Clyman, R.I., Wong, L., Heymann, M.A. and Rudolph, A.M. (1978) Prostaglandins 15, 325–331.
288 Änggård, E., Larsson, C. and Samuelsson, B. (1971) Acta Physiol. Scand. 81, 396–404.
289 Sun, F.F., Armour, S.B., Bockstanz, V.R. and McGuire, J.C. (1976) Adv. Prostaglandin Thromboxane Res. 1, 163–169.
290 Jarabak, J. (1972) Proc. Natl. Acad. Sci. USA 69, 533–534.
291 Schlegel, W. and Greep, R.O. (1975) Eur. J. Biochem. 56, 245–252.
292 Marrazzi, M.A. and Andersen, N.H. (1974) in The Prostaglandins, (Ramwell, P.W., ed.) Vol. 2, pp. 99–155, Plenum Press, New York.
293 Hansen, H.S. (1976) Prostaglandins 12, 647–679.
294 Leovey, E.M.K., Andersen, N.H. and Bissonette, P. (1979) Prostaglandins 17, 19–37.

295 Kindahl, H., Edqvist, L.-E., Bane, A. and Granström, E. (1976) Acta Endocrinol. (Kbh.) 82, 134–149.
296 Crutchley, D.J. and Piper, P.J. (1974) Br. J. Pharmacol. 52, 197–203.
297 Horton, E.W. and Jones, R.L. (1969) Br. J. Pharmacol. 37, 705–722.
298 Dawson, W., Lewis, R.L., McMahon, R.E. and Sweatman, W.J.F. (1974) Nature 250, 331–332.
299 Wilks, J.W. (1977) Prostaglandins 13, 161–170.
300 Hamberg, M. (1968) Eur. J. Biochem. 6, 135–146.
301 Nakano, J., Änggård, E. and Samuelsson, B. (1969) Eur. J. Bicohem. 11, 386–389.
302 Parkinson, T.W. and Schneider, J.C., Jr. (1969) Biochim. Biophys. Acta 176, 78–85.
303 Johnson, M., Davison, P. and Ramwell, P.W. (1972) J. Biol. Chem. 247, 5656–5658.
304 Hamberg, M. and Samuelsson, B. (1965) Biochim. Biophys. Acta 106, 215–217.
305 Taylor, P.L. and Kelly, R.W. (1974) Nature 250, 665–667.
306 Jonsson, H.T., Middleditch, B.S. and Desiderio, D.M. (1975) Science 187, 1093–1094.
307 Taylor, P.L. and Kelly, R.W. (1975) FEBS Lett. 57, 22–25.
308 Israelsson, U., Hamberg, M. and Samuelsson, B. (1969) Eur. J. Biochem. 11, 390–394.
309 Powell, W.S. (1978) J. Biol. Chem. 253, 6711–6716.
310 Powell, W.S. (1979) Biochim. Biophys. Acta 575, 335–349.
311 Theoharides, A.D. and Kupfer, D. (1981) J. Biol. Chem. 256, 2168–2175.
312 Okita, R.T., Parkhill, L.K., Yasukochi, Y., Siler Masters, B.S., Theoharides, A.D. and Kupfer, D. (1981) J. Biol. Chem. 256, 5961–5964.
313 Powell, W.S. (1980) Prostaglandins 19, 701–710.
314 Roberts, L.J., II, Sweetman, B.J. and Oates, J.A. (1981) J. Biol. Chem. 256, 8384–8393.
315 Hensby, C.N. (1974) Biochim. Biophys. Acta 348, 145–154.
316 Leslie, C.A. and Levine, L. (1973) Biochem. Biophys. Res. Commun. 52, 717–724.
317 Stone, K.J. and Hart, M. (1976) Prostaglandins 12, 197–207.
318 Lee, S.-C. and Levine, L. (1974) J. Biol. Chem. 249, 1369–1375.
319 Lee, S.-C., Pong, S.-S., Katzen, D., Wu, K.Y. and Levine, L. (1975) Biochemistry 14, 142–145.
320 Stone, K.J. and Hart, M. (1975) Prostaglandins 10, 273–288.
321 Hensby, C.N. (1975) Biochim. Biophys. Acta 409, 225–234.
322 Wong, P.Y.-K., Terragno, D.A., Terragno, N.A. and McGiff, J.C. (1977) Prostaglandins 13, 1113–1125.
323 Bishai, I. and Coceani, F. (1976) J. Neurochem. 26, 1167–1174.
324 Westbrook, C., Lin, Y.M. and Jarabak, J. (1977) Biochem. Biophys. Res. Commun. 76, 943–949.
325 Pace-Asciak, C. and Miller, D. (1974) Experienta 30, 590–591.
326 Pace-Asciak, C.R. (1975) J. Biol. Chem. 250, 2789–2794.
327 Pace-Asciak, C. and Domazet, Z. (1975) Biochim. Biophys. Acta 380, 338–343.
328 Hensby, C.N. (1974) Prostaglandins 8, 369–375.
329 Wong, P.Y.-K. (1981) Biochim. Biophys. Acta 659, 169–178.
330 Reingold, D.F., Kawasaki, A. and Needleman, P. (1981) Biochim. Biophys. Acta 659, 179–188.
331 van Dorp, D.A. (1971) Ann. N.Y. Acad. Sci. 180, 181–199.
332 Änggård, E., Bohman, S.-O., Griffin, J.E., III, Larsson, C. and Maunsbach, A.B. (1972) Acta Physiol. Scand. 84, 231–246.
333 Bosisio, E., Galli, C., Galli, G., Nicosia, S., Spagnuolo, C. and Tosi, L. (1976) Prostaglandins 11, 773–781.
334 Oliw, E., Lundén, I. and Änggård, E. (1978) Acta Pharmacol. Toxicol. 42, 179–184.
335 Granström, E. and Samuelsson, B. (1978) Adv. Prostaglandin Thromboxane Res. 5, 1–13.
336 Fitzpatrick, F.A., Aguirre, R., Pike, J.E. and Lincoln, F.H. (1980) Prostaglandins 19, 917–931.
337 Granström, E., Hamberg, M., Hansson, H. and Kindahl, H. (1980) Prostaglandins 19, 933–957.
338 Granström, E. and Kindahl, H. (1980) Adv. Prostaglandin Thromboxane Res. 6, 181–182.
339 Granström, E., Fitzpatrick, F.A. and Kindahl, H. (1982) Methods Enzymol. 86, 306–320.
340 Frölich, J.C., Wilson, T.W., Sweetman, B.J., Smigel, M., Nies, A.S., Carr, K., Watson, J.T. and Oates, J.A. (1975) J. Clin. Invest. 55, 763–770.
341 Seyberth, H.J., Sweetman, B.J., Frölich, J.C. and Oates, J.A. (1976) Prostaglandins 11, 381–397.

342 Edwards, N.S. and Pace-Asciak, C.R. (1982) Biochim. Biophys. Acta 711, 369–371.
342 a. Edwards, N.S. and Pace-Asciak, C.R. (1982) J. Biol. Chem. 257, 6339–6342.
343 Strömberg, P., Åkerlund, M., Forsling, M.L., Granström, E. and Kindahl, H. (1983) Acta Obstet. Gynecol. Scand., in press.
344 Kumlin, M., Kindahl, H. and Granström, E. (1983) Submitted for publication.
345 Frölich, J.C. (editor) (1978) "Methods in Prostaglandin Research" Adv. Prostaglandin Thromboxane Res., Vol. 5, pp. 1–236, Raven Press, New York.
346 Lands, W.E.M. and Smith, W.L. (1982) Methods Enzymol. 86, 3–667.
347 Moncada, S., Ferreira, S.H. and Vane, J.R. (1978) Adv. Prostaglandin Thromboxane Res. 5, 211–236.
348 Gréen, K., Hamberg, M., Samuelsson, B., Smigel, M. and Frölich, J.C. (1978) Adv. Prostaglandin Thromboxane Res. 5, 39–94.
349 Granström, E. and Kindahl, H. (1978) Adv. Prostaglandin Thromboxane Res. 5, 119–210.
350 Maclouf, J., de la Baume, H., Caen, J., Rabinovitch, H. and Rigaud, M. (1980) Anal. Biochem. 109, 147–155.
351 Jouvenaz, G.H., Nugteren, D.H., Beerthuis, R.K. and van Dorp, D.A. (1970) Biochim. Biophys. Acta 202, 231–234.
352 Gréen, K. and Samuelsson, B. (1971) Eur. J. Biochem. 22, 391–395.
353 Borgeat, P. and Samuelson, B. (1979) J. Biol. Chem. 254, 7865–7869.
354 Hansson, G., Dahlén, S.-E. and Granström, E. (1983) in The Prostaglandin System (Berti, F. and Velo, G.P., eds.) Vol. 54, pp. 65–80, Plenum Press, New York.
355 Turk, J., Weiss, S.J., Davis, J.E. and Needleman, P. (1978) Prostaglandins 16, 291–309.
356 Watkins, W.D. and Peterson, M.B. (1982) Anal. Biochem. 125, 30–40.
357 Fitzpatrick, F.A., Wynalda, M.A. and Kaiser, D.G. (1977) Anal. Chem. 49, 1032–1035.
358 Wickramasinghe, J.A.F. and Shaw, S.R. (1974) Bicohem. J. 141, 179–187.
359 Skrinska, V.A. and Butkus, A. (1978) Prostaglandins 16, 571–582.
360 Min, B.H., Pao, J., Garland, W.A., de Silva, J.A.F. and Parsonnet, M. (1980) J. Chromatogr. Biomed. Appl. 183, 411–419.
361 Blair, I.A., Barrow, S.E., Waddell, K.A., Lewis, P.J. and Dollery, C.T. (1982) Prostaglandins 23, 579–589.
362 Skrinska, V.A. (1983) Presented at the 1983 Winter Prostaglandin Conference, Keystone, Colorado, Jan. 4–8, 1983.
363 Ohki, S., Hanyu, T., Imaki, K., Nakasawa, N. and Hirata, F. (1974) Prostaglandins 6, 137–148.
364 Dray, F. (1982) Methods Enzymol. 86, 297–306.
365 Sautebin, L., Kindahl, H. and Granström, E. (1983) Manuscript in preparation.
366 Pickett, W.C. and Murphy, R.C. (1981) Anal. Biochem. 111, 115–121.
367 Leffler, C.W., Desiderio, D.M. and Wakelyn, C.E. (1981) Prostaglandins 21, 227–241.
368 Christ-Hazelhof, E. and Nugteren, D.H. (1981) Prostaglandins 22, 739–746.
369 Fitzpatrick, F.A., Gorman, R.R. and Wynalda, M.A. (1977) Prostaglandins 13, 201–208.
370 Verkade, P.E., Elzas, M., van der Lee, J. and de Wolff, H.H. (1933) Hoppe Seyler's Z. Phys. Chem. 215, 225–257.
371 Verkade, P.E. (1938) Soc. Chem. Ind. J. 57, 704–714.
372 Robbins, K.C. (1961) Fed. Proc. 20, 272.
373 Preiss, B. and Bloch, K. (1964) J. Biol. Chem. 239, 85–87.
374 Björkhem, I. and Danielsson, H. (1970) Eur. J. Biochem. 17, 450–459.
375 Lu, A.Y.H. and Coon, M.J. (1968) J. Biol. Chem. 243, 1329–1330.
376 Lu, A.Y.H., Junk, K.W. and Coon, M.J. (1969) J. Biol. Chem. 244, 3714–3721.
377 Lu, A.Y.H. and West, S.B. (1980) Pharmacol. Rev. 31, 277–295.
378 Maynert, E.W., Foreman, R.L. and Watabe, T. (1970) J. Biol. Chem. 245, 5234–5238.
379 Watabe, T., Ueno, Y. and Imazumi, J. (1971) Biochem. Pharmacol. 20, 912–913.
380 Hamberg, M. and Björkhem, I. (1971) J. Biol. Chem. 246, 7411–7416.
381 Ellin, Å., Jakobsson, S.V., Schenkman, J.B .and Orrenius, S. (1972) Arch. Biochem. Biophys. 150, 64–71.

382 Ichihara, K., Kusunose, E. and Kusunose, M. (1971) Biochim. Biophys. Acta 239, 178–189.
383 Arinc, E. and Philpot, R.M. (1976) J. Biol. Chem. 251, 3213–3220.
384 Ichihara, K., Yamakawa, I. Kusunose, E. and Kusunose, M. (1979) J. Biochem. 86, 139–146.
385 Jones, D.P., Orrenius, S. and Jakobson, S.W. (1980). in Extrahepatic Metabolism of Drugs and Other Foreign Compounds (Gram, T.E., ed.) pp. 123–158, Spectrum Publications, Inc., N.Y.
386 Björkhem, I. (1976) J. Biol. Chem. 251, 5259–5266.
387 Antony, G.J. and Landou, B.R. (1968) J. Lipid Res. 9, 267–269.
388 Wada, F. and Usami, M. (1977) Biochim. Biophys. Acta 487, 261–268.
389 Björkhem, I. (1973) Eur. J. Biochem. 40, 415–422.
390 Björkhem, I. (1976) J. Biol. Chem. 251, 5259–5266.
391 Pettersen, J.E. (1974) Diabetes 23, 16–20.
392 Kam, W., Kumaran, K. and Landou, B.R. (1978) J. Lipid Res. 19, 591–600.
393 Jakobsson, S., Thor, H. and Orrenius, S. (1970) Biochem. Biophys. Res. Commun. 39, 1073–1080.
394 Di Augustine, R.P. and Fouts, J.R. (1969) Biochem. J. 115, 547–554.
395 Oliw, E.H., Lawson, J.A., Brash, A.R. and Oates, J.A. (1981) J. Biol. Chem. 256, 9924–9931.
396 Oliw, E.H. and Oates, J.A. (1981) Biochim. Biophys. Acta 666, 327–340.
397 Oliw, E.H., Guengerich, F.P. and Oates, J.A. (1982) J. Biol. Chem. 257, 3771–3781.
398 Capdevila, J., Marnett, L.J., Chacos, N., Prough, R.A. and Estabrook, R.W. (1982) Proc. Natl. Acad. Sci. USA 79, 767–770.
399 Guengerich, F.P. and Martin, M.V. (1980) Arch. Biochem. Biophys. 205, 365–379.
400 Chacos, N., Falck, J.R., Wixtrom, C. and Capdevila, J. (1982) Biochem. Biophys. Res. Commun. 104, 916–922.
401 Oliw, E.H. and Oates, J.A. (1981) Prostaglandins 22, 863–871.
402 Oliw, E.H. and Moldéus, P. (1982) Biochim. Biophys. Acta 721, 135–143.
403 Ruettinger, R.T. and Fulco, A.J. (1981) J. Biol. Chem. 256, 5728–5734.
404 Oliw, E.H. (1983) J. Chromatogr. 275, 245–259.
405 Oliw, E.H. (1983) Biochim. Biophys. Res. Commun. 111, 644–651.
406 Navarro, J., Piccolo, D.E. and Kupfer, D. (1978) Arch. Biochem. Biophys. 191, 125–133.
407 Holman, R.T. (1978). in CRC Handbook Series in Nutrition and Food, Section E; Nutritional Disorders (Rechcigl, M., ed.) Vol. III, pp. 335–368, CRC Press, Cleveland, OH.
408 Leat, W.M.F. (1981). Trends Biochem. Sci. 6(4), IX–X.
409 Mathias, M.M. and Dupont, J. (1979). Lipids 14, 247–252.
410 Galli, C., Agradi, E., Petroni, A. and Tremoli, E. (1981). In Prostaglandin and Cardiovascular Disease. Johnsson Hegyeli, R., ed.) pp. 87–99, Raven Press, New York.
411 Mead, J.F. (1971); Progr. Chem. Fats Other Lipids 9, 159–192.
412 Carney, J.A., Slinger, S.J. and Walker, B.L. (1971) Lipids 6, 624.
413 Sinclair, A.J. and Crawford, M.A.J. (1972). J. Neurochem. 19, 1753–1758.
414 Sprecher, H. (1977). in Polyunsaturated Fatty Acids. (Kunan, W.H. and Holman, R.T., eds.) pp. 1–18, American Oil Chem. Soc. Champaign, IL.
415 Brenner, R.R. (1971). Lipids 6, 567–575.
416 Rivers, J.P.W., Sinclair, A.J. and Crawford, M.A. (1975). Nature 25, 171–173.
417 Nugteren, D.H., van Evert, W.C., Soeting, W.J. and Spuy, J.H. (1980). Adv. Prostaglandin Thromboxane Res. 8, 1793–1796.
418 Schoene, N.W., Ferretti, A. and Fiore, D. (1981). Lipids 16, 866–869.
419 Sullivan, L.M. and Mathias, M.M. (1982). Prostaglandins Leukotrienes Med. 9, 223–233.
420 ten Hor (1980). Nutr. Metab. 24 (suppl. 1), 162–180.
421 Friedman, Z. and Oates, J. (1981). in Prostaglandin and Cardiovascular Disease. (Johnsson Hegyeli, R., ed.) pp. 69–80, Raven Press, New York.
422 Adam, O., Wolfram, G. and Zöllner, N. (1982). Ann. Nutr. Metab. 26, 315–323.
423 Simpson, H.C.R., Barker, K., Carter, R.D., Cassels, E. and Mann, J.I. (1982). Br. Med. J. 285, 683–684.
424 Hassam, A.G., Rivers, J.P.W. and Crawford, J. (1977). J. Nutr. 107, 519–524.
425 Hassam, A.G. and Crawford, M.A. (1978). Lipids, 13, 801–803.

426 Danon, A., Heimberg, M. and Oates, J.A. (1975). Biochim. Biophys. Acta 388, 318–330.
427 Knapp, H.R., Oelz, O., Whorton, A.R. and Oates, J.A. (1978) Lipids 13, 804–808.
428 Oelz, O., Seyberth, H.J., Knapp, H.R., Sweetman, B.J. and Oates, J.A. (1976) Biochim. Biophys. Acta 431, 268–277.
429 Stone, K.J., Willis, A.L., Hart, M., Kirtland, S.J., Kernoff, P.B.A. and McNicol, G.P. (1979). Lipids 14, 174–180.
430 Kernoff, P.B.A., Willis, A.L., Stone, K.J., Davies, J.A. and McNicol, G.P. (1977). Brit. Med. J. 2, 1441–1444.
431 Seyberth, H.J., Oelz, C., Kennedy, T., Sweetman, B.J., Danon, A., Frölich, J.C., Heimberg, M. and Oates, J.A. (1973). Clin. Pharmacol. Ther. 18, 521–529.
432 Vergroesen, A.J. and de Boer, J. (1971). in Polyenfättsäuren. (Zöllner, N., ed.). pp. 22.
433 Dyerberg, J. and Bang, H.O. (1979). Haemostasis 8, 227–233.
434 Hwang, D.H. and Carroll, A.E. (1980). Am. J. Clin. Nutr. 33, 590–597.
435 Hornstra, G., Christ-Hazelhof, E., Haddeman, E., ten Hor, F. and Nugteren, D.H. (1981) Prostaglandins 21, 727–738.
436 Siess, W., Scherer, B., Böhlig, B., Roth, P., Kurzman, I. and Weber, P.C. (1980). Lancet i, 441–444.
437 Thorngren, M. and Gustafsson, A. (1981). Lancet ii, 1190–1193.
438 Needleman, P., Whitaker, M.O., Wyche, A., Watters, K., Sprecher, H. and Raz, A. (1980). Prostaglandins 19, 165–181.
439 Alling, C., Liljequist, S. and Engel, J. (1982) Med. Biol. 60, 149–154.
440 Chin, J.H., Goldstein, D.B. and Parson, L.M. (1979) Alcoholism 3, 47–49.
441 Sun, G.W. and Sun, A.Y. (1979) Res. Commun. Chem. Pathol. Pharmacol. 24, 405–408.
442 Littleton, J.M., John, G.R. and Grieve, S.J. (1979) Alcoholism 3, 50–56.
443 Alling, C., Aspenström, G., Dencker, S.J. and Svennerholm, L. (1979) Acta Med. Scand. (Suppl.) 631, 1–38.
444 Nervi, A.M., Peluffo, R.O., Brenner, R.R. and Leikin, A.L. (1980) Lipids 15, 263–268.
445 Änggård, E., Alling, C., Becker, W. and Jones, A.W. (1983) Adv. Prostaglandin Thromboxane Leukotriene Res. 12, 217–222.

CHAPTER 2

The thromboxanes

ELISABETH GRANSTRÖM, ULF DICZFALUSY
and MATS HAMBERG

*Department of Physiological Chemistry, Karolinska Institutet,
S-104 01 Stockholm, Sweden*

1. Introduction

The existence of endoperoxide intermediate(s) in prostaglandin biosynthesis was postulated in 1965 [1]. One year later strong evidence for prostaglandin endoperoxide(s) oxygenated at C-15 was presented [2,3]. In later studies two endoperoxide intermediates were detected [4,5] and isolated [6–8]. One compound formed from arachidonic acid carried a hydroxyl group at C-15 (prostaglandin H_2; PGH_2) whereas the other one had a hydroperoxy group at C-15 (prostaglandin G_2; PGG_2). The half life of the two endoperoxides in aqueous medium at 37°C was 4–5 min. In organic solvents, on the other hand, they were quite stable: they could be stored for months in dry acetone at −20°C. This made it possible to isolate milligram amounts of pure PGG_2 and PGH_2 needed for study of their chemical and biological properties.

Labelled endoperoxides were rapidly converted into prostaglandin E_2 (PGE_2) and prostaglandin $F_{2\alpha}$ ($PGF_{2\alpha}$) when incubated with homogenates of the sheep vesicular gland. In addition, formation of another stable prostaglandin, i.e. prostaglandin D_2 (PGD_2), could be studied with labelled endoperoxides: PGD_2 was formed enzymatically in e.g. rat brain homogenates [9] as well as non-enzymatically upon treatment with serum albumin [10] and Silica gel G [6].

The prostaglandin endoperoxides were potent stimulators of airway and vascular smooth muscle [6,11,12] and were found to cause irreversible aggregation of human blood platelets [7,13].

2. Discovery of the thromboxanes

The finding that the prostaglandin endoperoxides were potent stimulators of the isolated rabbit aorta [6,11] brought to mind the so-called "rabbit aorta contracting substance" (RCS) [14]. RCS was characterized in 1969 as an unstable factor released from guinea pig lung and causing contraction of the rabbit aorta. Its formation was inhibited by a number of non-steroidal anti-inflammatory drugs, and it thus appeared conceivable that the prostaglandin endoperoxide(s) were identical with RCS. However, in a careful study the half life of the factor responsible for the major part of the biological activity of RCS was found to be 30–40 s, i.e. much shorter than that of the endoperoxides (4–5 min) [15]. Furthermore, the content of endoperoxides in perfusates of guinea pig lung containing RCS activity was very small. The conclusion was that the major part of the rabbit aorta stimulating activity of RCS was due to a very unstable factor different from the prostaglandin endoperoxides [15].

The finding that the endoperoxides caused platelet aggregation made it of interest to study the transformations of arachidonic acid in suspensions of human platelets. Two pathways were identified [16]. The initial reaction of one of them was catalyzed by fatty acid cyclooxygenase and led to the formation of three major end-products, i.e. 12L-hydroxy-5,8,10-heptadecatrienoic acid (HHT), malondialdehyde, and a novel hemiacetal derivative named thromboxane B_2 (TXB_2). The other pathway consisted of conversion of arachidonic acid into 12L-hydroperoxy-5,8,10,14-eicosatetraenoic acid (12-HPETE) by a novel lipoxygenase. The hydroperoxide was subsequently converted into a stable end-product, 12L-hydroxy-5,8,10,14-eicosatetraenoic acid (12-HETE) by a glutathione peroxidase [16,17].

(a) Elucidation of the thromboxane structure

Treatment of suspensions of human platelets with aggregating agents led to formation and release of large amounts of TXB_2, HHT, and 12L-HETE, whereas the amounts of PGE_2, $PGF_{2\alpha}$ and of intact endoperoxides were approximately 2 magnitudes lower [18]. In subsequent studies filtrates of platelets incubated with arachidonic acid were found to contain a pro-aggregating factor which was active on untreated as well as indomethacin-treated platelets [19,20] (Fig. 1). Interestingly, the pro-aggregating factor was much more unstable than the prostaglandin endoperoxides ($t_{1/2}$ in aqueous medium at 37°C, 32 s) and was released in small amounts after incubation of platelets with PGG_2/PGH_2.

The factor was thus different from the endoperoxides, a conclusion independently supported by measurements of $PGG_2 + PGH_2$ in filtrates and the finding of only minute amounts of these endoperoxides, clearly insufficient to cause aggregation of the recipient platelets. Instead, strong evidence for the identity of a factor with that responsible for the major part of the biological activity of RCS was obtained [19,20].

In parallel with these experiments, studies on the mechanism of formation of TXB_2 were carried out [19]. It appeared conceivable that more than one reaction would be needed for the formation of the non-prostanoic acid structure of TXB_2 from PGG_2/PGH_2. An attractive sequence of reactions consisted of enzymatic formation of a bicyclic oxetane-oxane derivative followed by non-enzymatic hydrolysis of the oxetane ring to yield TXB_2. In order to test this possibility, short time incubations (30–60 s) of arachidonic acid with platelets were carried out. The

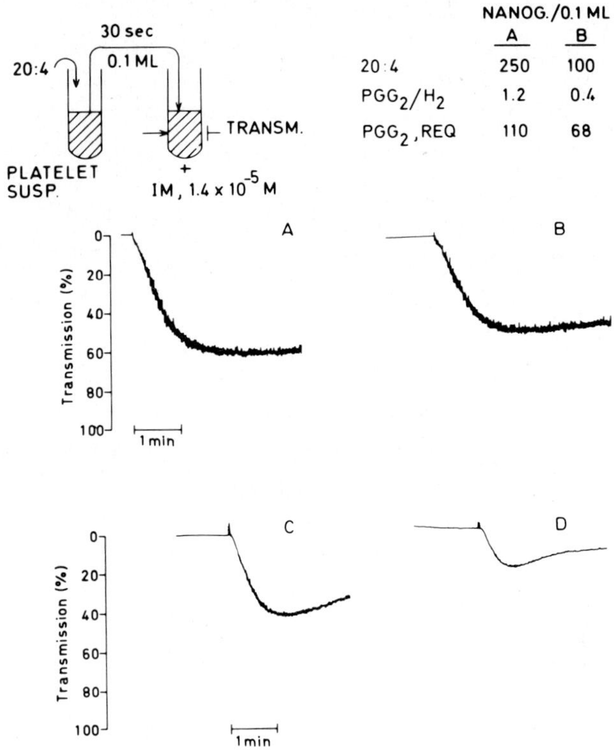

Fig. 1. Generation of proaggregating material (TXA_2) upon treatment of platelet suspensions with arachidonic acid (20:4). Platelet suspensions (1 ml) were stirred at 37°C for 30 s with 0.25–2.5 μg of arachidonic acid. Subsequently, 0.1 ml of the mixtures were rapidly transferred to aggregometer tubes which contained 0.5 ml of platelet suspensions preincubated with 14 μM indomethacin. The recipient platelets aggregated as shown by the aggregometer recordings A–D. Prostaglandin endoperoxides ($PGG_2 + PGH_2$) were measured in the 0.1 ml aliquots by $SnCl_2$-reduction followed by determination of $PGF_{2\alpha}$ by multiple ion analysis [15]. The contents of $PGG_2 + PGH_2$ in the aliquots that produced aggregation curves "A" and "B" (1.2 and 0.4 ng, respectively) were approximately 2 orders of magnitude lower than the amounts of PGG_2 needed to give equal responses. Prostaglandin endoperoxides could thus not explain the aggregation observed. Furthermore, since the recipient platelets were preincubated with indomethacin, the aggregatory responses could not be explained by transfer of arachidonic acid.

reaction was stopped by the addition of a large excess of methanol and the products were analyzed by thin layer radiochromatography. In addition to the products previously identified a pair of compounds less polar than TXB_2 appeared. These compounds were absent when arachidonic acid was incubated with platelets for a longer period of time (5 min) prior to addition of methanol. Structure determination showed that the compounds were epimeric mono-*O*-methyl derivatives (at the hemiactal group) of TXB_2. This was in agreement with the sequence of reactions proposed, methanol replacing H_2O as nucleophile in the second, non-enzymatic reaction. Analogous results were obtained using ethanol and sodium azide as

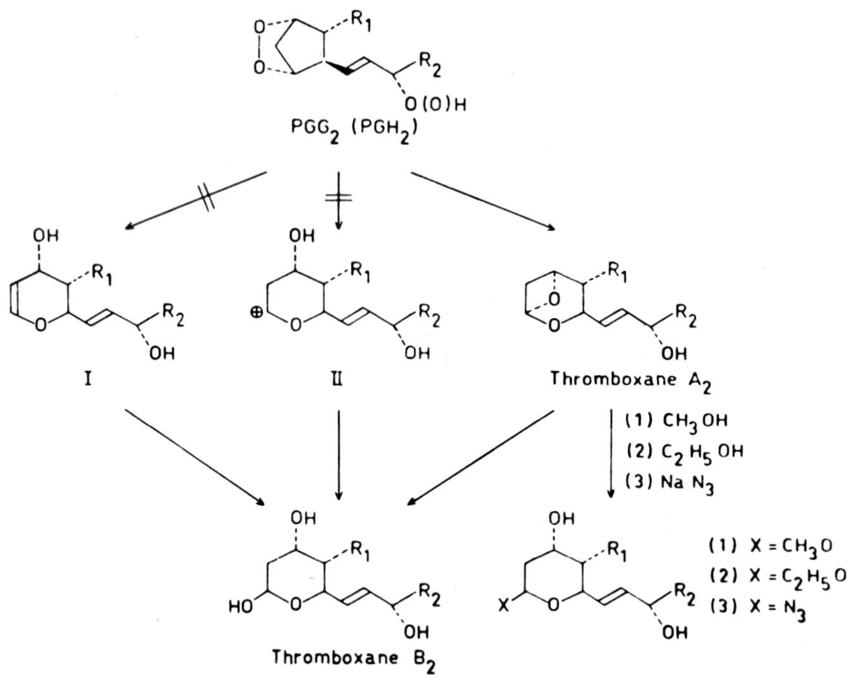

Fig. 2. Scheme of transformations of endoperoxides into thromboxane derivatives (Reproduced from Hamberg, M., Svensson, J. and Samuelsson, B. (1975) Proc. Natl. Acad. Sci. USA 72, 2994–2998, with permission from the publisher).

nucleophilic reagents. Two other structures of the unstable factor would give the same results upon trapping with nucleophiles, i.e. a dihydropyrane structure and a carbonium ion [19] (Fig. 2). The former structure could be excluded by experiments in which CH_3O^2H was used as the trapping agent and the finding that the epimeric mono-*O*-methyl TXB_2 derivatives were completely devoid of ^2H. The latter structure seemed extremely unlikely, taking into account the very short half life expected for a carbonium ion of this kind.

The factor which thus likely contained a fused oxetane-oxane ring system was called thromboxane A_2 (TXA_2). Synthesis of stable analogues of TXA_2 have been carried out (see below). The finding that such analogues have biological activity similar to that of TXA_2, i.e. stimulation of smooth muscle from vascular tissue and the respiratory tract and/or induction of platelet aggregation [19–21] support the oxetane-oxane structure proposed. Final proof for the structure of TXA_2, e.g. by NMR spectroscopy, would however require preparation of the pure compound, devoid of any other product. This has so far not been possible to achieve because of the pronounced instability of TXA_2.

(b) Nomenclature for thromboxanes

The discovery of the thromboxanes, and especially subsequent studies on the metabolism of TXB_2, made it necessary to introduce a nomenclature for the thromboxanes [22]. The basis for the nomenclature is the parent compound thrombane and corresponds to that in prostaglandin nomenclature [23] with the exception of the oxane oxygen which is designated "11a" (Fig. 3).

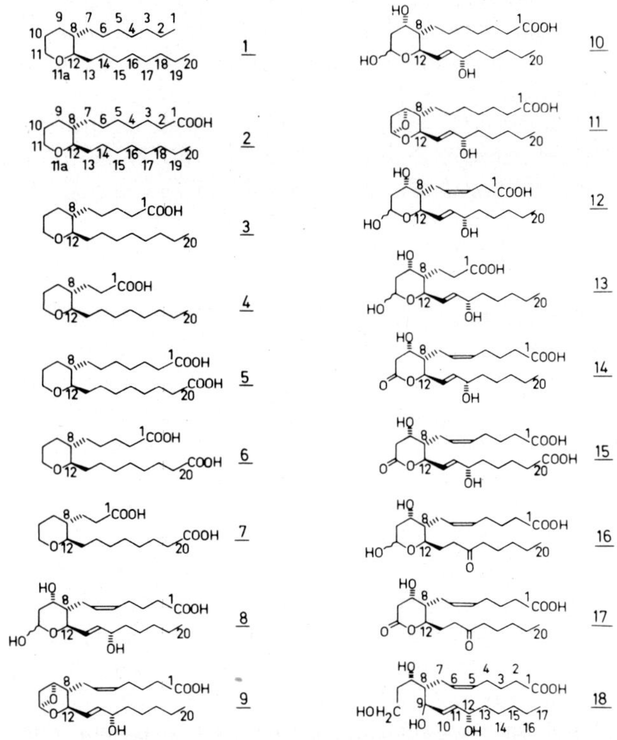

Fig. 3. Thromboxane nomenclature: 1. Thrombane. 2. Thrombanoic acid. 3. 2,3-Dinor-thrombanoic acid. 4. 2,3,4,5-Tetranor-thrombanoic acid. 5. Thrombane-1,20-dioic acid. 6. 2,3-Dinor-thrombane-1,20-dioic acid. 7. 2,3,4,5-Tetranor-thrombane-1,20-dioic acid. 8. 9α,11,15(S)-Trihydroxythromba-5Z,13E-dienoic acid (TXB_2). 9. 9α,11α-Epoxy-15(S)-hydroxythromba-5Z,13E-dienoic acid (TXA_2). 10. 9α,11,15(S)-Trihydroxy-thromb-13E-enoic acid (TXB_1). 11. 9α,11α-Epoxy-15(S)-hydroxythromb-13E-enoic acid (TXA_1); 12. 9α,11,15(S)-Trihydroxy-2,3-dinor-thromba-5Z,13E-dienoic acid. 13. 9α,11,15(S)-Trihydroxy-2,3,4,5-tetranor-thromb-13E-enoic acid. 14. 9α,15(S)-Dihydroxy-11-oxothromba-5Z,13E-dienoic acid. 15. 9α,15(S)-Dihydroxy-11-oxothromba-5Z,13E-diene-1,20-dioic acid. 16. 9α,11-Dihydroxy-15-oxothromb-5Z-enoic acid. 17. 9α-Hydroxy-11,15-dioxothromb-5Z-enoic acid. 18. 8-(1,3-dihydroxypropyl)-9,12(S)-Dihydroxy-5Z,10E-heptadecadienoic acid. (Reproduced from Samuelsson, B., Hamberg, M., Roberts II, L.J., Oates, J.A. and Nelson, N.A. (1978) Prostaglandins 16, 857–860, with permission from Geron-X, Inc. USA).

(c) Biological effects of thromboxanes

After the isolation of the pure prostaglandin endoperoxides PGG_2 and PGH_2, the biological activity of the compounds was investigated. It was found that the two compounds, apart from causing platelet aggregation and the platelet release reaction, stimulated smooth muscle from the respiratory tract and from blood vessels. Thus, PGG_2 and PGH_2 were found to be 80 and 210 times, respectively, more potent stimulators than PGE_2 of the isolated superfused rabbit aorta [11]. PGH_2 was also found to be a potent stimulator of the isolated swine coronary artery (16 and 50 times more potent than PGE_2 and $PGF_{2\alpha}$, respectively [12]). In contrast, dog coronary artery has been reported to be dilated by PGH_2 (and PGI_2) and to be unaffected by TXA_2 [24]. The human umbilical artery was contracted by low concentrations of PGG_2, and PGH_2 (threshold concentrations, 1–10 ng/ml in comparison with PGE_2, 200 ng/ml) [25].

The contractile effects of PGG_2 and PGH_2 on smooth muscle from the isolated guinea pig trachea was about 10 times stronger than that of $PGF_{2\alpha}$ [11]. In addition, when injected intravenously into anaesthetized, artificially ventilated guinea pigs, the endoperoxides (about 10 μg) caused a pronounced increase in the tracheal insufflation pressure. $PGF_{2\alpha}$ was found to be about 10 times less effective in this respect [11].

After the discovery of TXA_2, this compound was found to possess qualitatively similar properties as the endoperoxides: to some extent the endoperoxides may in fact partially exert their action by conversion into TXA_2 by the studied cell type or tissue. Thus, in addition to causing platelet aggregation and the release reaction (see below, Roles of thromboxane in platelet function), TXA_2 was found to stimulate the same type of smooth muscle organs as the endoperoxides, although its potency was greater [12,21]. In these studies TXA_2 was generated by incubation of suspensions of human platelets with arachidonic acid for 30 s. The mixture was rapidly filtered through a Millipore filter and aliquots of the clear filtrate (266 ± 46 ng/ml of TXA_2) were added to the test organs. The following potencies relative to PGH_2 were found: rabbit aorta, about 11; swine coronary artery, about 5; human umbilical artery, about 23; and guinea pig trachea, about 5. Like the endoperoxides, TXA_2 caused a pronounced increase of the tracheal insufflation pressure when injected intravenously into anaesthetized guinea pigs (about 37 times more potent than PGH_2). That the biological effects recorded for the filtrates really were due to TXA_2 was shown by addition of appropriate antagonists to the test systems. Routinely, the filtrates were also tested after an incubation period of 2.5 min. In these cases the response declined to about 6% of the original value. This is in agreement with the half life of TXA_2 in aqueous medium, i.e. 32 s [19].

Many other reports have been published concerning the effects of TXA_2 on various vessels, such as the aorta [14,15], coronary arteries [12,26–28] and the mesenteric and coeliac arteries [29,30].

Recently TXA_2 was also shown to be a potent constrictor of gastric vessels in the dog [31]. The vasoconstriction was followed by ulceration of the gastric mucosa.

These effects did not occur when the TXA_2 generating system, i.e. platelets incubated with arachidonic acid, had been pretreated with indomethacin or the thromboxane synthetase inhibitor, 1-benzylimidazole, which indicated that the active factor was indeed a thromboxane.

The vasoconstrictor and proaggregatory effects of TXA_2 suggest that the compound very probably plays a role in normal hemostasis in vivo, and possibly also in pathological conditions with increased tendencies to vasospasm, ulcerations and/or thrombosis. Several reviews have been written on the biological effects and possible roles of thromboxane in vivo (e.g. refs. 32, 33).

As mentioned above, TXA_2 was also found to be a potent contractile agent in airways [21]. This effect is demonstrable both in vitro and in vivo, and this discovery together with other findings led to the hypothesis that TXA_2 might be a mediator of broncho-constriction in asthma. The possible roles of the thromboxanes in the respiratory system, as well as their interactions with the even more potent leukotrienes, are discussed more in detail below (see Thromboxanes and the lung).

Although most interest has been focussed on the effects of TXA_2 on vascular and respiratory smooth muscle, other types of smooth muscle also react to the compound. Thus, uterine smooth muscle from the guinea pig appears to be stimulated by PGH_2 and TXA_2 [34]. Interestingly, the two compounds had little or no effect on rat uterine smooth muscle.

Evidence has been presented that TXA_2 mediates augmented adhesiveness of polymorphonuclear leukocytes [35]. This is another area where thromboxane and leukotrienes may act as agonists. The cyclooxygenase inhibitor, indomethacin, as well as the thromboxane synthetase inhibitors imidazole, 9,11-azoprosta-5,13-dienoic acid, and 1-benzylimidazole, suppressed the stimulation of adherence by 74, 31, 66 and 83%, respectively. Exogenous PGE_1, PGE_2, and $PGF_{2\alpha}$ did not increase polymorphonuclear leukocyte adherence. However, adherence induced by arachidonic acid was abolished by inhibitors of cyclooxygenase or thromboxane synthetase. Furthermore, augmented leukocyte adherence was accompanied by release of TXB_2. Finally, specific rabbit antibodies to TXB_2 inhibited enhanced adherence, strongly suggesting a primary role for TXA_2 as the mediator of augmented adherence.

Most studies on thromboxane bioactivities have dealt with TXA_2. There are however also reports on structurally related compounds as well. Recently 15-hydroperoxythromboxane A_2 was prepared by incubation of PGG_2 with purified thromboxane synthetase from human platelets [36]. The hydroperoxythromboxane was about 25 times more potent than PGG_2 in causing platelet aggregation and 30 times more potent than PGG_2 as a stimulator of rabbit aorta smooth muscle [37]. PGH_3 and TXA_3, formed from 5,8,11,14,17-eicosapentaenoic acid, were found to be somewhat less active on arterial smooth muscle than the corresponding compounds of the 2-series [38]. Surprisingly, when their effects on platelets were studied, they were found to increase platelet cyclic AMP and thus act as anti-aggregatory compounds [39]. This effect was however interpreted as caused by the presence of PGD_3, a break-down product of PGH_3 and a powerful anti-aggregating compound.

The stable hydrolysis product of TXA_2 is TXB_2, which was originally considered biologically inactive. Recently, however, this compound has also been shown to possess some activity. In relatively large doses it exerts some constrictor action in vivo on bronchial smooth muscle and pulmonary vasculature of the dog and cat [40,41]. TXB_2 and PGE_2 were found to have comparable pressor effects due to constriction of the pulmonary veins, although $PGF_{2\alpha}$ was more potent in this respect [41]. In this connection it may also be mentioned that TXB_2 has been reported to inhibit the pulmonary inactivation of PGE_2 in the dog [42].

TXB_2 has also been found to contract several smooth muscle preparations of the rat: the strongest effect was registered with the aorta [43]. Even a weak chemotactic activity of TXB_2 has been demonstrated [44].

3. *Biosynthesis of thromboxanes*

(a) Occurrence of thromboxane synthetase

Following the characterization of TXA_2 as the proaggregatory substance formed from PGH_2 in platelets [19], and the demonstration that the main component of "rabbit aorta contracting substance", RCS, [14] consisted of TXA_2 [19], great interest arose in screening other tissues for thromboxane synthesizing capacity.

Homogenates from the lung and spleen from guinea pigs produced large amounts of TXB_2 and 12-hydroxy-5,8,10,14-eicosatetraenoic acid (12-HETE) from endogenous arachidonic acid upon incubation at 37°C for 30 min [45]. Thromboxane synthesis was also demonstrated in lung from many other species, i.e. sheep [46], cattle [47], cat [48], rabbit [49,50] and rat [443]. However, the capacity for the transformation of arachidonic acid into TXA_2 is different in tissues from different species. It was shown that in this respect human and rat lung were less effective than guinea pig [51].

Thromboxane is synthesized by the kidney [52] and the production is enhanced in many situations leading to renal failure, i.e. uretereal obstruction (in the rabbit [53], in the rat [54]), renal vein constriction [55] and glycerol induced renal failure [56]. TXA_2 is the major metabolite of arachidonic acid in human cortical hydronephrotic tissue [57].

A number of other cell types and tissues have also been shown to possess thromboxane synthesizing capacity. Thus in rat heart myocytes incubated with [^{14}C]arachidonic acid, the main products formed were PGE_2 and PGA_2; however, PGI_2, TXB_2 and $PGF_{2\alpha}$ were also found. In contrast, dog heart myocytes synthesized mainly PGI_2 and PGD_2 [58]. Thromboxane biosynthesis has also been demonstrated in the brain [9,59–62]. Bone marrow from Rhesus monkey was reported to convert exogenous PGH_2 into TXA_2 [49]. Thromboxane formation was also observed in leukocytes, macrophages and lymphocytes [63–68]. The monocyte/macrophage can generate TXB_2 as well as PGE_2 [69]. Purified human lymphocytes have the capacity of synthesizing 5-hydroxy-eicosatetraenoic acid, 12-hydroxy-eicosatetraenoic acid and TXB_2 as shown by incubation of ^{14}C-labelled arachidonic acid. Since phytohemagglutinin (PHA) releases cell bound arachidonic acid, it appears likely that the products mentioned above are formed upon PHA stimulation [70].

Thromboxane production was determined in cultured fibroblasts from mouse embryo, baby hamster kidney [71] and lung [72,73]. Both rabbit [74,75] and human ocular tissues (anterior uvea) [76,77] are capable of synthesizing TXA_2. Human anterior uvea also synthesized PGI_2, $PGF_{2\alpha}$, PGE_2 and PGD_2 from [^{14}C]PGH_2 [77]. Vascular tissue was demonstrated to possess thromboxane synthesizing capacity [78,79]. Incubation of isolated human umbilical artery in organ bath produced TXA_2 in the bath medium, indicating thromboxane generation by the umbilical artery [25].

Furthermore, thromboxane synthesis has also been reported in the urinary bladder [80–83], the gastrointestinal tract [84–86], endometrial tissue [87], decidual tissue and amniotic fluid [88–90] as well as in inflamed tissues [91–94]. The information on species differences in these tissues is scanty.

(b) Purification of thromboxane synthetase

Thromboxane synthetase of lyzed human platelets was localized in the microsomal fraction, sedimenting between $12\,000 \times g$ and $100\,000 \times g$ [95]. When this fraction was treated with the non-ionic detergent Triton X-100, the enzymes required for the conversion of arachidonic acid into TXB_2 were solubilized. Chromatography of the solubilized material on a DE-52 column resolved two enzyme activities, one that converts arachidonic acid into PGH_2 and another one converting PGH_2 into TXB_2. These two enzymes, prostaglandin endoperoxide synthetase and thromboxane synthetase, respectively, showed similar subcellular distribution, and since prostaglandin endoperoxide synthetase has earlier been localized to the dense tubular system, this was also suggested to be the site of thromboxane synthetase [95]. Similar procedures resolved the two enzymes from bovine platelets [96], bovine lung [47] and sheep lung [46]. In an experiment with human and bovine platelets, Tween 20, which is a more hydrophilic detergent that Triton X-100, was found to be less effective than Triton X-100 in solubilizing the endoperoxide and thromboxane synthetases [97]. The solubilized thromboxane synthetase was stable for weeks at $+4°C$ [97].

Porcine lung microsomes were solubilized with the detergent Lubrol PX [98]. The solubilized material was treated with DEAE-cellulose in a batchwise manner; this resulted in the removal of a substantial amount of inactive proteins. The residual fraction was adsorbed to Affi-Gel Blue, from which thromboxane synthetase was eluted by washing with a buffer containing 2 M KCl. The eluate was dialyzed; in the fraction so obtained, a purification of 16.6 times compared to that of the lung microsomes was achieved. This purified enzyme preparation was stable for 1 month at $-80°C$ [98].

(c) Properties of thromboxane synthetase

The biosynthesis of TXA_2 from its precursor fatty acid, arachidonic acid, proceeds via the intermediate prostaglandin endoperoxides [19]. Studies on the kinetics of this reaction sequence indicated that the formation of the prostaglandin endoperoxides is the rate limiting step [99]. Variations in the pH of the incubation medium between pH 5 and pH 8 did not influence the reaction rate appreciably [95,100,101].

Quantitation of the three major metabolites of arachidonic acid in platelets, 12-hydroxy-5,8,10,14-eicosatetraenoic acid (12-HETE), 12-hydroxy-5,8,10-heptadecatrienoic acid (HHT) and TXB_2 revealed that approximately equal amounts of HHT and TXB_2 were formed after stimulation with thrombin [18]. In a study on the effect of thromboxane synthetase inhibitors on PGH_2 metabolism in platelet microsomes it was found that the TXB_2 and HHT formation were always inhibited concomitantly and to the same extent by all the inhibitors examined. Both products disappeared upon boiling of the platelet microsomes, indicating their enzymatic origin. It was suggested that these two compounds, HHT and TXB_2, were both formed by the same enzyme, thromboxane synthetase [102]. Experiments involving the addition of a large excess of methanol to the incubation mixture after different incubation times supported the idea that HHT is not a breakdown product of TXA_2 but is formed independently [102]. Addition of methanol converts the labile TXA_2 into *O*-methyl TXB_2, whereas TXB_2 is not influenced [19]. After an incubation period of 10 s, 55% of the recovered radioactivity from [^{14}C]PGH_2 was present as HHT, 21% as *O*-methyl TXB_2 and 22% in the form of TXB_2. When the incubation time was prolonged to 2 min, HHT still represented 55% of the recovered radioactivity, however, *O*-methyl TXB_2 accounted for less than 3% and TXB_2 had increased to

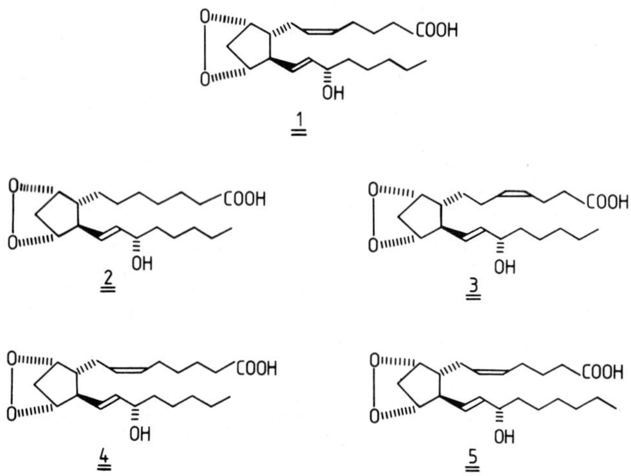

Fig. 4. Structures of prostaglandin H_2 and analogues: precursors of thromboxanes: (1) Prostaglandin H_2, (2) Prostaglandin H_1, (3) Δ^4-Prostaglandin H_1, (4) α-homo Prostaglandin H_2, (5) ω-homo Prostaglandin H_2.

42%. Thus, it appears that in the system used, TXA_2 was decomposed exclusively to TXB_2. A hypothetical reaction mechanism was outlined where PGH_2 is first protonated at the C-9 oxygen. The cation so formed can then either isomerize to TXA_2 or decompose to HHT [102,103]. An alternative mechanism in which TXA_2 is the common intermediate for HHT and TXB_2 has also been discussed [103]. Based on kinetic evidence, it has been proposed that the formation of TXA_2 should be a bimolecular reaction rather than an isomerization [104].

PGH_1, which lacks the Δ^5-double bond of PGH_2 (Fig. 4), is converted in human platelets to TXA_1 [105]. The conversion is however poor and the predominant product formed is 12-hydroxy-8,10-heptadecadienoic acid (HHD) [100]. An analogue of PGH_2 in which the Δ^5-double bond had been moved one methylene unit closer to the carboxyl group, i.e. Δ^4-PGH_1 (Fig. 4), was prepared and incubated with human platelet microsomes. The main product obtained was 12-hydroxy-4,8,10-heptadecatrienoic acid, and only minute amounts of thromboxane were formed [100]. These experiments suggested that the position of the double bond in the carboxyl side chain is important for the transformation of the endoperoxide into a thromboxane. Additional experiments were carried out to reveal the structural requirements for the conversion to thromboxanes. Two C_{21}-endoperoxides were prepared, α-homo-PGH_2 and ω-homo-PGH_2 (Fig. 4), and both these PGH_2-analogues were converted into thromboxane and hydroxy acids by platelet thromboxane synthetase. The product pattern was very similar to that of PGH_2 [106]. Both side chains of the endoperoxides could thus be elongated without disturbing the transformation into thromboxanes. Both C_{21}-endoperoxides, however, had a double bond in the carboxyl side chain at the same distance from the cyclopentane ring as PGH_2.

Incubation of 5,8,11,14,17-eicosapentaenoic acid (EPA, timnodonic acid) with human platelet thromboxane synthetase yielded only little TXA_3 [107]. This was not due to poor conversion of PGH_3 into TXA_3 but rather poor conversion of the precursor fatty acid into PGH_3 [38,39,107].

Human platelet thromboxane synthetase does not possess peroxidase activity, since the two hydroperoxides, 12-hydroperoxy-5,8,10-heptadecatrienoic acid and 15-hydroperoxy TXB_2 were detected in incubates from PGG_2 with partially purified thromboxane synthetase which was devoid of cyclooxygenase activity [36].

(d) Modulation of thromboxane synthesis

i. Inhibition

Shortly after the discovery of the thromboxane pathway, reports began to appear describing different agents with inhibitory effect on thromboxane synthetase.

Benzydamine was examined for inhibitory action on the transformation of PGG_2 into TXA_2 by horse platelet microsomes [108]. The concentration required for 50% inhibition (IC_{50}) was determined to be 100 μg/ml. The conversion of arachidonic acid into prostaglandin endoperoxides by ram seminal vesicle microsomes was also affected. However, some selectivity was achieved, since the IC_{50} of the latter reaction was 250 μg/ml [108]. Incubation of benzydamine with a human platelet microsomal fraction at concentrations $< 1 \times 10^{-3}$ M did not interfere with thromboxane biosynthesis [109].

A phenyl phosphonate, sodium *p*-benzyl-4-(1-oxo-2-(4-chlorobenzyl)-3-phenyl propyl) phenyl phosphonate (N-0164), inhibited thromboxane biosynthesis in human platelet microsomes with an IC_{50} of 2.2×10^{-5} M [110,111]. However, this compound also acts as a prostaglandin receptor antagonist [112,113].

The non-acidic anti-inflammatory compound 2-isopropyl-3-nicotinylindole (L-8027) inhibits thromboxane biosynthesis [114–116] with simultaneous inhibition of PGE formation, indicating that the compound is not a specific inhibitor of thromboxane synthetase [117]. Metopyrone (2-methyl-1,2-di-3-pyridyl-1-propanone), which shares some structural features with L-8027, was reported to inhibit thromboxane formation in microsomes from human platelets and bovine lung [118].

As the inhibitory effect appeared to be dependent on the nicotinyl moiety, a study was undertaken to see if the potency and specificity could be increased by replacing this group with a more basic imidazoylmethyl group. A series of 3-(1-imidazolylmethyl) indoles were synthesized, and two of these, 2-isopropyl-3(1-imidazolylmethyl) indole (UK-34787) and 3-(1-imidazoylmethyl) indole showed almost complete selectivity against thromboxane synthetase with an IC_{50} of 2×10^{-8} M [119,120].

Imidazole was shown to selectively inhibit thromboxane synthetase with an IC_{50} of 5.5×10^{-4} M [121–123]. Of several imidazole derivatives tested, 1-methyl-imidazole, was found to be more potent than imidazole itself [122]. This finding initiated extensive research on substituted imidazoles. A number of reports appeared, describing various substituted imidazoles as thromboxane synthetase inhibitors, e.g. 1-*n*-butyl-imidazole [124], 1-(3-phenyl-2-propenyl)-1H-imidazole (SQ 80,338) [125] and 1-(1-*O*-chlorophenyl-1,1-diphenylmethyl) imidazole (clotrimazole) [126]. A study of a series of substituted imidazoles showed that substitution at the 1-position retained the inhibitory activity of imidazole while substitution at other positions rendered the compound inactive. It seems that the nitrogen at the 3-position must be sterically unhindered for inhibitory activity. In a study of a series of 1-substituted imidazoles it was shown that the potency of the compounds increased with increasing chain length of the substituent. Thus 1-nonylimidazole was the most potent inhibitor tested, with an IC_{50} of 0.01 μM [127]. However, nonylimidazole did not inhibit thromboxane formation in guinea-pig platelet rich plasma at concentrations which blocked platelet aggregation, and it was therefore questioned whether this compound should be considered a specific thromboxane synthetase inhibitor [117]. In another study [128], it was shown that 1-alkylimidazoles, with a chain length of 8 to 16 carbon atoms, inhibited prostaglandin endoperoxide synthetase. In contrast to 1-alkylimidazoles, 1-carboxyalkylimidazoles with a chain length between 7 and 10 carbon atoms inhibited thromboxane formation without interfering with either prostaglandin endoperoxide synthetase, PGD_2- or PGI_2-isomerase. 1-Carboxyheptylimidazole was the most potent inhibitor investigated with an IC_{50} of 0.14 μM [128].

The histamine H_2-receptor antagonist burimamide, a derivative of imidazole, was shown to be equipotent to imidazole as a thromboxane synthetase inhibitor. Other histamine H_2-receptor antagonists of related structure, such as metiamide and cimetidine, exhibited only weak inhibitory activity. Selectivity studies showed that at concentrations 20 to 100 times IC_{50} of that of thromboxane synthetase, neither cyclooxygenase (of sheep seminal vesicle microsomes) nor prostacyclin synthetase was inhibited. The thromboxane inhibiting activity of burimamide was not related to its histamine H_2-receptor blocking properties [50,129,130].

The imidazole derivative, 4-(2-(1H-imidazol-1-yl)ethoxy) benzoic acid hydrochloride (UK-37,248), a thromboxane synthetase inhibitor, was given orally to healthy volunteers. Thromboxane B_2 levels in venous blood were measured, and it was found that the production of TXB_2 was inhibited in a dose-related manner [131]. After ingestion of 200 mg of the compound, arachidonic acid induced platelet aggregation was completely inhibited [132].

Among other heterocyclic compounds tested for thromboxane inhibiting activity, pyridine and some pyridine derivatives were found to be active [133,134]. Pyridine was equipotent to imidazole in this respect. Substitution in the 3- or 4-position with a hydrophobic group increased the inhibitory potency, while substitution in the 2-position rendered the molecule inactive [134,135]. Nicotinic acid (pyridine-3-carboxylic acid) had a weak inhibitory effect on thromboxane synthetase but it was less potent than pyridine [133,136].

The synthetic pyridine derivative, β-(4-(2-carboxy-1-propenyl)benzyl) pyridine hydrochloride (OKY-1555) inhibited thromboxane formation selectively and had an IC_{50} of 3 nM [135]. Also the corresponding sodium salt (OKY-1581) was a potent and selective inhibitor of thromboxane synthetase [137,138].

Three vasodilating agents, hydralazine, dipyridamole and diazoxide, were reported to be weak inhibitors of thromboxane biosynthesis in human platelets [50,139–141]. Dipyridamole has also been shown to inhibit 3′:5′-cyclic AMP phosphodiesterase of platelets [142].

Synthetic stable analogues of prostaglandin endoperoxides and TXA_2 were early considered potential inhibitors, agonists and antagonists (see below). Replacement of one of the endoperoxide oxygens by a methylene group, as in 9,11-epoxymethano-15-hydroxyprosta-5,13-dienoic acid and in 9,11-methanoepoxy-15-hydroxyprosta-5,13-dienoic acid, yielded stable analogues of PGH_2 [143]. The 9,11-epoxymethano analogue inhibited thromboxane formation in human platelet microsomes with an IC_{50} of 2×10^{-5} M [109]. The 11,9-epoxymethano analogue was not active in the concentration range studied [109], while 9,11-epoxymethanoprostanoic acid was a potent inhibitor with an IC_{50} of 7 μM [101]. Another, still more powerful inhibitor was found in 9,11-azo-15-hydroxyprosta-5,13-dienoic acid ($IC_{50} = 2$ μM) [109]. This compound mimicked the actions of the prostaglandin endoperoxides with respect to platelet aggregation and the platelet release reaction [144]. The corresponding 15-deoxy compound, 9,11-azoprosta-5,13-dienoic acid, was a selective thromboxane synthetase inhibitor, which also inhibited platelet aggregation [145–147]. In preparations of the corpus luteum, however, this compound inhibited prostacyclin synthetase [49]. The prostaglandin endoperoxide analogue 9,11-azo-13-oxa-15-hydroxy-prostanoic acid was a potent inhibitor of thromboxane synthetase ($IC_{50} = 1 \times 10^{-6}$ M) and, in addition, it showed PGH_2/TXA_2 receptor blocking properties [148,149].

Substitution of one of the endoperoxide oxygens of PGH_2 for an imino group, as in 9,11-iminoepoxyprosta-5,13-dienoic acid, yielded a selective thromboxane synthetase inhibitor [150,151]. The corresponding 9,11-epoxyimino analogue was devoid of thromboxane inhibiting activity but acted as a thromboxane antagonist [152]. The 9,11-iminomethano analogue of PGH_2 inhibited thromboxane biosynthesis in platelet suspensions and was reported to be 830 times more potent than imidazole [153].

Some stable thromboxane A_2 analogues with thromboxane synthetase inhibiting properties have also been synthesized [154–156], but these compounds exhibited agonistic or antagonistic properties as well (see below).

A protease inhibitor, L-1-tosylamido-2-phenylethyl chloromethyl ketone (TPCK), specific for chymotrypsin, has been shown to exert a number of effects on platelet processes. This compound also interferes with arachidonic acid metabolism in platelets. The 12-lipoxygenase was inhibited by TPCK, but the main effect was an irreversible inhibition of thromboxane synthetase [157].

Several reviews dealing with the screening and evaluation of thromboxane synthetase inhibitors have been published together with a number of related articles of more general character [158–162].

ii. Potentiation of thromboxane biosynthesis

Several factors are known to enhance the formation of thromboxanes, although their site of action may not necessarily be the enzyme, thromboxane synthetase. Some of these factors may be involved in the regulation of thromboxane biosynthesis in vivo. Thus, they may be of importance for the development of certain diseases: a number of pathological conditions are known that seem to involve an increase in the thromboxane production by platelets or other cell types. These will be covered more in detail below (see section on Thromboxane production in pathological conditions).

Heparin has been found to increase TXA_2 synthesis in human platelet rich plasma [163]. Administration of heparin to patients with angina pectoris also markedly increased the synthesis and release of thromboxane [164]. There was no correlation between the simultaneously increased plasma levels of free fatty acids and plasma TXB_2, suggesting that the cause of increase in TXB_2 levels was indirect [164–166].

Cholesterol was found to enhance the conversion of released arachidonic acid into TXB_2 [167]. This stimulation was believed to occur primarily at the level of the cyclooxygenase rather than the thromboxane synthetase.

Calcium ionophores, such as A23187 and X538A, are known to stimulate thromboxane biosynthesis in platelets [168]. These compounds mobilize calcium from intracellular storage sites, leading to an increased calcium concentration in the cytosol. This in turn stimulates the release of arachidonic acid from its esterified storage form, and the subsequent conversion into prostaglandins and thromboxanes is thus increased [168].

Other factors known to stimulate thromboxane formation by various cell types are norepinephrine (brain tissue [59]), vasopressin (toad urinary bladder [81]), and estrogens in oral contraceptives (platelets [169]). The mode of action of these compounds is not known.

iii. Dietary manipulations of thromboxane biosynthesis

A lower incidence of death from cardiovascular disease has been observed among Eskimos from western Greenland who consume a diet rich in $\omega 3$ polyunsaturated fatty acids. Analysis of their platelet lipids revealed higher percentages of eicosapentaenoic acid and docosahexaenoic acid than in a Danish control group and considerably less arachidonic acid. A significantly longer bleeding time was also observed among the Eskimos, due to reduced platelet aggregation and even a bleeding tendency. It has therefore been suggested that dietary enrichment of eicosapentaenoic acid can reduce the incidence of thrombotic disorders [170,171]. Eicosapentaenoic acid does not induce platelet aggregation [172]. It is a poor substrate for fatty acid cyclooxygenase but has a high binding affinity for the enzyme, thereby inhibiting arachidonic acid conversion into the pro-aggregatory thromboxane A_2 [39,107]. Human platelets can convert eicosapentaenoic acid into thromboxane A_3 [107], but this compound does not induce platelet aggregation. Eicosapentaenoic acid, however, gives rise to prostaglandin I_3, a potent anti-aggregatory substance [39].

The effect of dietary supplementation of fish oil, rich in eicosapentaenoic acid, on experimentally induced myocardial infarction in dogs was studied, and it was shown that the size of the infarction was reduced in oil-fed dogs [173]. Dietary supplement of fish-oil also had a protective effect on focal cerebral infarction [174].

A group of volunteers were put on a mackerel diet corresponding to a daily intake of 7–11 g of eicosapentaenoic acid. Analysis of their platelet lipids after six days on the diet showed a five-fold increase in eicosapentaenoic acid, while the arachidonic acid fraction decreased considerably. A decrease in collagen induced platelet aggregation was found that correlated with diminished TXB_2 formation and with an increase in the eicosapentaenoic acid to arachidonic acid ratio in platelet phospholipids [175].

Dietary supplement of cod liver oil was studied in another group of men. A daily dose of 20 ml of cod liver oil, corresponding to 1.8 g eicosapentaenoic acid and 2.2 g docosahexaenoic acid, was given. The proportions of eicosapentaenoic acid and docosahexaenoic acid in platelet lipids were increased mainly at the expense of $\omega 6$ unsaturated fatty acids. After three weeks with cod liver oil supplement, the mean bleeding time was significantly prolonged [176].

A hypothetical combined therapy consisting of an eicosapentaenoic acid rich diet with the addition of a thromboxane synthetase inhibitor has been discussed [177]. This combination might abolish the production of the pro-aggregatory TXA_2 and enhance the formation of the anti-aggregatory prostacyclin.

Dihomo-γ-linolenic acid has also received some attention as a potential antithrombotic substance [177–179]. This compound does not give rise to a pro-aggregatory thromboxane but is the precursor of the anti-aggregatory prostaglandin E_1 [180–182].

Among common foodstuffs, onion and garlic have been reported to contain a heat-stable, lipid soluble factor that inhibits platelet aggregation [183–186]. This factor inhibits thromboxane synthesis in platelets from exogenous [^{14}C]arachidonic acid. Along with the decreased thromboxane formation, a new metabolite of arachidonic acid appeared, 10-hydroxy-11,12-epoxy-5,8,14-eicosatrienoic acid, probably via the platelet lipoxygenase pathway [185].

The influence of cholesterol on thromboxane biosynthesis was briefly mentioned above. Cholesterol-rich platelets were shown to release more arachidonic acid than cholesterol-depleted ones upon stimulation with thrombin, and the subsequent conversion of the precursor into TXB_2 was also higher in the cholesterol-rich platelets [167]. An increased thromboxane production from platelets in vivo in the rabbit has also been demonstrated after a cholesterol-rich diet [187].

4. *Metabolism of thromboxanes*

Thromboxane metabolism has attracted great interest since the thromboxane pathway was discovered in 1975. The potent TXA_2 was already then known to be rapidly hydrolyzed into the almost inactive TXB_2 with a $t_{1/2}$ of about 30 s in buffer solution at pH 7.4 and at 37°C [19]. It was then erroneously assumed that this hydrolysis of TXA_2 always occurred to completion under all circumstances, and most studies of thromboxane metabolism have thus dealt with the further transformations of TXB_2 [188–195].

Metabolic studies were first undertaken because of the necessity to find an alternative to TXB_2 for monitoring, particularly in the circulation. A stable, major plasma metabolite was looked for, which should not be formed as an artifact during collection and handling of the blood sample. In analogy with the prostaglandin transformations, this expected metabolite was 15-keto-13,14-dihydro-TXB_2. However, incubations using crude preparations of 15-hydroxyprostanoate dehydrogenase from liver, kidney [194,195] or lungs failed to yield the expected metabolite, and the conclusion was that TXB_2 was not a substrate for this enzyme. Furthermore, intravenous injection of [^{3}H]TXB_2 into monkeys did not result in the appearance of 15-keto-13,14-dihydro-TXB_2 as a metabolite in plasma [188] or in urine [188–190]. In the circulation, [^{3}H]TXB_2 itself remained as the dominating compound for a considerable time and was only slowly replaced by more polar compounds [188].

Before being excreted into urine, TXB_2 is degraded mainly by β-oxidation. The major urinary metabolite was identified as dinor-TXB_2 in the guinea pig, monkey and man, [188–192,194,195]; in the rat, however, the major product was tetranor-TXB_2 [193]. In the simian and human species, a number of additional metabolites were identified [190,195], which have been formed by various combinations of well-known metabolic reactions such as β-oxidation and ω-oxidation. Several metabolites, however, had the saturated keto structure in the side chain, and it was proposed that some of the break-down products were better substrates for the 15-hydroxy dehydrogenase than TXB_2 itself, or alternatively, that any formed

15-keto-13,14-dihydro TXB_2 was immediately further metabolized into more degraded products [190,195].

Three primary pathways of metabolism were identified in primates [190,195]. The major pathway retained the original hemiacetal ring of TXB_2: degradation occurred exclusively by β-oxidation, leading first to the dominating urinary metabolite, dinor-TXB_2, and subsequently to the less abundant tetranor product. Another major pathway of metabolism involved dehydrogenation of the hemiacetal alcohol group at C-11 of TXB_2, leading to a series of metabolites with a δ-lactone instead of the oxane ring. These two pathways were about equal in importance in man [195]. A third, minor pathway involved an initial reduction of the hemiacetal ring, leading to acyclic compounds with alcohol groups at C-11 and C-12. The enzymes responsible for the latter two pathways were localized to the soluble fraction of guinea pig liver homogenates [195].

For quantitation of thromboxane formation in vivo, it seemed preferable to monitor the major urinary metabolite, dinor-TXB_2, instead of a circulating compound. A mass spectrometric method for this compound was developed and used for a quantitative study in the guinea pig [192]. The basal excretion of this metabolite was very low. Surprisingly, when anaphylaxis was induced in sensitized guinea pigs by challenge with the immunogen, no increase at all was seen in the excretion of dinor-TXB_2. This was difficult to explain, as anaphylactic lungs are known to produce large amounts of TXA_2 [14,196]. A possible explanation was that the released TXA_2 was metabolized by a different pathway than by hydrolysis into TXB_2 and later β-oxidation into dinor-TXB_2. This has also been supported by findings from perfusion experiments with anaphylactic guinea pig lungs [197–199]. The anticipated thromboxane metabolite, 15-keto-13,14-dihydro-TXB_2, was identified in the perfusate [197,198,200] and was later also quantitated together with several other products [199]. In non-sensitized lungs it occurred in small amounts, but the importance of this metabolic pathway increased after sensitization, and after repeated challenges 15-keto-dihydro-TXB_2 was by far the major metabolite [199, cf. also 201,202]. The explanation for the different results in these two quantitative studies on sensitized guinea pigs [192,199] may thus be that the wrong compound was monitored in the former study. TXA_2 is hydrolyzed into TXB_2 in buffer solution in vitro, but this may in complex biological systems, such as the anaphylactic lung, be preceded by the actions of 15-hydroxy prostanoate dehydrogenase and Δ^{13}-reductase. Whether the 15-keto-dihydro metabolite is normally a major circulating metabolite of TXA_2 in vivo, and thus the proper target for plasma measurements, is not known yet.

TXA_2 metabolism has been shown to be unexpectedly complicated also in simpler systems, such as in platelet rich plasma (PRP) in vitro. As no metabolizing enzymes are present in such a system, TXB_2 was supposed to be the only end product. However, it was discovered that released TXA_2 is extensively trapped by proteins, mainly albumin, in the presence of plasma [203–205]. It is conceivable that this reaction takes place also with TXA_2 released from platelets in vivo.

Albumin binding of TXA_2 has been noticed earlier [206,207]; however, in those studies a different phenomenon was seen: the half-life of this very unstable compound was considerably prolonged in the presence of albumin. This was apparently caused by the common, non-covalent binding by albumin, which considerably protected the compound against hydrolysis. Thus, albumin seems to exert two opposite actions: one protective and one destructive action. The relative importance of these two phenomena and their functions in vivo is not known at present.

The metabolic fates of TXA_2 thus seem to be very complicated. A few years ago, TXB_2 was almost automatically considered the end product of TXA_2 formation and a reliable parameter for monitoring thromboxane biosynthesis. Now it has become clear that under many circumstances it is only a minor and insignificant product. TXA_2 seems to be metabolized partially via different pathways and forms covalent derivatives with proteins, or is converted via the 15-hydroxy dehydrogenase pathway. The further fates of these products are not known. It is also possible that thromboxane formed in different cell types may undergo different fates.

5. *Assay methods for thromboxanes*

The biosynthesis and release of thromboxanes by a biological system can be monitored using several different approaches and a number of different types of assay methods. Many review articles discussing these problems have been published recently; most of them describing assay for prostaglandins as well as thromboxanes (see e.g. refs. 208–215).

Measurement of thromboxane biosynthesis is generally done either by assay of the immediate product, TXA_2, (as such or as a derivative), or of the subsequently formed hydrolysis product, TXB_2. Both these approaches can be used to monitor thromboxane produced from either endogenous or exogenous precursors, but may give somewhat different information, as discussed below. A common approach in many studies is to measure only the conversion of exogenous substrate by the studied biological system: in this case a convenient method is the use of radiolabeled precursor and monitoring the formed labeled thromboxanes [19,101,216–218]. In certain cases neither TXA_2 nor TXB_2 may be reliable as an indicator of thromboxane formation: the best target for measurements may then instead be a metabolite. As was pointed out in the preceding section, it is of great importance to establish which compound is the proper target for measurements in each biological situation: monitoring the wrong compound may lead to quite erroneous results (see above, Metabolism of thromboxanes).

(a) Assay of TXA_2

Since TXA_2 is an extremely unstable, highly potent compound, immediate bioassay is the only possible method for the assay of the intact compound. The most commonly employed assay organs are various vascular preparations, such as the rabbit aorta, mesenteric artery or celiac artery [15,19,20,29,30,108]. Other possibilities are the rabbit inferior caval vein [29], the rat aorta [219] and the bovine and porcine coronary arteries [12,26,220,221]. A frequently used non-vascular assay organ is the guinea pig lung parenchymal strip, which is highly sensitive to TXA_2 [15]. Platelet aggregation is also commonly employed as a sensitive bioassay for TXA_2.

One draw-back of bioassay however is its inherent non-specificity. Reactions to bioactive substances not related to this field of biochemistry can generally be blocked by pretreatment of the assay organ with specific antagonists and inhibitors [212]. However, even using these precautions, many bioassay systems for detection and assay of TXA_2 are not entirely specific for this compound but react in a similar fashion also to the endoperoxides. This is the case with two of the most frequently used systems: platelets and the rabbit aorta. Since endoperoxides may be present in parallel with TXA_2 in many biological situations, this non-specificity may create a problem. One possible solution is to use an assay more specific for TXA_2: the rabbit mesenteric artery, for example, has been reported to be contracted only by TXA_2 [215].

The specificity of the bioassay for TXA_2 can also be increased by insertion of a delay coil since TXA_2 has a short half life [212]. Such a modification would reveal the presence of a highly unstable compound such as TXA_2 in the analyzed material. However in a situation where two antagonistic and unstable compounds are present such as TXA_2 and PGI_2, the delay coil is not a solution. This situation would arise for example when perfusates from lungs are studied, since the lung can produce large amounts of both these compounds. Obviously, the formed quantities of TXA_2 would be grossly underestimated if they were assayed using only such assay systems in which the TXA_2 effects would be counteracted by the simultaneous presence of PGI_2. A delay coil would probably not be of much use in this situation, since both compounds are highly unstable. A combination of several different assay organs with different specificities for these compounds in a so-called cascade type of assay might solve the problem [212,215].

An alternative solution is to abandon bioassay entirely and use a more specific approach instead. One such approach in TXA_2 assay is based on the rapid conversion of this unstable compound into a stable derivative by trapping with excess methanol or some other nucleophilic reagent (see above, Elucidation of the thromboxane structure). If methanol is used, the formed products are two epimers of mono-*O*-methyl TXB_2 (Fig. 2). These compounds are biologically inactive but are instead suitable for assay by methods requiring chemical stability of the measured compound, such as gas chromatography mass spectrometry or radioimmunoassay.

The first quantitation method based on this trapping procedure was developed for TXA_2 formed from exogenous precursor and was a double isotope dilution method [19]. Later a radioimmunoassay was developed for the major epimer of mono-*O*-methyl TXB_2 [222]. This method allowed the assay of TXA_2 formed from endogenous precursor [e.g. 223].

It should be pointed out, however, that although the measured concentrations of mono-*O*-methyl TXB_2 will reflect the amount of TXA_2 present in the sample at the instant the methanol was added, the levels of the derivative will not be a reliable indicator of the *total* amount of TXA_2 formed by the system. A great part of this has already been hydrolyzed into TXB_2, and some further conversion of $TXA_2 \rightarrow TXB_2$ can perhaps also take place even in excess methanol. A better indication of the total TXA_2 is obtained by the sum of formed TXB_2 and the two epimers of mono-*O*-methyl TXB_2 (see also below, Pitfalls in thromboxane assay).

Methanol treatment of aliquots removed from the TXA_2 synthesizing system, followed by the assay of the formed mono-*O*-methyl TXB_2, gives excellent information about the kinetics of appearance and disappearance of TXA_2 in such a system. Fig. 5 demonstrates the differences in information obtained when TXA_2 (assayed as mono-*O*-methyl TXB_2 after methanol treatment) or its stable degradation product, TXB_2, were monitored after addition of arachidonic acid to a platelet suspension. Small aliquots were removed with very short intervals before and after this addition; they were added to 25 volumes of methanol. As soon as aggregation had occurred, the platelets were removed by filtration (to exclude any later biosynthesis of TXA_2 in the system) and aliquots were then continuously removed from the filtrate. Assay of TXB_2 by a specific radioimmunoassay demonstrated a sharp rise immediately after the addition of arachidonic acid; a high level was reached which remained constant during the rest of the experiment. Assay of mono-*O*-methyl TXB_2 however showed a different pattern. A maximal level was obtained within the first minute after the substrate was added; the level then rapidly declined, indicating a rapid disappearance of the precursor of this derivative, i.e. TXA_2. When the results were corrected for cross-reaction with the very high levels of TXB_2 present at this stage, a straight line was found in the semi-logarithmic diagram. The half-life of the precursor was 32 s calculated from this diagram: this is in perfect agreement with earlier reported data for TXA_2 [15,19].

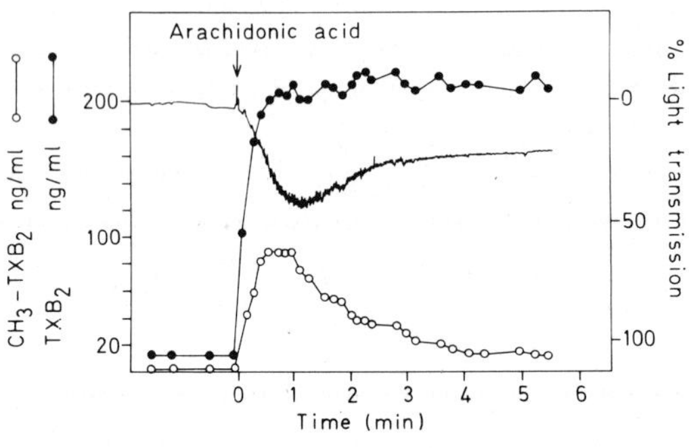

Fig. 5. Mono-*O*-methyl TXB_2 (○——○) and TXB_2 (●——●) levels (measured by radioimmunoassay) after addition of arachidonic acid to washed human platelets at 37°C. Light transmission was recorded simultaneously in an aggregometer. Arrow indicates addition of arachidonic acid. (Reproduced from Granström, E., Kindahl, H. and Samuelsson, B. (1976) Prostaglandins 12, 929–941, with permission from Geron-X Inc., USA).

(b) Assay of TXB_2

The great majority of quantitative studies in this field concern the measurement of TXB_2 rather than TXA_2. Although some biological activity has been found also for TXB_2 (see above), bioassay is normally not employed for this compound. Since it is chemically very stable, it is suitable for other types of quantification methods, such as gas chromatography mass spectrometry or radioimmunoassay.

The first method developed for TXB_2 was a gas chromatography mass spectrometry method, utilizing $[^2H_8]TXB_2$ as a carrier [18]. This was later followed by others of the same type [59,210,217,224]. A related gas chromatographic method was based on the electron capture technique [225]; a liquid chromatographic method utilizing fluorescent derivatives of TXB_2 has also been published [226].

By far the most common method in this field is radioimmunoassay. After the first radioimmunoassay for TXB_2 was published [227], a very large number of similar assays were developed [e.g. 217,228–232]. This type of measurement has been used for detection and/or quantification of thromboxane synthesis in platelet preparations, tissue homogenates, organ perfusates, cell culture media, various exudates or other biological material; it has also been used in monitoring enzyme activity of thromboxane synthetase during purification procedures.

(c) Pitfalls in thromboxane assay

Each type of assay method (e.g. bioassay, gas chromatography mass spectrometry, radioimmunoassay) suffers from certain sources of error, which may seriously influence the final results. Some bioassay problems, specific for TXA_2 measurements, were briefly discussed above. In addition to such sources of error, however, there are also other pitfalls in the three different approaches to thromboxane measurements described above (i.e. direct and indirect assay of TXA_2, and assay of TXB_2, respectively).

In order to increase the specificity of TXA_2 quantitation, some researchers have introduced an extraction step before bioassay of the compound [31,38,108]. This is performed at pH 7.4 using ether as the organic solvent. Under these conditions, the precursors, the endoperoxides and arachidonic acid, are also extracted to some extent. Since the latter compounds are considerably more stable, their relative amounts would increase during the subsequent evaporation step, which unfortunately degrades a major portion of the unstable TXA_2. Hence, quantitative data based on such a procedure would underestimate the true amounts of TXA_2 originally present in the sample, and if endoperoxides were present their bioactivities would prevail in the ensuing bioassay.

However, the pronounced instability of TXA_2 is well known, and quantitative data concerning this compound are generally interpreted with caution. This is unfortunately not the case in many studies where the stable hydrolysis product, TXB_2, has been monitored instead. The serious sources of error associated with TXB_2 measurements are often overlooked, because this stable product of the thromboxane pathway is generally regarded as a reliable indicator of thromboxane biosynthesis. In fact, it is often regarded as *the* degradation product of TXA_2, automatically reflecting all TXA_2 preexisting in the sample, or released into the blood stream, etc.

This concept may however be far from true:

First, as is the well known case with prostaglandins, artifactual formation of thromboxane may occur rapidly and extensively from e.g. blood cells during collection and processing of a blood sample. Reported TXB_2 levels in plasma are generally unrealistically high: it is unlikely that they reflect the endogenous biological situation.

Second, even if this artifactual contribution could somehow be prevented, it is not necessarily certain that TXA_2 formed in the body, in tissues or other biologic material, is quantitatively hydrolyzed into TXB_2. This hydrolysis may sometimes be a very minor pathway of TXA_2 degradation. It has for example been demonstrated that in samples containing albumin, such as platelet rich plasma, the major part of formed TXA_2 is not converted into TXB_2 but instead covalently bound to albumin [203–205], and will thus escape detection by conventional assay methods for TXB_2.

Third, it has been demonstrated in metabolic studies that after i.v. injection of $[^3H]TXB_2$ into monkeys, the highest attained plasma level of the compound (1 min after the injection) was only about 10% of the theoretical maximum, indicating a rapid uptake of TXB_2 by tissues [188]. Thus, even if TXB_2 was the only product formed from TXA_2 released into the blood stream, and if it could be measured reliably, it might only represent a minor fraction of the actually formed TXA_2.

That measurements of the TXB_2 formation may be totally misleading as an indicator of TXA_2 biosynthesis was mentioned above (Metabolism of Thromboxanes). It was found that TXA_2 formed in sensitized (and possibly to some extent also in normal) guinea pig lungs was extensively metabolized into 15-keto-13,14-dihydro-TXB_2 [197–199]. Thus, measurement of only a TXB_2 metabolite following guinea pig anaphylaxis failed to reveal any thromboxane biosynthesis during this condition [192, cf. 14,199].

(d) Assay of thromboxane metabolites

The uncertainties and practical difficulties involved in thromboxane assay when monitoring either TXA_2 or TXB_2 have prompted some groups to develop methods for further degraded metabolites instead. The major urinary metabolite of TXB_2, in most species dinor-TXB_2 (see above), has been monitored in the urine of the guinea pig [192] and man [194]. As mentioned above, however, it is by no means certain that the TXB_2 pathway reliably reflects TXA_2 biosynthesis, for example after pulmonary anaphylaxis. This condition could probably be better studied by measurement of some 15-keto-13,14-dihydro products instead [197–199], either 15-keto-dihydro-TXB_2 itself in the circulation or one of the more degraded products of this pathway found in urine.

The first quantitative study monitoring 15-keto-dihydro-TXB_2 utilized gas chromatography mass spectrometry of exudates of anaphylactic guinea pig lungs: the results were briefly described above [199]. Later, a radioimmunoassay was developed for the same compound [201]; the assay was recently improved to obtain higher sensitivity [202]. This method was also used to follow thromboxane release during guinea pig anaphylaxis, in this case in vivo.

6. Thromboxane agonists and antagonists

(a) Agonists

The discovery of the prostaglandin endoperoxides and thromboxane A_2, compounds with pronounced biological activity but short half-life under physiological conditions, initiated a search for stable synthetic compounds that mimic the actions of the labile arachidonate metabolites. Several of these synthetic compounds are structural analogues to PGH_2.

Replacement of one or the other of the endoperoxide oxygens in PGH_2 by a methylene group resulted in stable compounds that were biologically active [143]. One of these, 11α,9α-epoxy-methano-15-hydroxyprosta-5,13-dienoic acid (U46619) was 3.7 times more potent than PGG_2 in inducing platelet aggregation and 6.2 times more active than PGH_2 in contracting isolated rabbit aorta [233]. Cascade superfusion experiments suggested that U46619 is a selective TXA_2-like agonist [234]. Another structural analogue of PGH_2 which is biologically active was obtained by replacing both endoperoxide oxygens with an azo-group [144,235]. This 9,11-azoprostanoid was more active than PGG_2 in inducing platelet aggregation and the platelet release reaction. It was also more active than PGH_2 in contracting isolated rabbit aorta [144]. The 9,11-etheno-analogue of PGH_2 induced aggregation in platelet-rich plasma although it was ten times less potent than PGG_2 in this respect. The analogue induced [^{14}C]serotonin release from labelled platelets at concentrations which resulted in platelet aggregation [236,237]. Substitution of the endoperoxide group for a dithio group yielded a compound that was 24 times more active than PGH_2 in contracting aorta strips; in addition, it caused rapid and irreversible platelet aggregation [238]. Platelet aggregation induced by arachidonic acid or collagen was not inhibited by this prostaglandin endosulfide [239].

A series of 9α-homo-9,11-epoxy prostanoic acid analogues, where the side chains correspond to the 1-series of prostaglandins, were synthesized and examined for various biological activities [240]. One of these analogues, GBR-30728, contracted smooth muscle and induced platelet aggregation in rat blood, but was approximately 5000 times less potent than ADP [240].

A more active thromboxane receptor agonist was found in the 9α-homo-9,11-epoxy-5,13-prostadienoic acid analogue, SQ 26,538. This compound was 200 times more potent than arachidonic acid in inducing platelet aggregation but was only 1/10 as potent as PGH_2. This effect was not blocked by inhibitors of cyclo-oxygenase or of thromboxane synthetase [241].

A derivative of prostaglandin $F_{2\alpha}$,17,18,19,20-tetranor-16-*p*-fluorophenoxy $PGF_{2\alpha}$ (ICI 79939) as well as its 11-oxo analogue mimicked the actions of 11,9-epoxymethano-PGH_2 on four endoperoxide sensitive preparations, namely human platelets, rabbit aortic strip, guinea pig tracheal chain and pig blood pressure [242]. ICI 79939 as well as a number of related analogues showed full agonist activity on a dog saphenous vein preparation [243]. Since replacement of the four terminal carbons at the ω-end with a *p*-fluorophenoxy group increased the thromboxane-like activity of $PGF_{2\alpha}$ and PGD_2, the 16-*p*-fluorophenoxy derivative of 9,11-etheno-PGH_2, structurally more closely related to PGH_2 than $PGF_{2\alpha}$ or PGD_2, was prepared. This compound caused a rapid and reversible aggregation of human platelets at 50–100 ng/ml and irreversible aggregation at higher concentrations. Like the 9,11-etheno-PGH_2 analogue, its 16-*p*-fluorophenoxy derivative contracted rabbit aortic strip but had a very long-lasting action [244].

Some compounds with thromboxane-like structure have been screened for agonist activity on thromboxane sensitive systems. Carbocyclic TXA_2 [155,245,246] behaved as a potent TXA_2 agonist on the vasculature (isolated cat coronary artery) but rather as an antagonist on arachidonic acid induced platelet aggregation. The TXA_1 analogue, 9α-homo-(11,12)-deoxa-(11,12)-methylene thromboxane A_1 showed weak TXA_2-like properties with respect to vasoconstriction but had no effect on platelet aggregation [247].

A sulphur analogue of TXA_2, DL-(9,11),(11,12)-dideoxa-(9,11)-methylene-(11,12)-epithio-thromboxane A_2 methyl ester, showed moderate contractile activity on isolated rat aorta. It did not induce platelet aggregation [248]. Sulphur substitution of the oxetane oxygen in TXA_2, as in the analogue DL-(9,11),(11,12)-dideoxa-(9,11)-epithio-(11,12)-methylene-thromboxane A_2, resulted in a compound with potent contractile activity on the isolated rat aorta. In addition, this compound caused platelet aggregation [249]. A third analogue, in which both ring oxygens of TXA_2 were replaced by sulphur, showed properties very similar to natural TXA_2. This analogue effectively contracted rat aorta and caused rapid and irreversible aggregation of human platelets [250].

(b) Antagonists

Ever since the discovery of TXA_2, much effort has been directed towards the search for compounds that either inhibit its formation or antagonize its actions, since TXA_2 has been postulated to be involved in a number of pathophysiological conditions. Some of the compounds that have been described as antagonists of thromboxane action are reviewed below.

One of the first antagonists described of the TXA_2 receptor in human platelets was 9,11-epoxyiminoprosta-5,13-dienoic acid (EIP) [152]. EIP antagonized TXA_2-mediated platelet aggregation without inhibiting thromboxane synthetase or fatty acid cyclo-oxygenase. However, EIP contracted rat aorta and thus acted as an agonist in this system.

The PGH_2 analogue, 9,11-azo-13-oxa-15-hydroxy-prostanoic acid, blocked the actions of 9,11-epoxymethano-PGH_2 and TXA_2 on human platelet-rich plasma, suggesting that it is a PGH_2/TXA_2 receptor antagonist [148,251]. This compound also inhibited thromboxane synthetase. Another nitrogen-containing compound, 13-aza-prostanoic acid, exhibited antagonistic properties on the platelet PGH_2/TXA_2-receptor. It inhibited platelet aggregation induced by arachidonic acid, PGH_2 and 9,11-epoxy-methano PGH_2. Neither primary aggregation induced by ADP or thrombin nor thromboxane synthetase was inhibited [252]. 13-Aza-prostanoic acid not only prevented arachidonic acid induced platelet aggregation, but also reversed aggregation once the process had been initiated. However, aggregation induced by ADP or epinephrine could not be reversed by 13-aza-prostanoic acid, suggesting that this deaggregating effect is specific for PGH_2- and TXA_2-mediated aggregation [253].

The compound [1α(Z),2β,5α]-methyl-7-[2-(4-morpholinyl)-3-oxo-5-(phenylmethoxy)cyclopentyl]-5-heptenoate (AH 19437) inhibited platelet aggregation and 5-hydroxytryptamine release without inhibiting fatty acid cyclo-oxygenase, thromboxane synthetase, cAMP phosphodiesterase or prostacyclin synthetase, consistent with the view that AH 19437 is a selective antagonist of platelet TXA_2 receptors [254–256].

A number of carbathromboxane analogues (analogues of thromboxane A_2 where one or both of the ring oxygens have been replaced by carbon) were recently synthesized [155,156,245,246,257–260]. Three of these, 11a-carbathromboxane A_2, 15-deoxy-15,16-dihydro-11a carbathromboxane A_2 and 9,11-epoxy-11a-carbathrombanoic acid, were examined for agonist/antagonist activity on TXA_2 receptors from human platelets and rat aortic strips [154]. All three compounds were shown to possess both thromboxane synthetase inhibiting activity and antagonistic activity on platelet TXA_2-receptors. Interestingly, none of the compounds exhibited agonist or antagonist activity on TXA_2-receptors from vascular smooth muscle [154]. Thus, it seems that there are different classes of thromboxane receptors with respect to binding characteristics. This is supported by experiments with another carbathromboxane analogue, carbocyclic thromboxane A_2 (CTA_2) [155,246]. This analogue is a potent coronary vasoconstrictor, which acts as a thromboxane agonist on the vasculature. However, CTA_2 acted as a TX-antagonist on platelet aggregation; in addition, it selectively inhibited thromboxane synthetase. In contrast, pinane thromboxane A_2 [156,261,262] showed antagonistic effects on TXA_2-receptors both in vascular smooth muscle and in human platelets. It also inhibited thromboxane synthetase. These properties make pinane thromboxane A_2 interesting as a potential antithrombotic agent [263,264].

The synthetic thromboxane analogue, 9α-homo-9,11-epoxy-5,13-prostadienoic acid analogue (SQ 26,536), inhibited arachidonic acid induced platelet aggregation without inhibiting the prostaglandin synthesizing activity of bovine seminal vesicles or thromboxane synthetase activity of lyzed human platelets [241]. This compound thus acted as an antagonist on the platelet TXA_2 receptor, while its 15R-epimer turned out to be an agonist.

A study was undertaken to find compounds with partial agonist activity on TXA_2

receptors [243]. The idea was that chemical modification of such a partial agonist could eventually produce an antagonist of the receptor. The 9,11-etheno analogue of PGH_2 was found to be a partial agonist, and chemical modification of this compound resulted in an antagonist of the thromboxane receptor. The modified compound (±)-5-endo-(6′-carboxyhex-2′Z-enyl)-6-oxo[*N*-(phenylcarbamoyl)-hydrazono-methyl]-bicyclo[2.2.1]heptane (EP 045) antagonized contraction of rabbit aorta and dog saphenous vein by TXA_2. Platelet aggregation induced by arachidonic acid or 11,9-epoxy-methano PGH_2 was inhibited, while thromboxane biosynthesis was unaffected [265].

A number of 7 oxabicyclo[2.2.1]heptane prostaglandin analogues were synthesized and evaluated as potential thromboxane synthetase inhibitors or thromboxane antagonists. Several of the compounds tested were shown to be TXA_2 antagonists, judged from platelet aggregation and thromboxane inhibition tests. Two of the compounds also inhibited arachidonic acid induced bronchoconstriction [266].

Dantrolene has been suggested to be a competitive antagonist of TXA_2 in muscle [268]. Phtalazinol (EG 626) was first reported to be a TXA_2 antagonist [268]. However, later it was shown that it is not a specific TXA_2 antagonist but has a general inhibitory effect on smooth muscle, possibly exerted by inhibition of phosphodiesterase [269].

7. Thromboxanes and the lung

In the guinea pig, the lung has a very high capacity for thromboxane biosynthesis compared with other tissues [45]. This is especially the case with sensitized lungs challenged with antigen [196]. In 1969 Piper and Vane found that perfused sensitized guinea pig lungs released a “rabbit aorta contracting substance” (RCS) during anaphylactic shock [14]. This substance also contracted the guinea pig trachea. The biologically active material in RCS was later shown to consist mainly of TXA_2 and smaller amounts of the prostaglandin endoperoxides, PGG_2 and PGH_2 [15,19]. TXA_2, which is a strong vasopressor, is also extremely potent in contracting respiratory smooth muscle. TXA_2 is about 50 times more potent than $PGF_{2\alpha}$ in contracting the isolated guinea pig trachea and 600 times more potent than $PGF_{2\alpha}$ in causing bronchoconstriction in guinea pigs in vivo [21]. Two metabolites of TXA_2, i.e. TXB_2 and 15-keto-13,14-dihydro-TXB_2, on the other hand display little or no contractile activity on respiratory smooth muscle [197].

Most studies on pulmonary thromboxane biosynthesis have been performed with homogenates of lungs, or with perfused normal or sensitized lungs, generally from the guinea pig. In whole homogenates of normal guinea pig lungs the major products of exogenous arachidonic acid were TXB_2 and HHT (about 20% of each compound) whereas PGE_2 and $PGF_{2\alpha}$ were found only in small amounts [2–3%) [270]. Similar results were obtained when guinea pig lung microsomes were incubated with PGH_2 [49]. TXB_2 was the major metabolite of arachidonic acid or PGH_2 also in lung homogenates from other species, such as cattle [271,272], rabbit [49,271], and sheep

[271,273]. There were, however, apparent species differences in the obtained metabolite spectra from the cyclo-oxygenase pathway. Thus the bovine, rabbit, rat and sheep lungs had a lower capacity for conversion of arachidonic acid into TXB_2 than lungs of guinea pigs [49,51,271,272,274]. No thromboxane formation was detected at all in homogenates from human or monkey lung [49,276]. Furthermore, in homogenates of bovine, rabbit, sheep or cat lungs, the stable product of the prostacyclin pathway, 6-keto-$PGF_{1\alpha}$, was also found. The conversion via this pathway was strongly favoured over thromboxane biosynthesis at low substrate concentrations [48,49].

During the fetal development bovine, rabbit and sheep lung were shown to have a poor capacity for thromboxane synthesis compared with the adult lung. The fetal lung was instead quite active in converting arachidonic acid into PGE_2 [271,272,275].

When intact, normal guinea pig lungs were perfused with arachidonic acid, similar results were obtained as in incubations with lung homogenates. Thus, large amounts of TXB_2 were detected in the perfusate, whereas only small amounts of PGE_2 and $PGF_{2\alpha}$ were found [270]. Normal guinea pig lungs, perfused with arachidonic acid, were later shown to produce also 15-keto-13,14-dihydro-TXB_2 together with relatively large amounts of 6-keto-$PGF_{1\alpha}$ and the corresponding metabolite, 6,15-diketo-13,14-dihydro-$PGF_{1\alpha}$ [199]. When sensitized guinea pig lungs were employed instead, the release of TXB_2 and especially 15-keto-13,14-dihydro-TXB_2 increased, while the production of 6-keto-$PGF_{1\alpha}$ and 6,15-diketo-13,14-dihydro-$PGF_{1\alpha}$ correspondingly decreased.

During antigen challenge of sensitized guinea pig lungs, thromboxane biosynthesis from endogenous substrate was increased several-fold [196]. The main cyclo-oxygenase metabolite in pooled perfusates from anaphylactic guinea pig lungs was now 15-keto-13,14-dihydro-TXB_2, followed by TXB_2 [197,201]. The relative amounts of the 15-keto-dihydro metabolite progressively increased with repeated immunological challenges [199]. 15-Keto-13,14-dihydro-TXB_2, formed from endogenous precursor during anaphylaxis, constituted up to 85% of the total amount of cyclo-oxygenase products in the perfusate after repeated challenges with the antigen [199]. Anhut et al. [201] reported that the TXB_2 concentration in the perfusate was highest 0–3 min after challenge, while the 15-keto-13,14-dihydro-TXB_2 level reached a peak about 4–6 min after administration of the antigen. When the same events were studied in the guinea pig in vivo, the plasma levels of 15-keto-dihydro-TXB_2 were found to increase about 200 times during anaphylactic shock [202]. If guinea pigs were exposed to 100% O_2 before challenge of their isolated perfused lungs, the release of TXB_2 increased two-fold [277,278]. The amounts of the metabolite, 15-keto-dihydro-TXB_2, were not measured in this study; however, the enhanced TXB_2 production was interpreted as caused by inhibition of the enzyme 15-hydroxy-prostanoate dehydrogenase by O_2.

An increased release of thromboxanes was also demonstrated when normal or sensitized guinea pig lungs were challenged with certain mediators of anaphylaxis, such as slow reacting substance of anaphylaxis (SRS-A), histamine or bradykinin [14,279–281]. The thromboxane production induced by these mediators was more pronounced in sensitized lungs [282,283]. The increased release of TXA_2 induced by histamine or SRS-A was shown to be reduced by the β-adrenergic receptor agonists, isoproterenol and salbutamol [284]. This inhibiting effect could then be abolished by β-adrenoceptor blocking drugs, such as practolol or sotalol. Activation of α-adrenergic receptors by phenylephrine or of cholinergic receptors by carbachol did not modify the release of TXA_2 induced by histamine or SRS-A [284]. However, atropin and ipratropium bromide, a synthetic anticholinergic compound, were reported to inhibit the TXA_2 release, possibly by an action at the phospholipase site [283].

The generation of thromboxanes caused by histamine or SRS-A can be inhibited in the guinea pig by non-steroidal anti-inflammatory drugs [285], however without significantly reducing the bronchoconstriction [286]. On the other hand, these drugs prevented both the increased airway resistance and the thromboxane formation induced by bradykinin [286].

Recently SRS-A was identified as a mixture of certain novel lipoxygenase products of arachidonic acid, viz. leukotrienes C_4, D_4 and E_4 [287–292] (see also Chapter 4). When pure leukotrienes became available, it was confirmed that guinea pig lungs, when exposed to these potent airway constrictors, release TXA_2 [223,293–295]. This release was blocked by treatment with non-steroidal or steroidal anti-inflammatory drugs, thromboxane synthetase inhibitors, the SRS antagonist FPL 55712, and also by β_2 adrenoceptor stimulation [293–295], all of these drugs acting at their different and specific points of attack in the sequence of events leading to thromboxane release.

The bronchoconstrictor effect of the leukotrienes may thus be augmented by a secondary formation of TXA_2. There has been some controversy concerning the relative importance of such a mechanism. Thus, pretreatment with non-steroidal antiinflammatory drugs may abolish [293,294], leave unaffected [295], or enhance [296] the constrictor action of leukotrienes in guinea pig airways. Furthermore, the bronchoconstrictor effects of intravenously injected leukotrienes are antagonized by indomethacin, whereas the responses to aerosolized leukotrienes are enhanced by this drug [296–298]. Therefore, it is evident that the experimental design may favor TXA_2-dependent or independent leukotriene actions [299].

Gryglewski et al. [280] reported that histamine challenge of guinea pig lung strips generated TXA_2 in the lung parenchyma, probably from the interstitial cells. On the other hand, histamine stimulation of guinea pig trachea released mainly the bronchodilator, PGE_2, but no detectable amounts of TXA_2. The thromboxane release from the lung parenchyma was induced by stimulation of the histamine H_1 receptors [282], whereas the PGE_2 release from trachea was induced by stimulation of the histamine H_2 receptors [300]. The produced PGE_2 could then inhibit further release of histamine and SRS-A. This effect has been reported both during antigen challenge in chopped human lungs [301] and in perfused guinea pig lungs [302]. TXB_2, on the other hand, increased the release of SRS-A from challenged guinea pig lungs [198]. It might be mentioned in this context that TXB_2 has also been shown to inhibit the pulmonary degradation of PGE_2 when infused through the rat isolated lung [303] or administered to anesthetized dogs [42,304].

In human bronchial asthma a number of mediators, e.g. histamine, SRS-A, prostaglandins and thromboxanes, have been felt to play a role [305,306]. Asthmatic subjects were found to be markedly hyperresponsive to $PGF_{2\alpha}$ aerosols: they displayed an increase about 8000-fold in bronchial sensitivity compared with normals [307]. An enhanced release of $PGF_{2\alpha}$ metabolites in urine and plasma was demonstrated in asthmatic patients following inhalation of specific antigen [308–310]. A marked increase in plasma levels of the major $PGF_{2\alpha}$ metabolite and of TXB_2 was also registered in exercise-induced asthma [311]. Inhibition of the prostaglandin and thromboxane synthesis by the cyclo-oxygenase inhibitors, aspirin, indomethacin or other non-steroidal anti-inflammatory drugs, did not result in any significant reduction of the bronchoconstriction during asthmatic attacks [309,310,312]. In some asthmatic patients aspirin could instead induce bronchoconstriction [313–315]. The identification of the leukotrienes as extremely potent bronchoconstrictors [316,317], and the elucidation of their biosynthesis from polyunsaturated fatty acids via lipoxygenase catalyzed pathways, provided a likely explanation for these findings: the biosynthesis of these cyclo-oxygenase independent products is not inhibited by non-steroidal anti-inflammatory drugs. Since the cysteinyl-containing leukotrienes may be responsible for the major part of the bronchoconstriction during asthmatic attacks, it is not surprising that no alleviation of the symptoms was obtained by aspirin-like drugs. It is even possible that in "aspirin-sensitive asthma" inhibition of the cyclo-oxygenase might instead contribute to the symptoms by diverting the arachidonic acid metabolism into the leukotriene pathway, while at the same time the inhibiting effect of PGE_2 on histamine release is abolished [305,316,318].

As mentioned above, the bronchoconstrictor effect of the leukotrienes can be partially mediated by formation of TXA_2 in the guinea pig lung [223]. The human lung however has been reported to differ from the guinea pig lung in the activation and metabolism of arachidonic acid [51,276]. The capacity for thromboxane formation from endogenous arachidonic acid after stimulation by crude SRS-A was much lower in the human lung [51].

The interrelationship between the different arachidonic acid products, the prostaglandins, thromboxanes and leukotrienes, in the pathophysiology of human asthma is obviously complex, and extensive further studies are required to clarify the roles of these substances as well as of other mediators of the anaphylactic reaction.

8. Roles of thromboxanes in platelet function

The arachidonic acid derived prostaglandin endoperoxides PGG_2 and PGH_2 were found to induce platelet aggregation and the platelet release reaction in submicromolar concentrations [7,13]. Aspirin, a well-known inhibitor of platelet aggregation by e.g. collagen and arachidonic acid, and an inhibitor of the enzyme fatty acid cyclo-oxygenase in platelets [16,319], did not prevent endoperoxide induced aggregation [7]. TXA_2 formed from the endoperoxides in platelets was found to be a more potent inducer of platelet aggregation than the endoperoxides [19,20]. The question

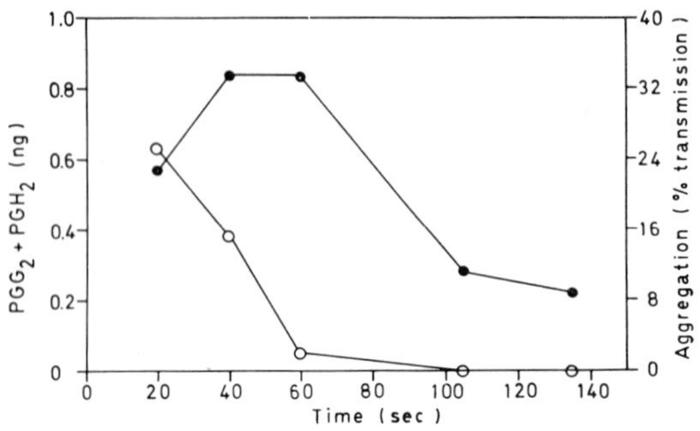

Fig. 6. Maximum aggregation induced by 0.1 ml suspensions of washed platelets incubated for different times with 120 ng of arachidonic acid (●———●). The content in these samples of $PGG_2 + PGH_2$ are also given (○———○). The platelet suspension in the aggregometer tube was preincubated for 2 min at 37°C with 14 μM indomethacin. (Reproduced from Svensson, J., Hamberg, M. and Samuelsson, B. (1976) Acta Physiol. Scand. 98, 285–294, with permission from the publisher).

whether or not TXA_2 is the sole aggregating agent normally formed from platelet arachidonic acid has not been settled. It seems likely, however, partly on the basis of experiments with inhibitors of thromboxane synthetase, that TXA_2 is the important mediator under physiological conditions and that the endoperoxides per se play a minor role [121,144,156] (cf. also Figs. 1 and 6).

The mechanism by which TXA_2 causes aggregation is not clearly understood. Endoperoxide- and TXA_2-induced aggregation is strongly inhibited in the presence of an ADP consuming enzyme system [320]. This suggests that TXA_2-induced aggregation is dependent upon the release from the very dense granules of ADP, a well-known pro-aggregating compound [321]. In addition, there is a release of other constituents of the very dense granules, e.g. Ca^{2+}. This ion appears to be required for the contractile process of the release reaction. In this connection, it may be mentioned that a related ion, i.e. Sr^{2+}, when added exogenously, is able to penetrate the platelet membrane and cause synthesis and release of TXA_2 as well as release of serotonin [322]. A third component of the very dense granules, i.e. serotonin, is also released upon stimulation with TXA_2 [20]. Recent studies have shown that a number of diseases such as aspirin-induced asthma and migraine [323] as well as endogenous depressive states [324] are accompanied by an abnormal transport of serotonin. It would thus be very interesting to study the TXA_2 formation in platelets from such patients.

When dealing with the mechanism of TXA_2 induced aggregation, it should be noted that TXA_2 may have an effect of its own, independent of the release of compounds from the very dense granules. Thus a number of studies have shown that platelets low in ADP or lacking ADP (storage pool disease) as well as degranulated platelets may be aggregated by TXA_2 [325,326]. It is known that some agents that induce platelet aggregation also lower the level of platelet cAMP, whereas other agents that inhibit aggregation increase platelet cAMP [327]. This relation is also true in case of the endoperoxides and TXA_2, i.e. incubation of platelets with these compounds leads to a decrease of cAMP. Furthermore, the level of cAMP influences the availability of free arachidonic acid necessary for TXA_2 formation, i.e. increasing platelet cAMP leads to inhibition of the liberation of phospholipid-bound arachidonic acid [328].

Arachidonic acid released from platelet phospholipids is not only converted into thromboxanes by way of fatty acid cyclo-oxygenase and thromboxane synthetase, but is also converted by a lipoxygenase into 12L-hydroperoxy-5,8,10,14-eicosatetraenoic acid and its stable end-product, 12L-hydroxy-5,8,10,14-eicosatetraenoic acid [16]. The role of the lipoxygenase pathway is largely unknown. It appears likely, however, that there is an intimate relation between the lipoxygenase and the cyclo-oxygenase/thromboxane synthetase pathways. This is suggested by the weak inhibitory effect of 12-hydroperoxy-5,8,10,14-eicosatetraenoic acid on thromboxane synthetase [95] as well as by the activation of the lipoxygenase by prostaglandin endoperoxides [329].

In recent work the origin and mechanism of formation of free arachidonic acid on stimulation of platelets have been studied. Initially, phospholipase A_2 was thought to play a key role in the liberation of free arachidonic acid from various platelet phospholipids. Recently, a new concept implicating phospholipase C catalyzed degradation of a specific phospholipid, i.e. phosphatidylinositol, has emerged [330,331]. It appears that the substrate is attacked by the enzyme to form a diglyceride. Subsequent hydrolysis catalyzed by a diglyceride lipase gives rise to a monoglyceride and free arachidonic acid. Finally, the liberated arachidonic acid is converted into inter alia TXA_2 by way of the enzymes fatty acid cyclo-oxygenase and thromboxane synthetase. This mechanism is attractive from a purely theoretical point of view, since it is another example of the so-called "PI-response" which occurs upon stimulation of a large number of tissues [332,333].

In addition to TXA_2 another factor, viz. PGI_2 or prostacyclin, which is formed from arachidonic acid and PGH_2 in the endothelial layer of the vessels, is of importance in influencing platelet aggregation [32]. PGI_2 gives rise to an increased level of platelet cAMP and thus inhibits aggregation. Although the physiological role of PGI_2 is under dispute [334,335], an imbalance between the rate of synthesis of TXA_2 and PGI_2 appears to exist in a number of pathological conditions, e.g. in cardiovascular and cerebrovascular diseases. An imbalance between TXA_2 and PGI_2 synthesis also appears to exist in diabetes mellitus. Thus platelets from rats rendered diabetic by streptozotocin treatment showed markedly increased liberation of arachidonic acid following stimulation with thrombin [336]. Also, a decreased production of PGI_2 in vascular tissue was found.

In the human, diabetic subjects have an enhanced synthesis of platelet TXA_2 [337,338]. Interestingly, no significant difference in the production of TXA_2 (measured as TXB_2) was found when normal subjects were compared with diabetic subjects without apparent vascular damage [337]. On the other hand, when vascular lesions were present in the diabetic subjects a significant increase in the synthesis of platelet TXA_2 was noted. In addition, platelets from diabetic subjects (with or without vascular damage) had a lower threshold for aggregation in response to ADP as well as collagen.

A few platelet disorders involving defective formation or action of prostaglandin endoperoxides/TXA_2 have been described. The first case reported was a young man with a mild bleeding tendency and a slight increase in the bleeding time [13]. The defect could be tracked to deficient platelet cyclo-oxygenase ("PCO-deficiency"), i.e. the deficient platelets were unable to convert arachidonic acid into TXA_2 and 12L-hydroxy-5,8,10-heptadecatrienoic acid. Aggregation was elicited by PGG_2 but not by arachidonic acid and collagen. Recently, a similar case was reported [335]. In this case, vein biopsies were taken and the cyclo-oxygenase normally present in the vessel wall was found to be deficient. The patient thus offered a possibility to evaluate the relative roles of TXA_2 from platelets and PGI_2 from the vessel wall in normal subjects. The findings that the patient lacking capacity for biosynthesis of TXA_2 as well as PGI_2 had a mild bleeding tendency and a prolonged bleeding time indicate the importance of TXA_2 formation for normal hemostasis. Another type of bleeding disorder due to defective action of TXA_2 has also been described [339,340]. In this case, the TXA_2 formation was essentially normal. However, the response of TXA_2 was impaired, possibly due to inability of TXA_2 to act as a calcium ionophore [cf. 341]. This type of platelet disorder is reminiscent of dog platelets where aggregation cannot be induced by arachidonic acid, endoperoxides or TXA_2, although formation of TXA_2 from arachidonic acid proceeds undisturbed [342].

9. Thromboxane formation in pathological conditions

There are numerous pathological conditions in which derangements in thromboxane biosynthesis are supposed to contribute to the development of the symptoms. The well-known effects of TXA_2, bronchoconstriction, vasoconstriction and induction of platelet aggregation, suggest the possible involvement of the compound in various pulmonary and cardiovascular events. The roles of thromboxanes in some respiratory diseases as well as in certain platelet disorders have already been discussed.

Thromboxane production has been detected in several inflammatory conditions; in inflamed joints such as urate arthritis [343] and rheumatoid arthritis [92]; in carageenin induced pleurisy [91]; and in burns [93,94,344]. The involvement of thromboxanes in burns has attracted particular attention. TXB_2 has been demonstrated both in burn blister fluid and in lymph from the scalded limb [93,344] as well as in burned tissue [94]; and the formation of the biologically active precursor, TXA_2, has been postulated as one factor responsible for the progressive dermal ischemia seen after burn injury, which may lead to extensive skin necrosis [94,344]. The effects of three inhibitors of thromboxane biosynthesis on dermal ischemia were studied [345]. All compounds were found to increase dermal perfusion after scalding injury compared to untreated animals, which supports the theory of the deleterious influence of TXA_2 upon dermal circulation in burned tissues.

The renal production of thromboxanes seems to be very low normally. In certain conditions, however, the capacity of the kidney for thromboxane biosynthesis increases greatly. Thus, ureteral obstruction led to the appearance of TXA_2 as well as of large amounts of PGE_2 in the venous effluent of the affected kidney [346,347]. This biosynthesis was demonstrated both in the cortex and the medulla. The interplay between the enhanced production of the vasodilatory PGE_2 and the vasoconstrictive TXA_2 was believed to be of importance for regulating the in vivo renal perfusion pressure in the hydronephrotic kidney.

Renal vein constriction for 1–2 days also markedly increased the biosynthesis of both TXA_2 and PGE_2 by the kidney [55]. Acute renal failure induced by glycerol in the rabbit also led to a pronounced TXA_2 production by the kidney [56].

However, most pathological conditions, believed to involve derangements in the thromboxane biosynthesis – or in the thromboxane/prostacyclin balance – concern the cardiovascular system. A large number of diseases affecting this organ system have been studied in this respect, i.e. atherosclerosis, myocardial infarction, coronary artery disease with angina of various etiologies, thrombotic disorders, hemostatic defects, circulatory shock, ulcerative diseases, and so on. The possible roles of thromboxane and prostacyclin in the cardiovascular system have been discussed in several reviews, e.g. refs. 32, 33, 348–354.

Atherosclerosis is a condition with a probably very complex etiology. Platelets are known to play important roles in the development of this disease [33,354–356]. Hyperaggregability of platelets is known to occur in this condition, not only in vivo – which may be partially explained by the damaged vascular endothelium having lost its protective PGI_2 production – but also in vitro [33,354,356]. Increased production of TXA_2 has been detected in platelets from patients with atherosclerosis [357,358].

When the coronary arteries are affected, intravascular platelet aggregation may not only aggravate the atherosclerosis with time [361]. The simultaneous release of the vasoconstrictive TXA_2 may also be one underlying cause for the transient attacks of chest pains in angina [12,26,28]. Several types of angina have been found to be associated with release of TXA_2 during attacks, such as pacing induced angina, effort angina and vasotonic or Prinzmetal's variant angina [166,362–367]. This release was found to be increased after heparin treatment [164,165]. Other factors must however also be involved; aspirin in a dose sufficiently high to abolish all thromboxane as well as prostacyclin biosynthesis actually aggravated the condition [368].

Related studies have shown an increased thromboxane and prostaglandin generation following myocardial infarction [369,370]. Animal studies further point to the possible role of TXA_2 in this disease: experimental heart attacks have been induced in rabbits by TXA_2 [371], and inhibition or antagonism of thromboxane was found to have a beneficial effect on ischemic myocardium [262,372].

Other conditions with an increased risk for arterial thrombosis may also be associated with hyperaggregability of the platelets and increased TXA_2 production, or at least an altered balance between pro- and anti-aggregatory arachidonate metabolites. This has for example been found in subjects taking oral contraceptives [169], and in diabetics, which was briefly discussed in the section on platelets and thromboxanes (see above). Many studies now indicate that platelets of diabetic patients as well as of diabetic experimental animals have an increased capacity for thromboxane biosynthesis; in some studies a decreased PGI_2 synthesis by vessel walls has been found as well [336–338,373–377].

The stimulatory effect of cholesterol on thromboxane formation in platelets was mentioned in the section on modulation of thromboxane biosynthesis. This effect has been found both in vitro [167] and in vivo [378]; in a study on patients with type IIa hypercholesterolemia a linear relationship was found between the serum cholesterol level and the capacity for TXB_2 production by the platelets [378]. The importance of these findings is obvious: many conditions with an increased tendency to thrombosis may also be associated with elevated serum cholesterol levels, such as atherosclerosis and diabetes.

Some of the profound hemodynamic changes seen in endotoxin induced shock, viz. pulmonary hypertension, platelet aggregation and systemic hypotension, have also been correlated with an increased thromboxane biosynthesis [379–384]. Mortality in endotoxic shock was significantly reduced following administration of the thromboxane synthetase inhibitors, imidazole and carboxyheptyl-imidazole, as well as of the thromboxane A_2 antagonist, 13-azaprostanoic acid [380,381]. However, the increased PGI_2 production associated with the systemic arterial hypotension is more likely the cause of the often fatal outcome of this event [384].

Certain ulcerative diseases may be caused by overproduction of the vasoconstrictive TXA_2 and/or underproduction of the vasodilatory PGI_2. The role of TXA_2 for tissue necrosis in burn injury was mentioned above; the possible involvement of TXA_2 production in atherosclerotic ulcerations is also obvious. The latter condition has sometimes been successfully treated with PGI_2 infusions [385,386]. Ulcerations in the gastric mucosa by TXA_2 have also been reported [31]: endogenous TXA_2 produced by platelets was postulated to be involved in the pathogenesis of certain ulcerative disorders of the stomach.

Finally, other pathological conditions believed to be associated with derangements in thromboxane formation, or an abnormal response to this compound, are for example uremia [387], leukemia [388,389], schizophrenia [390,391] and myeloproliferative disorders [392].

10. Alteration of thromboxane–prostacyclin balance in vivo: approaches in thrombosis prevention

The anti-platelet effects of acetylsalicyclic acid, both in vitro and in vivo, were recognized long before the biochemical details of arachidonic acid metabolism in platelets had been elucidated, and before the inhibitory effects of aspirin on cyclo-oxygenase were known (reviews, refs. 348–353). The drug had even been employed in large clinical trials as an anti-thrombotic agent, for example in attempts to prevent secondary myocardial infarction or stroke (for reviews, see e.g. refs.

393–397). In view of the prominent roles platelets are believed to play in such conditions, and the strong inhibitory effects of aspirin on crucial events in platelet function, the success of these trials was unexpectedly modest.

This lack of success seemed even more difficult to explain when the biochemical details behind the aspirin inhibition of platelet function were unravelled. Aspirin was found to irreversibly inhibit the cyclo-oxygenase by acetylation of a serine residue at the active site [398–400]. Since platelets lack a nucleus, they have very little capacity for de novo protein biosynthesis, and thus the inhibition of the cyclo-oxygenase lasts for the entire life span of the platelet, i.e. about 7–10 days [398], and the effects of aspirin are overcome only by the gradual replacement of these damaged cells by new ones. It seemed likely that the use of such an efficient drug should give more pronounced clinical results than was actually the case.

However, after the discovery of the antagonistic prostacyclin [349,350], formed in the vessel wall from the same precursor as thromboxane, an explanation for this discrepancy was obtained. Obviously, the biosynthesis of this anti-aggregatory vasodilating substance is also inhibited after ingestion of aspirin, and thus the net effect of such a treatment is negligible.

Recently, it has been postulated that even using the common inhibitor aspirin it should nonetheless be possible to interfere more or less selectively with the thromboxane biosynthesis by platelets. The inhibition of the vessel wall cyclo-oxygenase was found to be of shorter duration than that in platelets [401,402]; this is expected since the nucleated endothelial cells can rapidly synthesize new enzyme. Furthermore, it has been demonstrated that the platelet cyclo-oxygenase is much more sensitive to aspirin, requiring both lower concentration and shorter exposure to the drug for complete inhibition than does the vascular enzyme [403].

Thus it is possible that the reason for the apparent inefficiency of aspirin as an antithrombotic agent in the clinical trials was that the drug had been given in too high amounts and/or with too short intervals. In the abovementioned trials, doses of 1–1.5 g/day had generally been used: thus, also the protective PGI_2 biosynthesis had inadvertantly been kept suppressed continuously.

The hypothesis arose that it might be possible to employ aspirin as an efficient anti-thrombotic agent, if the drug was given in very low doses and/or with long intervals instead [348–353]. This hypothesis was based on data indicating that single high doses of aspirin had a paradoxical effect, i.e. actually shortened the bleeding time in man compared with lower doses [405,406], or had a thrombogenic effect in animals [407,408]. Conflicting data have however also been reported [409–411].

Amezcua et al. [404] studied the temporal changes in bleeding time during one week after a single high dose of aspirin. Initially, no change was seen, which reflected the simultaneous inhibition of vessel wall prostacyclin and platelet thromboxane biosynthesis. After 1–3 days, bleeding time was significantly prolonged: this was interpreted as due to the faster recovery of the endothelial cyclo-oxygenase. After one week the bleeding time was again normal. All the damaged platelets had then been replaced by new ones, and the balance between the prostacyclin and TXA_2 formation was reestablished.

After the different reactions of the platelet and the vessel wall cyclo-oxygenase became known, a very large number of studies on this phenomenon were carried out. Animal models have been employed in some of these studies (e.g. refs. 407, 708, 411–415) whereas others have been carried out in the human (e.g. refs. 404–406, 409, 410, 413, 416–420). The results of these studies are difficult to compare, since their designs as well as the measured parameters differ considerably. For example, aspirin was given in single doses in some studies, and daily or even several times daily in others. Its effects were measured after 2 h in some studies, or after 1 week in others, etc. Parameters monitored were bleeding time, platelet aggregation in response to various stimuli, PGI_2 biosynthesis by vessel biopsies, levels of TXB_2, malondialdehyde and 6-keto-$PGF_{1\alpha}$, and so on.

The human studies have generally been carried out with the aim of identifying the lowest possible aspirin dose or the best dose schedule for successful use of this drug in thrombosis prevention. This problem has been subject to considerable debate recently (e.g. refs. 421–424). The lowest daily dose suggested is 20 mg [399,425]; other investigators recommend 40 mg [426], about 80 mg [413,427] or 100 mg [428]; others consider 150–200 mg of aspirin a "low dose" [417,420]. Still others do not go below 300–400 mg in their studies: this may however be too high for a clear differential effect on thromboxane and prostacyclin biosynthesis (cf. refs. 418, 426). Some even draw the line between "low" and "high" doses of aspirin at 1 g of the drug. Judging from the extent of acetylation of the platelet cyclo-oxygenase, 20 mg (giving 60% inhibition [399]) or a slightly higher dose may well prove sufficient.

As a general criticism to many of these studies, one might point out the fact that there are large individual variations in the absorption and metabolism of aspirin. Despite this, the vast majority of studies have not included any attempts to measure the resulting acetylsalicylic acid concentrations in plasma after oral ingestion, or its rate of disappearance from the circulation after oral ingestion: the actual concentration that the platelets are exposed to, as well as the exposure time must be much more relevant than the given dose (cf. refs. 403, 429). Related to this problem is also the fact that different preparations of the drugs are metabolized differently: the "slow release preparations" carry a higher risk of hydrolysis of the active drug to its metabolite, salicyclic acid, before absorption. This break-down product not only does not inhibit the cyclo-oxygenase but in fact counteracts the normal inhibition by aspirin [430–435]. The actual preparation used was however reported only in a few of the studies. A minimum requirement at least is that the given dose of the drug had been related to the body weight of the subject taking it [413,418]; in most studies however only the absolute amounts of acetylsalicylic acid were reported.

Despite these uncertainties, there seems to be a general tendency in the reported studies to support the hypothesis that low doses of aspirin may be more effective in anti-thrombotic therapy than the conventional doses. As mentioned, the results of these studies vary somewhat in terms of definite recommendations of the lowest, clinically useful dose of the drug for prevention of thrombosis, possibly due to the factors discussed above. Perhaps an even better solution would be to use long intervals between doses: preferably the drug should not be given more often than

1–2 times/week (cf. refs. 416, 417). Several investigators have shown a 24–48 hrs delay after a single dose of aspirin before new, unacetylated platelets can be detected in the circulation [399,416,436,437]. This has been interpreted as caused by an effect of aspirin also on the megakaryocytes (cf. however ref. 438). If this is the case, it seems superfluous – or even harmful, due to the effect of this drug on PGI_2 biosynthesis – to give aspirin with intervals shorter than 48 h.

This area has however become even more complex by the abovementioned discovery that salicyclic acid, the major metabolite of aspirin in vivo, counteracts the inhibitory actions of aspirin [430–435]. Salicyclic acid has a much longer half-life in blood than its parent compound and may readily accumulate to plasma concentrations where this anti-inhibitory effect occurs. To complicate matters even further, it has recently been found in the rat that this anti-inhibitory or protective effect of salicyclic acid is considerably greater for the vascular cyclo-oxygenase than for the platelet enzyme [439].

Thus, in view of the complexity of the pharmacology of aspirin, and the fact that it acts on a step common to PGI_2 and TXA_2 biosynthesis, a better approach in anti-thrombotic therapy might be to employ inhibitors specific for the thromboxane synthetase. As has already been discussed in this chapter, a large number of such inhibitors have been found. The most promising of these are derivatives of imidazole [121,122], such as 1-*n*-butyl-imidazole [124] and 4-[2-(1H-imidazole-1-yl)ethoxy]benzoic acid hydrochloride (UK 37248) [131,132].

There are several advantages with the use of a selective thromboxane synthetase inhibitor in thrombosis prevention. First, PGI_2 biosynthesis is generally not inhibited at the doses necessary for thromboxane inhibition. Second, the biosynthesis of anti-aggregatory substances may actually increase when thromboxane synthesis is impaired: the endoperoxides which may accumulate when the further transformation into TXA_2 is blocked may instead be converted into antiaggregatory prostaglandins (mainly PGD_2 and PGI_2). This has been demonstrated in several studies in vivo as well as in vitro [131,132,440,441].

It should be mentioned that using this approach it may not necessarily be possible to detect any inhibition of platelet aggregation in vitro, particularly when working with washed platelet suspensions [442]. The final effects depend on the combined actions of the platelets, the vessel wall and the plasma; the accumulated endoperoxides are strongly proaggregatory in themselves and may thus mask even a total inhibition of the thromboxane biosynthesis, if platelets alone are studied.

Finally, the inhibition of thromboxane biosynthesis at a later step eliminates the risk of channelling arachidonic acid into the lipoxygenase pathways instead. It should be noted that many biologically active arachidonic acid metabolites have recently been detected, that are not formed via the common cyclo-oxygenase pathway initially, but originate in lipoxygenase catalyzed reactions instead. Some of these, the leukotrienes, are extremely potent compounds. Their formation is not inhibited by aspirin or related drugs: in fact cyclo-oxygenase inhibitors may stimulate their biosynthesis, presumably by directing released arachidonic acid into the lipoxygenase catalyzed pathways instead (see above, section on Thromboxanes and the lung). This may be a possibility that should be kept in mind whenever a cyclo-oxygenase inhibitor is considered.

Acknowledgement

Part of this review was supported by grants from the Swedish Medical Research Council, proj. no 03P-5804 and O3X-05170.

References

1 Samuelsson, B. (1965) J. Am. Chem. Soc. 87, 3011–3013.
2 Hamberg, M. and Samuelsson, B. (1966) J. Am. Chem. Soc. 88, 2349–2350.
3 Nugteren, D.H., Beerthuis, R.K. and van Dorp, D.A. (1966) Rec. Trav. Chim. Pays-Bas 85, 405–419.
4 Nugteren, D.H. (1972) Presented at the 15th Int. Conf. on the Biochemistry of Lipids, The Hague.
5 Hamberg, M. and Samuelsson, B. (1972) Presented at the Int. Conf. on Prostaglandins, Vienna.
6 Hamberg, M. and Samuelsson, B. (1973) Proc. Natl. Acad. Sci .USA 70, 899–903.
7 Hamberg, M., Svensson, J., Wakabayashi, T. and Samuelsson, B. (1974) Proc. Natl. Acad. Sci. USA 71, 345–349.
8 Nugteren, D.H. and Hazelhof, E. (1973) Biochim. Biophys. Acta 326, 448–461.
9 Abdel-Halim, M.S., Hamberg, M., Sjöquist, B. and Änggard, E. (1977) Prostaglandins 14, 633–643.
10 Hamberg, M. and Fredholm, B.B. (1976) Biochim. Biophys. Acta 431, 189–193.
11 Hamberg, M., Hedqvist, P., Strandberg, K., Svensson, J. and Samuelsson, B. (1975) Life Sci. 16, 451–462.
12 Svensson, J. and Hamberg, M. (1976) Prostaglandins 12, 943–950.
13 Malmsten, C., Hamberg, M., Svensson, J. and Samuelsson, B. (1975) Proc. Natl. Acad. Sci. USA 72, 1446–1450.
14 Piper, P.J. and Vane, J.R. (1969) Nature 223, 29–35.
15 Svensson, J., Hamberg, M. and Samuelsson, B. (1975) Acta Physiol. Scand. 94, 222–228.
16 Hamberg, M. and Samuelsson, B. (1974) Proc. Natl. Acad. Sci. USA 71, 3400–3404.
17 Nugteren, D.H. (1975) Biochim. Biophys. Acta 380, 299–307.
18 Hamberg, M., Svensson, J. and Samuelsson, B. (1974) Proc. Natl. Acad. Sci. USA 71, 3824-3828.
19 Hamberg, M., Svensson, J. and Samuelsson, B. (1975) Proc. Natl. Acad. Sci. USA 72, 2994–2998.
20 Svensson, J., Hamberg, M. and Samuelsson, B. (1976) Acta Physiol. Scand. 98, 285–294.
21 Svensson, J., Strandberg, K., Tuvemo, T. and Hamberg, M. (1977) Prostaglandins 14, 425–436.
22 Samuelsson, B., Hamberg, M., Roberts, L.J. II, and Oates, J.A. (1978) Prostaglandins 16, 857–860.
23 Nelson, N.A. (1974) J. Med. Chem. 17, 911–918.
24 Wang, H.H., Kulkarni, P.S. and Eakins, K.E. (1980) Eur. J. Pharmacol. 66, 31–41.
25 Tuvemo, T., Strandberg, K., Hamberg, M. and Samuelsson, B. (1976) Acta Physiol. Scand. 96, 145–149.
26 Ellis, E.F., Oelz, O., Roberts, L.J. II, Payne, N.A., Sweetman, B.J., Nies, A.S. and Oates, J.A. (1976) Science 193, 1135–1137.
27 Needleman, P., Kulkarni, P.S. and Raz, A. (1977) Science, 195, 409–412.
28 Terashita, Z., Fukkui, H., Nishikawa, K., Hirata, M. and Kikuchi, S. (1978) Eur. J. Pharmacol. 53, 49–56.
29 Bunting, S., Moncada, S. and Vane, J.R. (1976) Br. J. Pharmacol. 57, 462–463.
30 Moncada, S., Gryglewski, R., Bunting, S. and Vane, J.R. (1976) Nature 263, 663–665.
31 Whittle, B.J.R., Kauffman, G.L. and Moncada, S. (1981) Nature 292, 472–474.
32 Moncada, S. and Vane, J.R. (1979) Pharmacol. Rev. 30, 293–331.

33 Gryglewski, R.J., Dembinska-Kiec, A. and Korbut, R. (1978) Acta Biol. Med. Ger. 37, 715–723.
34 Coleman, R.A., Kennedy, I., Whalley, E.T. and White, S.K. (1981) Br. J. Pharmacol. 73, 222P.
35 Spagnuolo, P.J., Ellner, J.J., Hassid, A. and Dunn, M.J. (1980) J. Clin. Invest. 66, 406–414.
36 Hammarström, S. (1980) J. Biol. Chem. 255, 518–521.
37 Hammarström, S. (1980) Prostaglandins Med. 4, 297–302.
38 Needleman, P., Minkes, M.S. and Raz, A. (1976) Science 193, 163–165.
39 Needleman, P., Raz, A., Minkes, M.S., Ferrendelli, J.A. and Sprecher, H. (1979) Proc. Natl. Acad. Sci. USA 76, 944–948.
40 Friedman, L.S., Fitzpatrick, T.M., Bloom, M.F., Ramwell, P.W., Rose, J.C. and Kot, P.A. (1979) Circ. Res. 44, 748–751.
41 Kadowitz, P.J. and Hyman, A.L. (1980) J. Pharmacol. Exp. Ther. 213, 300–305.
42 Fitzpatrick, T.M., Friedman, L.S., Kot, P.A. and Ramwell, P.W. (1980) Br. J. Pharmacol. 70, 295–299.
43 Sirois, P., Borgeat, P. and Jeanson, A. (1981) J. Pharm. Pharmacol. 33, 466–468.
44 Kitchen, E.A., Boot, J.R. and Dawson, W. (1978) Prostaglandins 16, 239–244.
45 Hamberg, M. (1976) Biochim. Biophys. Acta 431, 651–654.
46 Tai, H. and Yuan, B. (1977) Fed. Proc. 36, 309.
47 Wlodawer, P and Hammarström, S. (1978) Biochem. Biophys. Res. Commun. 80, 525–532.
48 She, H.S., McNamara, D.B., Spannhake, E.W., Hyman, A.L. and Kadowitz, P.J. (1981) Prostaglandins 21, 531–541.
49 Sun, F.F., Chapman, J.P. and McGuire, J.C. (1977) Prostaglandins 14, 1055–1074.
50 Ahnfelt-Ronne, I. and Arrigoni-Martelli, E. (1979) Agents Actions, Suppl. 4, 110–119.
51 Al-Ubaidi, F. and Bakhle, Y.S. (1980) Eur. J. Pharmacol. 62, 89–96.
52 Zenser, T.V., Herman, C.A., Gorman, R.R. and Davis, B.B. (1977) Biochem. Biophys. Res. Commun. 79, 357–363.
53 Morrison, A.R., Nishikawa, K. and Needleman, P. (1977) Nature 27, 259–260.
54 Yarger, W.E., Schocken, D.D. and Harris, R.H. (1980) J. Clin. Invest. 65, 400–412.
55 Zipser, R., Myers, S. and Needleman, P. (1980) Circ. Res. 47, 231–237.
56 Benabe, J.E., Klahr, S., Hoffman, M.K. and Morrison, A.R. (1980) Prostaglandins 19, 333–347.
57 Morrison, A.R., Thornton, F., Blumberg, A. and Vaughan, E.D. (1981) Prostaglandins 21, 471–481.
58 Bolton, H.S., Chanderbhan, R., Bryant, R.W., Bailey, J.M., Weglicki, W.B. and Vahouny, G.V. (1980) J. Mol. Cell Cardiol. 12, 1287–1298.
59 Wolfe, L.S., Rostworoski, K. and Marion, J. (1976) Biochem. Biophys. Res. Commun. 70, 907–913.
60 Anhut, H., Jackisch, R. and Peskar, B.A. (1979) Pol. J. Pharmacol. Pharm. 31, 381–386.
61 Spagnuolo, C., Sautebin, L., Galli, G., Racagni, G., Galli, C., Mazzari, S. and Finesso, M. (1979) Prostaglandins 18, 53–61.
62 Steinhauer, H.B., Anhut, H and Hertting, G. (1979) Naunyn Schmiedeberg's Arch. Pharmacol. 310, 53–58.
63 Davidson, E.M., Doig, M.V., Ford-Hutchinson, A.W. and Smith, M.J. (1980) in Advances in Prostaglandin and Thromboxane Research (Samuelsson, B., Ramwell, P. and Paoletti, R., eds.) Vol. 8, pp. 1661–1663, Raven Press, New York.
64 Goldstein, I.M., Malmsten, C.L., Kindahl, H., Kaplan, H.B., Radmark, O., Samuelsson, B. and Weissman, G. (1978) J. Exp. Med. 148, 787–792.
65 Morley, J., Bray, M.A., Jones, R.W., Nugteren, D.H. and van Dorp, D.A. (1979) Prostaglandins 17, 729–746.
66 Murota, S.I., Kawamura, M. and Morita, I. (1978) Biochim. Biophys. Acta 528, 507–511.
67 Weidmann, M.J., Peskar, B.A., Wrogemann, K., Rietschel, E.T., Staudinger, H. and Fisher, H. (1978) FEBS Lett. 89, 136–140.
68 McGuire, J.C. and Sun, F.F. (1980) in Advances in Prostaglandin and Thromboxane Research (Samuelsson, B., Ramwell, P. and Paoletti, R. eds.) Vol. 8, pp. 1665–1667, Raven Press, New York.
69 Kennedy, M.S., Stobo, J.D. and Goldyne, M.E. (1980) Prostaglandins 20, 135–145.
70 Parker, C.W., Stenson, W.F., Huber, M.G. and Kelly, J.P. (1979) J. Immunol. 122, 1572–1577.
71 Ali, A.E., Barrett, J.C. and Eling, T.E. (1980) Prostaglandins 20, 667–688.

72 Bryant, R.W., Feinmark, S.J., Makheja, A.N. and Bailey, J.M. (1978) J. Biol. Chem. 253, 8134–8142.
73 Hopkins, N.K., Sun, F.F. and Gorman, R.R. (1978) Biochem. Biophys. Res. Commun. 85, 827–836.
74 Bhattacherjee, P., Kulkarni, P.S. and Eakins, K.E. (1979) Invest. Ophthamol, Vis. Sci. 18, 172–178.
75 Kass, M.A. and Holmberg, N.J. (1979) Invest. Ophthamol. Vis. Sci. 18, 166–171.
76 Kulkarni, P.S. and Eakins, K.E. (1977) Prostaglandins 14, 601–605.
77 Kulkarni, P.S. (1981) Exp. Eye Res. 32, 197–204.
78 Hagen, A.A., White, R.P. and Robertson, J.T. (1979) Stroke 10, 306–309.
79 Salzman, P.M., Salmon, J.A. and Moncada, S. (1980) J. Pharmacol. Exp. Ther. 215, 240–247.
80 Burch, R.M., Knapp, D.R. and Halushka, P.V. (1979) J. Pharmacol. Exp. Ther. 210, 344–348.
81 Burch, R.M., Knapp, D.R. and Halushka, P.V. (1980) in Advances in Prostaglandin and Thromboxane Research (Samuelsson, B., Ramwell, P. and Paoletti, R., eds.) Vol. 6, pp. 505–509, Raven Press, New York.
82 Burch, R.M. and Halushka, P.V. (1980) J. Clin. Invest. 66, 1251–1257.
83 Bisordi, J.E., Schlondorff, D. and Hays, R.M. (1980) J. Clin. Invest. 66, 1200–1210.
84 Ali, M., Zamecnik, J., Cerskus, A.L., Stoessl, A.J., Barnett, W.H. and McDonald, J.W.D. (1977) Prostaglandins 14, 819–827.
85 LeDuc, L.E. and Needleman, P. (1979) J. Pharmacol. Exp. Ther. 211, 181–188.
86 Ali, M. and McDonald, J.W.D. (1980) Prostaglandins 20, 245–254.
87 Liggins, G.C., Campus, G.A., Roberts, C.M. and Skinner, S.J. (1980) Prostaglandins 19, 461–477.
88 Williams, K.I. and Downing, I. (1977) Prostaglandins 14, 813–817.
89 Poyser, N.L. and Scott, F.M. (1980) J. Reprod. Fert. 60, 33–40.
90 Ölund, A., Kindahl, H., Oliw, E., Lindgren, J.Å. and Larsson, B. (1980) Prostaglandins 19, 791–803.
91 Katori, M., Harada, Y., Tanaka, K., Miyazaki, H., Ishibashi, M. and Yamashita, Y. (1980) in Advances in Prostaglandin and Thromboxane Research (Samuelsson, B., Ramwell, P. and Paoletti, R., eds.) Vol. 8, pp. 1733–1737, Raven Press, New York.
92 Blotman, F., Chaintreuil, J., Poubelle, P., Flandre, O., Crastes de Paulet, A. and Simon, L. (1980) in Advances in Prostaglandin and Thromboxane Research (Samuelsson, B., Ramwell, P. and Paoletti, R., eds.) Vol. 8, pp. 1705–1708, Raven Press, New York.
93 Jonsson, C.E., Granström, E. and Hamberg, M. (1979) Scand. J. Plast. Reconstr. Surg. 13, 45–47.
94 Heggers, J.P., Loy, G.L. Robson, M.C. and Del Beccaro, E.J. (1980) J. Surg. Res. 28, 110–117.
95 Hammarström, S. and Falardeau, P. (1977) Proc. Natl. Acad. Sci USA 74, 3691–3695.
96 Yoshimoto, T., Yamamoto, S., Okuma, M. and Hayaishi, O. (1977) J. Biol. Chem. 252, 5871–5874.
97 Dutilh, C.E., Haddeman, E., Jouvenaz, G.H., ten Hoor, F. and Nugteren, D.H. (1979) Lipids 14, 241–246.
98 Hall, E.R. and Tai, H.H. (1981) Biochim. Biophys. Acta 665, 498–503.
99 Tai, H.H. and Yuan, B. (1978) Biochim. Biophys. Acta 531, 286–294.
100 Diczfalusy, U. and Hammarström, S. (1979) FEBS Lett. 105, 291–295.
101 Sun, F.F. (1977) Biochem. Biophys. Res. Commun. 74, 1432–1440.
102 Diczfalusy, U., Falardeau, P. and Hammarström, S. (1977) FEBS Lett. 84, 271–274.
103 Raz, A., Aharony, D. and Kenig-Wakshal, R. (1977) Eur. J. Biochem. 86, 447–454.
104 Anderson, M.W., Crutchley, D.J., Tainer, B.E. and Eling, T.E. (1978) Prostaglandins 16, 563–570.
105 Falardeau, P., Hamberg, M. and Samuelsson, B. (1976) Biochim. Biophys. Acta 441, 193–200.
106 Diczfalusy, U. and Hammarström, S. (1980) Biochem. Biophys. Res. Commun. 94, 1417–1423.
107 Hamberg, M. (1980) Biochim. Biophys. Acta 618, 389–398.
108 Moncada, S., Needleman, P., Bunting, S. and Vane, J.R. (1976) Prostaglandins 12, 323–335.
109 Diczfalusy, U. and Hammarström, S. (1977) FEBS Lett. 82, 107–110.
110 Eakins, K.E. and Kulkarni, P.S. (1977) Br. J. Pharmacol. 60, 135–140.
111 Kulkarni, P.S. and Eakins, K.E. (1976) Prostaglandins 12, 465–469.
112 Eakins, K.E., Rajadhyaksha, V. and Schroer, R. (1976) Br. J. Pharmacol. 58, 333–339.
113 MacIntyre, D.E. and Cordinm, J.L. (1977) Thromb. Res. 11, 705–713.
114 Gryglewski, R.J. (1977) Naunyn-Schmiedeberg's Arch. Pharmacol. 297, S85–S88.
115 Gryglewski, R.J., Zmuda, A., Dembinska-Kiec, A. and Krecioch, E. (1977) Pharmacol. Res. Commun. 9, 109–116.

116 Gryglewski, R.J., Zmuda, A., Korbut, R., Krecioch, E. and Bieron, K. (1977) Nature 267, 627–628.
117 Prancan, A.V., Lefort, J., Chignard, M., Gerozissis, K., Dray, F. and Vargaftig, B.B. (1979) Eur. J. Pharmacol. 60, 287–297.
118 Tai, H.H., Tai, C.L. and Lee, N. (1979) Fed. Proc. 38, 407.
119 Cross, P.E., Dickinson, R.P., Parry, M.J. and Randall, M.J. (1981) Agents Actions 11, 274–280.
120 Heptinstall, S., Bevan, J., Cockbill, S.R., Hanley, S.P. and Parry, M.J. (1980) Thromb. Res. 20, 219–230.
121 Needleman, P., Raz, A., Ferrendelli, J.A. and Minkes, M. (1977) Proc. Natl. Acad. Sci. USA 74, 1716–1720.
122 Moncada, S., Bunting, S., Mullane, K., Thorogood, P., Vane, J.R., Raz, A. and Needleman, P. (1977) Prostaglandins 13, 611–618.
123 Nijkamp, F.P., Moncada, S., White, H.L. and Vane, J.R. (1977) Eur. J. Pharmacol. 44, 179–186.
124 Blackwell, G.J., Flower, R.J., Russell-Smith, N., Salmon, J.A., Thorogood, P.B. and Vane, J.R. (1978) Br. J. Pharmacol. 64, 435P.
125 Harris, D.N., Greenberg, R., Phillips, M.B., Osman Jr., G.H. and Antonaccio, M.J. (1980) in Advances in Prostaglandin and Thromboxane Research (Samuelsson, B., Ramwell, P. and Paoletti, R., eds.) Vol. 6, pp. 437–441, Raven Press, New York.
126 Ladd, N. and Lewis, G.P. (1980) Br. J. Pharmacol. 69, 3–5.
127 Tai, H.H. Yuan, B. (1978) Biochem. Biophys. Res. Commun. 80, 236–242.
128 Yoshimoto, T., Yamamoto, S. and Hayaishi, O. (1978) Prostaglandins 16, 529–540.
129 Allan, G. and Eakins, K.E. (1978) Prostaglandins 15, 659–661.
130 Allan, G., Eakins, K.E., Kulkarni, P.S. and Levi, R. (1980) Br. J. Pharmacol. 71, 157–164.
131 Tyler, H.M., Saxton, C.A.P.D. and Parry, M.J. (1981) Lancet i, 629–632.
132 Vermylen, J., Carreras, L.O., van Schaeren, J., Defreyn, G., Machin, S.J. and Verstraete, M. (1981) Lancet i, 1073–1075.
133 Tai, H.H., Lee, N., and Tai, C.L. (1980) in Advances in Prostaglandin and Thromboxane Research (Samuelsson, B., Ramwell, P. and Paoletti, R., eds.) Vol. 6, pp. 447–452, Raven Press, New York.
134 Tai, H.H., Tai, C.L. and Lee, N. (1980) Arch. Biochem. Biophys. 203, 758–763.
135 Miyamoto, T., Taniguchi, K., Tanouchi, T. and Hirata, F. (1980) in Advances in Prostaglandin and Thromboxane Research (Samuelsson, B., Ramwell, P. and Paoletti, R., eds.) Vol. 6, pp. 443–445, Raven Press, New York.
136 Vincent, J.E. and Zijlstra, F.J. (1978) Prostaglandins 15, 629–636.
137 Smith, J.B and Jubiz, W. (1981) Prostaglandins 22, 353–362.
138 Feuerstein, N. and Ramwell, P.W. (1981) Eur. J. Pharmacol. 69, 533–534.
139 Ally, A.I., Manku, M.S., Horrobin, D.F., Morgan, R.O., Karmazyn, M. and Karmali, R.A. (1977) Prostaglandins 14, 607–609.
140 Greenwald, J.E., Wong, L.K., Rao, M., Bianchine, J.R. and Panganamala, R.V. (1978) Biochem. Biophys. Res. Commun. 84, 1112–1118.
141 Greenwald, J.E., Wong, L.K., Alexander, M. and Bianchine, J.R. (1980) in Advances in Prostaglandin and Thromboxane Research (Samuelsson, B., Ramwell, P. and Paoletti, R., eds.) Vol. 6, pp. 293–295, Raven Press, New York.
142 Mills, D.C.B. and Smith, J.B. (1971) Biochem. J. 121, 185–196.
143 Bundy, G.L. (1975) Tetrahedron Lett. 24, 1957–1960.
144 Corey, E.J., Nicolaou, K.C., Machida, Y., Malmsten, C.L. and Samuelsson, B. (1975) Proc. Natl. Acad. Sci. USA 72, 3355–3358.
145 Fitzpatrick, F.A. and Gorman, R.R. (1978) Biochim. Biophys. Acta 539, 162–172.
146 Gorman, R.R., Bundy, G.L., Peterson, D.C., Sun, F.F., Miller, O.V. and Fitzpatrick, F.A. (1977) Proc. Natl. Acad. Sci. USA 74, 4007–4011.
147 Gorman, R.R., Fitzpatrick, F.A. and Miller, O.V. (1977) Biochem. Biophys. Res. Commun. 79, 305–313.
148 Kam, S., Portoghese, P.S., Gerrard, J.M. and Dunham, E.W. (1979) J. Med. Chem. 22, 1402–1408.
149 Kam, S., Portoghese, P.S., Dunham, E.W. and Gerrard, J.M. (1979) Prostaglandins Med. 3, 279–290.
150 Fitzpatrick, F., Gorman, R., Bundy, G., Honohan, T., McGuire, J. and Sun, F. (1979) Biochim. Biophys. Acta 573, 238–244.

151 Bundy, G.L. and Peterson, D.C. (1978) Tetrahedron Lett. 1, 41–44.
152 Fitzpatrick, F.A., Bundy, G.L., Gorman, R.R. and Honohan, T. (1978) Nature 275, 764–766.
153 Corey, E.J., Niwa, H., Bloom, M. and Ramwell, P.W. (1979) Tetrahedron Lett. 8, 671–674.
154 Gorman, R.R., Maxey, K.M. and Bundy, G.L. (1981) Biochem. Biophys. Res. Commun. 100, 184–190.
155 Nicolaou, K.C., Magolda, R.L. and Claremon, D.A. (1980) J. Am. Chem. Soc. 102, 1404–1409.
156 Nicolaou, K.C., Magolda, R.L., Smith, J.B., Aharony, D., Smith, E.F. and Lefer, A.M. (1979) Proc. Natl. Acad. Sci. USA 76, 2566–2570.
157 Yahn, D.M. and Feinstein, M.B. (1981) Prostaglandins 21, 243–254.
158 Gorman, R.R. (1980) in Advances in Prostaglandin and Thromboxane Research (Samuelsson, B., Ramwell, P. and Paoletti, R., eds.) Vol. 6, pp. 417–425, Raven Press, New York.
159 Gryglewski, R.J. (1978) Adv. Lipid Res. 16, 327–344.
160 Gryglewski, R.J. (1979) Agents Actions, Suppl. 4, 82–95.
161 Hammarström, S. and Diczfalusy, U. (1979) in Advances in Inflammation Research (Weissmann, G., Samuelsson, B. Paoletti, R., eds.) Vol. 1, pp. 431–438, Raven Press, New York.
162 Vane, J.R. (1978) in Advances in Prostaglandin and Thromboxane Research (Coceani, F. and Olley, P.M., eds.) Vol. 4, pp. 27–44, Raven Press, New York.
163 Anderson, W.H., Mohammad, S.F., Chuang, H.Y. and Mason, R.G. (1980) in Advances in Prostaglandin and Thromboxane Research (Samuelsson, B., Ramwell, P. and Paoletti, R., eds.) Vol. 6, pp. 287–295, Raven Press, New York.
164 Lewy, R.I., Wiener, L., Smith, J.B., Walinsky, P. and Silver, M.J. (1979) Lancet i, 97.
165 Lewy, R.I. (1980) Haemostasis 9, 134–140.
166 Lewy, R.I., Smith, J.B., Silver, M.J., Saia, J., Walinsky, P. and Wiener, L. (1979) Prostaglandins Med. 5, 243–248.
167 Stuart, M.J., Gerrard, J.M. and White, J.G. (1980) New Engl. J. Med. 302, 6–10.
168 Knapp, H.R., Oelz, O., Roberts, L.J.II., Sweetman, B.J., Oates, J.A. and Reed, P.W. (1977) Proc. Natl. Acad. Sci. USA 74, 4251–4255.
169 Schorer, A.E., Gerrard, J.M., White, J.G. and Krivit, W. (1978) Prostaglandins Med. 1, 5–11.
170 Dyerberg, J. and Bang, H.O. (1979) Lancet i, 433–435.
171 Dyerberg, J., Bang, H.O., Stoffersen, E., Moncada, S. and Vane, R. (1978) Lancet ii, 117–119.
172 Silver, M.J., Smith, J.B., Ingerman, C. and Kocsis, J.J. (1973) Prostaglandins 4, 863–875.
173 Culp, B.R., Lands, W.E.M., Lucchesi, B.R., Pitt, B. and Romson, J. (1980) Prostaglandins 20, 1021–1031.
174 Black, K.L., Culp, B., Madison, D., Randall, O.S. and Lands, W.E.M. (1979) Prostaglandins Med. 3, 257–268.
175 Siess, W., Roth, P., Scherer, B., Kurzmann, I., Böhlig, B. and Weber, P.C. (1980) Lancet i, 441–444.
176 Sanders, T.A.B., Vickers, M. and Haines, A.P. (1981) Clinical Sci. 61, 317–324.
177 Needleman, P., Whitaker, M.O., Wyche, A., Watters, K., Sprecher, H. and Raz, A. (1980) Prostaglandins 19, 165–181.
178 Kernoff, P.B.A., Willis, A.L., Stone, K.J., Davies, J.A. and McNicol, G.P. (1977) Br. Med. J. 2, 1441–1444.
179 Sim, A.K. and McCraw, A.P. (1977) Thrombosis Res. 10, 385–397.
180 Bergström, S., Danielsson, H. and Samuelsson, B. (1964) Biochim. Biophys. Acta 90, 207–210.
181 van Dorp, D.A., Beerthuis, R.K., Nugteren, D.H. and Vonkeman, H. (1964) Biochim. Biophys. Acta 90, 204–207.
182 Kloeze, J. (1967) in Nobel Symposium 2, Prostaglandins (Bergström, S. and Samuelsson, B., eds.) pp. 241–252, Almqvist and Wiksell, Stockholm.
183 Bordia, A. (1978) Atherosclerosis 30, 353–360.
184 Makheja, A.N., Vanderhoek, J.Y. and Bailey, J.M. (1979) Prostaglandins Med. 2, 413–414.
185 Makheja, A.N., Vanderhoek, J.Y., Bryant, R.W. and Bailey, J.M. (1980) in Advances in Prostaglandin and Thromboxane Research (Samuelsson, B., Ramwell, P. and Paoletti, R., eds.) Vol. 6, pp. 309–312, Raven Press, New York.
186 Vanderhoek, J.Y., Makheja, A.N. and Bailey, J.M.. (1980) Biochem. Pharmacol. 29, 3169–3173.

187 Shimamoto, T., Kobayashi, M., Takanashi, T., Takashima, Y., Sakamoto, M. and Morooka, S. (1978) Jpn Heart J. 19, 748–753.
188 Kindahl, H. (1977) Prostaglandins 13, 619–629.
189 Roberts, L.J.II, Sweetman, B.J., Morgan, J., Payne, N. and Oates, J.A. (1977) Prostaglandins 13, 631–647.
190 Roberts, L.J.II, Sweetman, B.J. and Oates, J.A. (1978) J. Biol. Chem. 253, 5305–5318.
191 Roberts, L.J.II, Sweetman, B.J., Payne, N. and Oates, J.A. (1977) J. Biol. Chem. 252, 7415–7417.
192 Svensson, J. (1979) Prostaglandins 17, 351–365.
193 Pace-Asciak, C.R. and Edwards, N. (1980) Biochem. Biophys. Res. Commun. 97, 81–86.
194 Oates, J.A., Roberts, L.J.II, Sweetman, B.J., Maas, R.N., Gerkens, J.F. and Taber, D.F. (1980) in Advances in Prostaglandin and Thromboxane Research (Samuelsson, B., Ramwell, P. and Paoletti, R., eds.) Vol. 6, pp. 35–41, Raven Press, New York.
195 Roberts, L.J.II, Sweetman, B.J. and Oates, J.A. (1981) J. Biol. Chem. 256, 8384–8393.
196 Hamberg, M., Svensson, J., Hedqvist, P., Strandberg, K. and Samuelsson, B. (1976) in Advances in Prostaglandin and Thromboxane Research (Samuelsson, B. and Paoletti, R., eds.) Vol. 1, pp. 495–501, Raven Press, New York.
197 Dawson, W., Boot, J., Cockerill, A., Mallen, D. and Osborne, D. (1976) Nature 262, 699–702.
198 Boot, J., Dawson, W., Cockerill, A., Mallen, D. and Osborne, D. (1977) Prostaglandins 13, 927–932.
199 Boot, J., Cockerill, A., Dawson, W., Mallen, D. and Osborne, D. (1978) Int. Arch. Allergy Appl. Immunol. 57, 159–164.
200 Mallen, D.N., Osborne, D.J., Cockerill, A.F., Boot, J.R. and Dawson, W. (1978) Biomed. Mass Spectrometry 5, 449–452.
201 Anhut, H., Peskar, B.A. and Bernauer, W. (1978) Naunyn Schiedeberg's Arch. Pharmacol. 305, 247–252.
202 Peskar, B.A. and Holland, A. (1979) Agents Action Suppl. 6, 51–56.
203 Fitzpatrick, F.A. and Gorman, R.R. (1977) Prostaglandins 14, 881–889.
204 Maclouf, J., Kindahl, H., Granström, E. and Samuelsson, B. (1980) in Advances in Prostaglandin and Thromboxane Research (Samuelsson, B., Ramwell, P. and Paoletti, R., eds.) Vol. 6, pp. 283–286, Raven Press, New York.
205 Maclouf, J., Kindahl, H., Granström, E. and Samuelsson, B. (1980) Eur. J. Biochem. 109, 561–566.
206 Smith, J.B., Ingerman, C. and Silver, M. (1976) J. Clin. Invest. 58, 1119–1122.
207 Folco, G.C., Granström, E. and Kindahl, H. (1977) FEBS Lett. 82, 321–325.
208 Granström, E. and Samuelsson, B. (1978) in Advances in Prostaglandin and Thromboxane Research (Frölich, J.C., ed.) Vol. 5, pp. 1–13, Raven Press, New York.
209 Green, K., Hamberg, M., Samuelsson, B. and Frölich, J.C. (1978) in Advances in Prostaglandin and Thromboxane Research (Frölich, J.C., ed.) Vol. 5, pp. 15–37, Raven Press, New York.
210 Green, K., Hamberg, M., Samuelsson, B., Smigel, M. and Frölich, J.C. (1978) in Advances in Prostaglandin and Thromboxane Research (Frölich, J.C., ed.) Vol. 5, pp. 39–94, Raven Press, New York.
211 Granström, E. and Kindahl, H. (1978) in Advances in Prostaglandin and Thromboxane Research (Frölich, J.C., ed.) Vol. 5, pp. 119–210, Raven Press, New York.
212 Moncada, S., Ferreira, S.H. and Vane, J.R. (1978) in Advances in Prostaglandin and Thromboxane Research (Frölich, J.C., ed.) Vol. 5, pp. 211–236, Raven Press, New York.
213 Granström, (1980) in Advances in Prostaglandin and Thromboxane Research (Samuelsson, B., Paoletti, R. and Ramwell, P., eds.) Vol. 6, pp. 69–76, Raven Press, New York.
214 Granström, E. (1980) in The Prostaglandin System (Berti, F. and Velo, G.P., eds.) pp. 67–72, Plenum Press, New York.
215 Gryglewski, R.J. (1980) in The Prostaglandin System. (Berti, F., and Velo, G.P., eds.) pp. 73–84, Plenum Press, New York.
216 Ho, P.P.K., Walters, P. and Sullivan, H.R. (1976) Prostaglandins 12, 951–971.
217 Sors, H., Pradelles, P., Dray, F., Rigaud, M., Maclouf, J. and Bernard, P. (1978) Prostaglandins 16, 277–290.

218 Vincent, J.E., Zijlstra, F.J. and Van Vliet, H. (1980) Prostaglandins Med. 5, 79–84.
219 Hemker, D.P. and Aiken, J.W. (1979) Prostaglandins 17, 239–248.
220 Dusting, G.J., Moncada, S. and Vane, J.R. (1977) Prostaglandins 13, 3–15.
221 Omini, C., Moncada, S. and Vane, J.R. (1977) Prostaglandins 14, 625–632.
222 Granström, E., Kindahl, H. and Samuelsson, B. (1976) Prostaglandins 12, 929–941.
223 Folco, G.C., Hansson, G. and Granström, E. (1981) Biochem. Pharmacol. 30, 2491–2493.
224 Ali, M., Cerskus, A.L., Zamecnik, J. and McDonald, J.W.D. (1977) Thrombosis Res. 11, 485–496 (1977).
225 Fitzpatrick, F.A., Gorman, R.R. and Wynalda, M.A. (1977) Prostaglandins 13, 201–209.
226 Turk, J., Weiss, S.J., Davis, J.E. and Needleman, P. (1978) Prostaglandins 16, 291–309.
227 Granström, E., Kindahl, H. and Samuelsson, B. (1976) Anal. Lett. 9, 611–627.
228 Fitzpatrick, F.A., Gorman, R.R., McGuire, J.C., Kelly, R.C., Wynalda, M.A. and Sun, F.F. (1977) Anal. Biochem. 82, 1–7.
229 Anhut, H., Bernauer, W. and Peskar, B.A. (1977) Eur. J. Pharmacol. 44, 85–88.
230 Tai, H.H. Yuan, B. (1978) Anal. Biochem. 87, 343–349.
231 Koh, H., Inoue, A., Mashimo, N., Numano, F. and Maezawa, H. (1980) Thrombosis Res. 17, 403–413.
232 Patrono, C., Ciabattoni, G., Pugliese, F., Pinca, E., Castrucci, G., De Salvo, A., Satta, M.A., Parachini, M. (1980) in Advances in Prostaglandin and Thromboxane Research (Samuelsson, B., Paoletti, R. and Ramwell, P., eds.) Vol. 6, pp. 187–191, Raven Press, New York.
233 Malmsten, C. (1976) Life Sci. 18, 169–176.
234 Coleman, R.A., Humphrey, P.P.A., Kennedy, I., Lewy, G.P. and Lumley, P. (1980) Br. J. Pharmacol. 68, 127P–128P.
235 Corey, E.J., Narasaka, K. and Shibasaki, M. (1976) J. Am. Chem. Soc. 98, 6417–6418.
236 Corey, E.J., Shibasaki, M., Nicolaou, K.C., Malmsten, C.L. and Samuelsson, B. (1976) Tetrahedron Lett. 10, 737–740.
237 Shimomura, H., Sugie, A., Katsube, J. and Yamamoto, H. (1976) Tetrahedron Lett. 45, 4099–4102.
238 Miyake, H., Iguchi, S., Itoh, H. and Hayashi, M. (1977) J. Am. Chem. Soc. 99, 3536–3537.
239 Okuma, M., Yoshimoto, T. and Yamamoto, S. (1977) Prostaglandins 14, 891–896.
240 Hall, D.W.R., Funcke, A.B.H. and Jaitly, K.D. (1979) Prostaglandins 18, 317–330.
241 Harris, D.N., Phillips, M.B., Michel, I.M., Goldenberg, H.J., Heikes, J.E., Sprague, P.W. and Antonaccio, M.J. (1981) Prostaglandins 22, 295–307.
242 Jones, R.L. and Marr, C.G. (1977) Br. J. Pharmacol. 61, 694–696.
243 Jones, R.L. and Wilson, N.H. (1980) in Advances in Prostaglandin and Thromboxane Research (Samuelsson, B., Ramwell, P. and Paoletti, R., eds.) Vol. 6, pp. 467–475, Raven Press, New York.
244 Jones, R.L. and Wilson, N.H. (1978) Br. J. Pharmacol. 63, 362P.
245 Ohuchida, S., Hamanaka, N. and Hayashi, M. (1979) Tetrahedron Lett. 38, 3661–3664.
246 Lefer, A.M., Smith III, E.F., Araki, H., Smith, J.B., Aharony, D., Claremon, D.A., Magolda, R.L. and Nicolaou, K.C. (1980) Proc. Natl. Acad. Sci. USA 77, 1706–1710.
247 Ansell, M.F., Caton, M.P.L. and Mason, J.S. (1981) Tetrahedron Lett. 22, 1141–1142.
248 Kosuge, S., Hamanaka, N. and Hayashi, M. (1981) Tetrahedron Lett. 22, 1345–1348.
249 Ohuchuda, S., Hamanaka, N. and Hayashi, M. (1981) Tetrahedron Lett. 22, 1349–1352.
250 Ohuchida, S., Hamanka, N. and Hayashi, M. (1981) J. Am. Chem. Soc. 103, 4597–4599.
251 Kam, S. and Portoghese, P.S. (1979) Prostaglandins Med. 3, 279–290.
252 Le Breton, G.C., Venton, D.L., Enke, S.E. and Halushka, P.V. (1979) Proc. Natl. Acad. Sci. USA, 76, 4097–4101.
253 Le Breton, G.C. and Venton, D.L. (1980) in Advances in Prostaglandin and Thromboxane Research (Samuelsson, B., Ramwell, P. and Paoletti, R., eds.) Vol. 6, pp. 497–503, Raven Press, New York.
254 Coleman, R.A., Humphrey, P.P.A., Kennedy, I., Levy, G.P. and Lumley, P. (1980) Br. J. Pharmacol. 73, 258P.
255 Coleman, R.A., Collington, E.W., Geisow, H.P., Hornby, E.J., Humphrey, P.P.A. Kennedy, I., Levy, G.P., Lumley, P., McCabe, P.J. and Wallis, C.J. (1981) Br. J. Pharmacol. 72, 524P–525P.
256 Geisow, H.P., Hornby, E.J and McCabe, P.J. (1981) Br. J. Pharmacol. 73, 219P–220P.

257 Ansell, M.F., Caton, M.P.L., Palfreyman, M.N., Stuttle, K.A.J., Tuffin, D. and Walker, J.L. (1980) in Advances in Prostaglandin and Thromboxane Research (Samuelsson, B., Ramwell, P. and Paoletti, R., eds.) Vol. 6, pp. 485–487, Raven Press, New York.
258 Ansell, M.F., Caton, M.P.L., Palfreyman, M.N. and Stuttle, K.A.J. (1979) Tetrahedron Lett. 46, 4497–4498.
259 Maxey, K.M. and Bundy, G.L. (1980) Tetrahedron Lett. 21, 445–448.
260 Corey, E.J., Ponder, J.W. and Ulrich, P. (1980) Tetrahedron Lett. 21, 137–140.
261 Aharony, D., Smith, J.B., Smith, E.F., Lefer, A.M., Magolda, R.L. and Nicolaou, K.C. (1980) in Advances in Prostaglandin and Thromboxane Research (Samuelsson, B., Ramwell, P. and Paoletti, R., eds.) Vol. 6, pp. 489–492, Raven Press, New York.
262 Nicolaou, K.C., Magolda, R.L. and Claremon, D.A. (1980) in Advances in Prostaglandin and Thromboxane Research (Samuelsson, R., Ramwell, P. and Paoletti, R., eds.) Vol. 6, pp. 481–483, Raven Press, New York.
263 Schrör, K., Smith, E.F. III, Bickerton, M., Smith, J.B., Nicolaou, K.C. Magolda, R. and Lefer, A.M. (1980) Am. J. Physiol. 238, H87–H92.
264 Lefer, A.M., Araki, H., Smith, J.B., Nicolaou, K.C. and Magolda, R.L. (1979) Prostaglandins Med. 3, 139–146.
265 Jones, R.L. and Wilson, N.H. (1981) Br. J. Pharmacol. 73, 220P–221P.
266 Sprague, P.W., Heikes, J.E., Harris, D.N. and Greenberg, R. (1980) in Advances in Prostaglandin and Thromboxane Research (Samuelsson, B., Ramwell, P. and Paoletti, R., eds.) Vol. 6, pp. 493–496, Raven Press, New York.
267 Ally, A.I., Horrobin, D.F., Manku, M.S., Morgan, R.O., Karmazyn, M., Karmali, R.A. and Cunnane, S.C. (1978) Can. J. Physiol. Pharmacol. 56, 520–523.
268 Shimamoto, T., Takashima, Y., Kobayashi, M., Moriya, K. and Takahashi, T. (1976) Proc. Japan Acad. 52, 591–594.
269 Harada, Y., Tanaka, K. and Katori, M. (1979) Prostaglandins 17, 957–966.
270 Hamberg, M. and Samuelsson, B. (1974) Biochem. Biophys. Res. Commun. 61, 942–949.
271 Powell, W.S. and Solomon, S. (1978) Prostaglandins 15, 351–364.
272 Powell, W.S. and Solomon, S. (1978) in Advances in Prostaglandin and Thromboxane Research (Coceani, F. and Olley, P.M., eds.) Vol. 4, pp. 61–74, Raven Press, New York.
273 Tai, H.-H., Yuan, B. and Wu, A.T. (1978) Biochem. J. 170, 441–444.
274 Alabaster, V.A. (1980) Br. J. Pharmacol. 69, 479–489.
275 Sun, F.F. and McGuire, J.C. (1978) in Advances in Prostaglandin and Thromboxane Research (Coceani, F. and Olley, P.M., eds.) Vol. 4, pp. 75–85, Raven Press, New York.
276 Hamberg, M., Hedqvist, P. and Radegran, K. (1980) Acta Physiol. Scand. 110, 219–221.
277 Crutchley, D.J., Boyd, J.A. and Eling, T.E. (1980) in Advances in Prostaglandin and Thromboxane Research (Samuelsson, B., Ramwell, P. and Paoletti, R., eds.) Vol. 8, pp. 1751–1753, Raven Press, New York.
278 Crutchley, D.J., Boyd, J.A. and Eling, T.E. (1980) Am. Rev. Respir. Dis. 121, 695–699.
279 Engineer, D.M., Morris, H.R., Piper, P.J. and Sirois, P. (1978) Br. J. Pharmacol. 64, 211–218.
280 Gryglewski, R.J., Dembinska-Kiec, A. and Grodzinska, L. (1977) in Prostaglandins and Thromboxanes (Berti, F., Samuelsson, B. and Velo, G.P., eds.) pp. 165–178, Plenum Press, New York.
281 Palmer, M.A., Piper, P.J. and Vane, J.R. (1973) Br. J. Pharmacol. 49, 226–242.
282 Berti, F., Folco, G., Nicosia, S., Omini, C. and Pasargiklian, R. (1979) Br. J. Pharmacol. 65, 629–633.
283 Berti, F., Folco, G., Giachetti, A., Malandrino, S., Omini, C. and Vigano, T. (1980) Br. J. Pharmacol. 68, 467–472.
284 Folco, G., Omini, C., Vigano, T., Iantorno, G. and Berti, F. (1980) in Advances in Prostaglandin and Thromboxane Research (Samuelsson, B., Ramwell, P. and Paoletti, R., eds.) Vol. 7, pp. 917–923, Raven Press, New York.
285 Engineer, D.M., Niederhauser, U., Piper, P.J. and Sirois, P. (1978) Br. J. Pharmacol. 62, 61–66.
286 Rossoni, G., Omini, C., Vigano, T., Mandelli, V., Folco, G. and Berti, F. (1980) Prostaglandins 20, 547–557.
287 Samuelsson, B., Hammarström, S., Murphy, R.C. and Borgeat, P. (1980) Allergy 35, 375–381.

288 Samuelsson, B., Borgeat, P., Hammarström, S. and Murphy, R.C. (1980) in Advances in Prostaglandin and Thromboxane Research (Samuelsson, B., Ramwell, P. and Paoletti, R., eds.) Vol. 6, pp. 1–18, Raven Press, New York.
289 Örning, L., Hammarström, S. and Samuelsson, B. (1980) Proc. Natl. Acad. Sci. USA 77, 2014–2017.
290 Lewis, R.A., Austen, K.F., Drazen, J.M., Clark, D.A., Marfat, A. and Corey, E.J. (1980) Proc. Natl. Acad. Sci. USA 77, 3710–3714.
291 Morris, H.R., Taylor, G.W., Piper, P.J., Samhoun, M.N. and Tippins, J.R. (1980) Prostaglandins 19, 185–201.
292 Lewis, R.A., Drazen, J.M., Austen, K.F., Clark, D.A. and Corey, E.J. (1980) Biochem. Biophys. Res. Commun. 96, 271–277.
293 Folco, G.C., Omino, C., Vigano, T., Brunelli, G., Rossoni, G. and Berti, F. (1982) Adv. Prostaglandin Thromboxane Leukotriene Res. (Samuelsson, B. and Paoletti, R., eds.) vol. 9, pp. 153–167, Raven Press, New York.
294 Piper, P.J. and Samhoun, M.N. (1982) Br. J. Pharmacol. 77, 267–275.
295 Dahlén, S.-E., Hedqvist, P., Westlund, P., Granström, E., Hammarström, S., Lindgren, J.-Å. and Rådmark, O. (1983) Acta Physiol. Scand. 118, 393–403.
296 Weichman, B.M., Muccitelli, R.M., Osborn, R.R., Holden, D.A., Gleason, J.G. and Wasserman, M.A. (1982) J. Pharmacol. Exp. Ther. 222, 202–208.
297 Hamel, R., Masson, P., Ford-Hutchinson, A.W., Jones, T.R., Brunet, G. and Piechuta, H. (1982). Prostaglandins 24, 419–432.
298 Dahlén, S.-E. (1983) Acta Physiol. Scand. 118, 415–421.
299 Hedqvist, P. and Dahlén, S.-E. (1983) Adv. Prostaglandin Thromboxane Leukotriene Res. (Samuelsson, B., Ramwell, P.W. and Paoletti, R., eds.) vol. 11, pp. 27–32, Raven Press, New York.
300 Yen, S.S., Mathé, A.A. and Dugan, J.J. (1976) Prostaglandins 11, 227–239.
301 Tauber, A.I., Kaliner, M., Stechschulte, D.J. and Austen, K.F. (1973) J. Immunol. 111, 27–32.
302 Boot, J.R., Brockwell, A.D.J. Dawson, W. and Sweatman, W.J.F. (1977) Br. J. Pharmacol. 59, 444P–445P.
303 Boura, A.L.A. and Murphy, R.D. (1978) Clin. Exp. Pharmacol. Physiol. 5, 387–392.
304 Friedman, L.S., Fitzpatrick, T.M., Ramwell, P.W. and Kot, P.A. (1980) in Advances in Prostaglandin and Thromboxane Research (Samuelsson, B., Ramwell, P. and Paoletti, R., eds.) Vol. 7, pp. 981–983, Raven Press, New York.
305 Lichtenstein, L.M. (1977) in Asthma, Physiology, Immunopharmacology, and Treatment (Lichtenstein, L.M. and Austen, K.F., eds.) pp. 93–110, Academic Press, New York.
306 Hedqvist, P. and Mathé, A. (1977) in Asthma, Physiology, Immunopharmacology, and Treatment (Lichtenstein, L.M. and Austen, K.F., eds.) pp. 131–146, Academic Press, New York.
307 Mathé, A.A., Hedqvist, P., Holmgren, A. and Svanborg, N. (1973) Br. Med. J. 1, 193–196.
308 Svanborg, N., Hamberg, M. and Hedqvist, P. (1973) Acta Physiol. Scand. 89, Suppl. 396, 101.
309 Gréen, K., Hedqvist, P. and Svanborg, N. (1974) Lancet ii, 1419–1421.
310 Svanborg, N., Hedqvist, P. and Gréen, K. (1976) in Advances in Prostaglandin and Thromboxane Research (Samuelsson, B. and Paoletti, R., eds.) Vol. 1, pp. 439–447, Raven Press, New York.
311 Morris, H.G., Sherman, N.A., Shepperdson, F.T. and Selner, J.C. (1980) in Advances in Prostaglandin and Thromboxane Research (Samuelsson, B., Ramwell, P. and Paoletti, R., eds.) Vol. 8, pp. 1759–1764, Raven Press, New York.
312 Smith, A.P. and Cuthbert, M.F. (1976) in Advances in Prostaglandin and Thromboxane Research (Samuelsson, B. and Paoletti, R., eds.) Vol. 1, pp. 449–459, Raven Press, New York.
313 Gryglewski, R.J., Szczeklik, A. and Nizankowska, E. (1977) in Prostaglandins and Thromboxanes (Berti, F., Samuelsson, B. and Velo, G.P., eds.) pp. 191–203, Plenum Press, New York.
314 Parker, C.W. (1977) in Asthma, Physiology, Immunopharmacology, and Treatment (Lichtenstein, L.M. and Austen, K.F., eds.) pp. 301–313, Academic Press, New York.
315 Szczeklik, A., Gryglewski, R.J., Czerniawska-Mysik, G. and Nizankowska, E. (1980) in Advances in Prostaglandin and Thromboxane Research (Samuelsson, B., Ramwell, P. and Paoletti, R., eds.) Vol. 7, pp. 993–994, Raven Press, New York.
316 Dahlén, S.E., Hedqvist, P., Hammarström, S. and Samuelsson, B. (1980) Nature 288, 484–486.

317 Hedqvist, P., Dahlén, S.E., Gustafsson, L., Hammarström, S. and Samuelsson, B. (1980) Acta Physiol. Scand. 110, 331–333.
318 Morris, H.R., Piper, P.J., Taylor, G.W. and Tippins, J.R. (1980) Prostaglandins 19, 371–383.
319 Smith, J.B. and Willis, A.L. (1971) Nature 231, 235–237.
320 Claesson, H.-E. and Malmsten, C. (1977) Eur. J. Biochem. 76, 277–284.
321 Born, G.V.R. (1962) Nature 194, 927–929.
322 Bone, E.A., Best, L.C., Jones, P..B., Holland, T.K. and Russell, R.G. (1980) Biochem. Soc. Trans. 8, 530–531.
323 Malmgren, R., Olsson, P., Thornling, G. and Unge, G. (1980) Thromb. Res. 18, 733–741.
324 Malmgren, R., Åsberg, M., Olsson, P., Thornling, G. and Unge, G. (1981) Life Sci. 29, 2649–2658.
325 Kinlough-Rathbone, R.L., Reimers, H.J., Mustard, J.F. and Packham, M.A. (1976) Science 192, 1011–1012.
326 Meyers, K.M., Seachard, C.L., Holmsen, H., Smith, J.B. and Prieur, D.J. (1979) Nature 282, 331–333.
327 Salzman, E.W. (1979) Biochim. Biophys. Acta 449, 48–60.
328 Minkes, M., Stanford, N., Maggie, M.Y., Roth, G.J., Raz, A., Needleman, P. and Majerus, P.W. (1977) J. Clin. Invest. 59, 449–454.
329 Hamberg, M. and Hamberg, G. (1980) Biochem. Biophys. Res. Commun. 95, 1090–1097.
330 Bell, R.L., Kennerly, D.A., Stanford, N. and Majerus, P.W. (1979) Proc. Natl. Acad. Sci. USA 76, 3238–3241.
331 Rittenhouse-Simmons, S. (1980) J. Biol. Chem. 255, 2259–2262.
332 Michell, R.H. (1975) Biochim. Biophys. Acta 415, 81–147.
333 Michell, R.H. (1979) Trends Biochem. Sci. 4, 128–131.
334 Steer, M.L., MacIntyre, D.E., Levine, L. and Salzman, E.W. (1980) Nature 283, 194–195.
335 Pareti, F.I., Mannucci, P.M., D'Angelo, A., Smith, J.B., Sautebin, L. and Galli, G. (1980) Lancet i, 898–901.
336 Gerrard, J.M., Stuart, M.J., Rao, G.H., Steffes, M.W. Mauer, S.M., Brown, D.M. and White, J.G. (1980) J. Lab. Clin. Med. 95, 950–958.
337 Butkus, A., Skrinska, V.A. and Schumacher, O.P. (1980) Thromb. Res. 19, 211–223.
338 Halushka, P.V., Rogers, R.C., Loadhult, C.B. and Colwell, J.A. (1981) J. Lab. Clin. Med. 97, 87–96.
339 Lages, B., Malmsten, C., Weiss, H.J. and Samuelsson, B. (1981) Blood 57, 545–552.
340 Samama, M., Lecrubier, C., Conard, J., Hotchen, M., Berton-Gorius, J., Vargaftig, B., Chignard, M., Lagarde, M. and Dechavanne, M. (1981) Br. J. Haematol. 48, 293–303.
341 Gerrard, J.M., Townsend, D.W., Stoddard, S., Witkop, C.J. Jr. and White, J.C. (1977) Am. J. Pathol. 86, 99–115.
342 Chignard, M. and Vargaftig, B. (1976) Eur. J. Pharmacol. 38, 7–18.
343 Peskar, B.A., Glatt, M., Anhut, H. and Brune, K. (1978) Eur. J. Pharmacol. 50, 437–441.
344 Jonsson, C.E., Shimizu, Y., Fredholm, B.B., Granström, E. and Oliw, E. (1979) Acta Physiol. Scand. 107, 377–384.
345 Robson, M.C., DelBeccaro, E.J., Heggers, J.B. and Loy, G.L. (1980) J. Trauma 20, 722–725.
346 Morrison, A.R., Nishikawa, K. and Needleman, P. (1978) J. Pharmacol. Exp. Ther. 205, 1–8.
347 Sivakoff, M., Holmberg, S. and Needleman, P. (1980) in Advances in Prostaglandin and Thromboxane Research (Samuelsson, B., Ramwell, P. and Paoletti, R., eds.) Vol. 7, pp. 1175–1176, Raven Press, New York.
348 Smith, J.B. (1980) Am. J. Pathol. 99, 742–804.
349 Moncada, S. and Vane, J.R. (1979) Adv. Intern Med. 24, 1–22.
350 Moncada, S. and Amezcua, J.L. (1979) Haemostasis 8, 252–265.
351 Smith, J.B., Araki, H. and Lefer, A.M. (1980) Circulation 62, (suppl. V) 19–25.
352 Packham, M.A. and Mustard, J.F. (1980) Circulation 62, (suppl. V) 26–41.
353 Mustard, J.F., Kinlough-Rathbone, R.L. and Packham, M.A. (1980) Annu. Rev. Med. 31, 89–96.
354 McGiff, J.C. (1980) Adv. Intern Med. 25, 199–216.
355 Harker, L.A., Ross, R. and Glomset, J. (1976) Ann. N.Y. Acad. Sci. USA 275, 321–329.

356 Gryglewski, R.J. (1980) CRC Crit. Rev. Biochem. 7, 291–338.
357 Szczeklik, A., Gryglewski, R.J., Musial, J., Grodzinska, L., Serwonska, M. and Marcinkiewicz, E. (1978) Thrombos. Haemostas (Stuttg.) 40, 66–74.
358 Szczeklik, A., Gryglewski, R.J., Musial, J., Grodzinska, L., Serwonska, M., Wojcik-Switek, L. and Marcinkiewicz, E. (1978) Acta Biol. Med. Germ. 37, 741–742.
359 Gryglewski, R.J., Dembinska-Kièc, A., Zmuda, A. and Gryglewska, T. (1978) Atherosclerosis 31, 385–394.
360 Dembinska-Kièc, A., Rücker, W. and Schönhöfer, P.S. (1979) Atherosclerosis 33, 217–226.
361 Ross, R., Glomset, J., Kariya, B. and Harker, L. (1974) Proc. Natl. Acad. Sci. USA 71, 1207–1210.
362 Lewy, R.I. Wiener, L., Walinsky, P., Lefer, A.M., Silver, M.J. and Smith, J.B. (1980) Circulation 61, 1165–1171.
363 Kuzuya, T., Tada, M., Inoue, M., Kodama, K., Takeda, H., Mishima, M., Inui, M. and Abe, H. (1980) Am. J. Cardiol. 45, 454.
364 Tada, M., Kuzuya, T., Inoue, M., Kadama, K., Fukushima, M. and Abe, H. (1980) Adv. Myocardiol 2, 397–405.
365 Lewy, R.I., Wiener, L., Smith, J.B., Walinsky, P., Silver, M.J. and Saia, M. (1979) Clin. Cardiol. 2, 404–406.
366 Robertson, R.M., Robertson, D., Roberts, L.J. II, Maas, R.L., Fitzgerald, G.A., Friesinger, G.C. and Oates, J.A. (1981) N. Engl. J. Med. 304, 998–1003.
367 Sobel, M., Salzman, E.W., Davies, G.C., Handin, R.I., Sweeney, J., Plaetz, J. and Kurland, G. (1981) Circulation 63, 300–306.
368 Miwa, K., Kambara, H. and Kawai, C. (1981) Am. J. Cardiol. 47, 1210–1214.
369 Matthias, F.R. (1978) Haemostasis 7, 273–281.
370 Smith, E.F. III, Smith, J.B. and Lefer, A.M. (1979) Fed. Proc. 38, 1037.
371 Morooka, S., Kobayashi, M., Takahashi, T., Takashima, Y., Sakamoto, M. and Shimamoto, T. (1979) Exp. Mol. Pathol. 30, 449–457.
372 Smith, E.F. III, Lefer, A.M. and Smith, J.B. (1980) Can. J. Physiol. Pharmacol. 58, 294–300.
373 Ziboh, V.A., Maruta, H., Lord, J., Cagle, W.D. and Lucky, W. (1979) Eur. J. Clin. Invest. 9, 223–228.
374 Sarji, K.E., Kleinfelder, J., Brewington, R., Gonzales, J., Hempling, H. and Colwell, J.A. (1979) Thromb. Res. 15, 639–650.
375 Johnson, M., Reece, A.H. and Harrison, H.E. (1980) in Advances in Prostaglandin and Thromboxane Research (Samuelsson, B., Ramwell, P. and Paoletti, R., eds.) Vol. 8, pp. 1283–1286, Raven Press, New York.
376 Colwell, J.A. and Halushka, P.V. (1980) Br. J. Haematol. 44, 521–526.
377 Subbiah, M.T.R. and Dietemeyer (1980) Biochemical Med. 23, 231–235.
378 Tremoli, E., Folco, G.C., Agradi, E. and Galli, C. (1979) Lancet i, 107–108.
379 Bult, H. and Herman, A.G. (1979) Agents Actions, Suppl. 4, 147–155.
380 Cook, J.A., Wise, W.C. and Halushka, P.V. (1980) J. Clin. Invest. 65, 227–230.
381 Wise, W.C., Cook, J.A., Halushka, P. and Knapp, D.R. (1980) Circ. Res. 46, 854–859.
382 Bult, H., Beetens, J. and Herman, A.G. (1980) Eur. J. Pharmacol. 63, 47–56.
383 Frölich, J.C., Ogletree, M., Peskar, B.A. and Brigham, K.L. (1980) in Advances in Prostaglandin and Thromboxane Research (Samuelsson, B., Ramwell, P. and Paoletti, R., eds.) Vol. 7, pp. 745–750, Raven Press, New York.
384 Harris, R.H., Zmudka, M., Maddox, Y., Ramwell, P.W. and Fletcher, R.J. (1980) in Advances in Prostaglandin and Thromboxane Research (Samuelsson, B., Ramwell, P. and Paoletti, R., eds.) Vol. 7, pp. 843–849, Raven Press, New York.
385 Szczeklik, A., Nizankowski, R., Skawinski, S., Szczeklik, J., Gluszko, P. and Gryglewski, R.J. (1979) Lancet i, 1111–1114.
386 Olsson, A.G. and Nilsson, E. (1981) Prostaglandins Med. 6, 329–339.
387 Remuzzi, G., Marchesi, D., Livio, M., Cavenaghi, A.E., Mecca, G., Donati, M.B. and De Gaetano, G. (1978) Thromb. Res. 13, 1007–1015.
388 Gerrard, J.M., Stoddard, S.F., Shapiro, R.S., Coccia, P.F., Ramsay, M.K., Nesbit, M.E., Rao, G.H., Krivit, W. and White, J.G. (1978) Br. J. Haematol. 40, 597–607.

389 Russel, N.H., Keenan, J.P. and Bellingham, A.J. (1979) Br. J. Haematol. 41, 417–425.
390 Kafka, M.S., van Kammen, D.P. and Bunney, W.E. (1979) Am. J. Psych. 136, 685–687.
391 Rotrosen, J., Miller, A.D., Mandio, D., Traficante, L.J and Gershon, S. (1980) Arch. Gen. Psych. 37, 1047–1054.
392 Okuma, M. and Uchino, H. (1979) Blood 54, 1258–1271.
393 Jobin, F. (1978) Semin Thrombosis Haemostasis 4, 199–240.
394 McNicol, G.P. (1980) Lancet i, 736–738.
395 Editorial (1980) Lancet i, 1172–1173.
396 Garfield, E. (1981) Current Contents 24, 5–13.
397 The Canadian Cooperative Study Group (1978) N. Engl. J. Med. 299, 53–59.
398 Roth, G.J. and Majerus, P.W. (1975) J. Clin. Invest. 56, 624–632.
399 Burch, J.W., Stanford, N. and Majerus, P.W. (1978) J. Clin. Invest. 61, 314–319.
400 Roth, G.J., Ozols, J. and Siok, C.J. (1978) Clin. Res. 26, 356A.
401 Vargaftig, B.B. and Lefort, J. (1977) Eur. J. Pharmacol. 43, 125–141.
402 Jaffe, E.A. and Weksler, B.B. (1979) J. Clin. Invest. 63, 532–535.
403 Burch, J.W., Baenzinger, N.L., Stanford, N. and Majerus, P.W. (1978) Proc. Natl. Acad. Sci. USA 75, 5181–5184.
404 Amezcua, J.L., O'Grady, J., Salmon, J.A. and Moncada, S. (1979) Thrombosis Res. 16, 69–79.
405 O'Grady, J. and Moncada, S. (1978) Lancet ii, 780.
406 Rajah, S.M., Penny, A., Kester, R. (1978) Lancet ii, 1104.
407 Korbut, R. and Moncada, S. (1978) Thrombosis Res. 13, 489–500.
408 Kelton, J.G., Hirsch, J., Carter, C.J. and Buchanan, M.R. (1978) J. Clin. Invest. 62, 892–895.
409 Treacher, D.T., Warlow, C. and McPherson, K. (1978) Lancet ii: 1378.
410 Godal, H.C., Eika, C., Dybdahl, J.H., Daal, L. and Larsen, S. (1979) Lancet i, 1236.
411 Reyers, I., Mussoni, L., Donati, M.B. and de Gaetano, G. (1980) Thrombosis Res. 18, 669–674.
412 Basista, M., Dobranowski, J. and Gryglewski, R.J. (1978) Pharmacol. Res. Commun. 10, 759–763.
413 Ellis, E.F., Wright, K.F., Jones, P.S., Richardson, P.W. and Ellis, C.K. (1980) J. Cardiovasc. Pharmacol. 2, 387–397.
414 Villa, S., Livio, M. and de Gaetano, G. (1979) Br. J. Haematol. 42, 425–431.
415 Zimmerman, R., Thiessen, M., Mörl, H. and Weckesser, G. (1979) Thrombosis Res. 16, 843–846.
416 Szczeklik, A., Gryglewski, R.J., Grodzinska, L., Musial, J., Servonska, M. and Marcinkiewicz, E. (1979) Thrombosis Res. 15, 405–413.
417 Patrono, C., Ciabattoni, G., Pinca, E., Pugliese, F., Castrucci, G., de Salvo, A., Satta, M.A. and Peskar, B.A. (1980) Thrombosis Res. 17, 317–327.
418 Masotti, G., Galanti, G., Poggesi, L., Abbate, R. and Neri Serneri, G.G. (1979) Lancet ii, 1213–1216.
419 Shaikh, B.S., Bott, S.J. and Demers, L.M. (1980) Prostaglandins Med. 4, 439–447.
420 Preston, F.E., Whipps, S., Jackson, C.A., French, A.J., Wyld, P.J. and Stoddard, C.J. (1981) N. Engl. J. Med. 304, 76–79.
421 Paretti, F.J., D'Angelo, A., Mannucci, P.M. and Smith, J.B. (1980) Lancet i, 371–372.
422 O'Brien, J.R. (1980) Lancet i, 372–373.
423 Kern, D. (1981) Lancet i, 1173–1174.
424 Patrono, C. and Patrignani, P. (1981) Lancet i, 1174.
425 Patrignani, P., Cattani, P., Minuz, P. and Patrono, C. (1980) Clin. Res. 28, 636A.
426 Hanley, S.P., Bevan, J., Cockbill, S.R. and Heptinstall, S. (1981) Lancet i, 969–971.
427 Paccioretti, M.J. and Block, L.H. (1980) Clin. Pharmacol. Ther. 27, 803–809.
428 Lorenz, R., Seiss, W. and Weber, P. (1981) Eur. J. Pharmacol. 70, 511–518.
429 de Gaetano, G., Rajtar, G., Livio, M. and Merino, J. (1980) Naunyn-Schmiedeberg's Arch. Pharmacol. 312, 85–89.
430 Vargaftig, B.B. (1978) Eur. J. Pharmacol. 50, 231–241.
431 Vargaftig, B.B. (1978) J. Pharm. Pharmac. 30, 101–104.
432 Ali, M. and McDonald, J.W.D. (1979) Prostaglandins Med. 3, 327–332.
433 Smith, M.J.H., Ford-Hutchinson, A.W., Walker, J.R. and Slack, J.A. (1979) Agents Action 9, 483–487.

434 Merino, J., Livio, M., Rajtar, G. and de Gaetano, G. (1980) Biochem. Pharmacol. 29, 1093–1096.
435 Peterson, D.A., Gerrard, J.M., Rao, G.H.R. and White, J.G. (1981) Prostaglandins Med. 6, 161–164.
436 Kocsis, J.J., Hernandovich, J., Silver, M.J., Smith, J.B. and Ingerman, C. (1973) Prostaglandins 3, 141–144.
437 Jafari, E., Saleem, A., Shaikh, B.S. and Demers, L.M. (1976) Prostaglandins 12, 829–835.
438 Catalano, P.M., Smith, J.B. and Murphy, S. (1981) Blood 57, 99–105.
439 de Castellarnau, C., Cerletti, C., Dejana, E., Galletti, F., Latini, R., Livio, M. and de Gaetano, G. (1981) Thrombos. Haemostas. 45, 294.
440 Randall, M.J., Parry, M.J., Hawkeswood, E., Cross, P.E. and Dickinson, R.P. (1981) Thrombosis Res. 23, 145–162.
441 Flower, R.J., Russel-Smith, N.C., Salmon, J.A. and Thorogood, P. (1981) Br. J. Pharmacol. 74, 791P.
442 Bertele, V., Cerletti, C., Schiepatti, A., di Minno, G. and de Gaetano, G. (1981) Lancet i, 1057.
443 Pace-Asciak, C.R. and Rangaraj, G. (1977) Biochim. Biophys. Acta 486, 579–582.

CHAPTER 3

The prostacyclins

CECIL PACE-ASCIAK [a] and
RICHARD GRYGLEWSKI [b]

[a] *Research Institute, The Hospital for Sick Children, 555 University Avenue, Toronto, Canada and*
[b] *Department of Pharmacology, Copernicus Medical Academy, 31-531 Cracow, Grzegorzecka 16, Poland*

1. Introduction

A new prostaglandin pathway distinct from that which forms PGE_2 and $PGF_{2\alpha}$, now referred to as the prostacyclin pathway, was first described in 1970. At a time when a major effort was being directed towards investigating the biological role of PGE_2 and $PGF_{2\alpha}$ (PGD had just been discovered [1]), the importance of this other pathway was not immediately appreciated as biological activity data of products in this pathway were lacking. In a series of papers ranging from 1970 to 1976 Pace-Asciak and Wolfe described the isolation, chemical structures and biosynthetic mechanism involved in the formation from arachidonic acid of two unique bicyclic prostaglandins having an ether bridge between carbons 6 and 9 of the prostanoic acid skeleton [2–8]. The structures proposed were 6(9)-oxy-11,15-dihydroxy prosta-5,13-dienoic acid and its corresponding $\Delta^{7,13}$ isomer [2–5]. They were the major products formed by the rat stomach but were also formed by sheep seminal vesicles [5]. A collaborative effort between Pace-Asciak and the Chemistry section at the Upjohn Company led to a verification of the bicyclic nature of these structures through chemical synthesis of the hydrogenated product (U. Axen, personal communication), although synthetic attempts into the unsaturated structures proved mostly unsuccessful. At a Prostaglandin Winter Conference in January 1976, Pace-Asciak presented evidence of the rapid and almost exclusive conversion by rat stomach homogenates of purified prostaglandin endoperoxides, PGG_2 and PGH_2, into another new prostaglandin, 6-keto $PGF_{1\alpha}$ [9–11] which was shown to exist also in rat brain and sheep liver [12,13]. Around this time a potent antiaggregating substance (structure unknown) had just been discovered by scientists at Burroughs-Wellcome led by Moncada, Gryglewski and Vane which was rapidly formed from prostaglandin endoperoxides during incubation with aortic rings. The subsequent demonstration by these investigators that rat stomach microsomes also transformed endoperoxides into this antiaggregatory substance referred to as PGX [14], gave an important clue into its biosynthetic pathway and therefore its possible structure based on the biochemical studies of Pace-Asciak and Wolfe [2–5] and Pace-Asciak [9–13]. It had to be either 6-keto $PGF_{1\alpha}$ or one of its precursors derived from PGH_2 [4]. A collaboration between chemists at the Upjohn Company and Burroughs Wellcome now proved successful. This factor was shown in a December 1976 paper [15] to be 6(9)oxy-11,15-dihydroxyprosta-5,13-dienoic acid reported six years earlier by Pace-Asciak and Wolfe [4]. In separate studies Sih and Huang [16] later suggested that in the Δ^7 isomer reported by Pace-Asciak and Wolfe [4] the double bond had been assigned incorrectly, a suggestion which was supported by Sih and Graber [17] who synthesised the $\Delta^{7,13}$ bicyclic ether.

While Pace-Asciak and Wolfe described the biochemical aspects of this pathway [1–13] avoiding to a large extent biological activity measurements, scientists at Burroughs-Wellcome provided the much needed biological relevance by demonstrating that products in this pathway were indeed biologically active and in fact prostacyclin has turned out to be a powerful antiaggregating substance through its capacity to stimulate adenylate cyclase [14,15,18].

With the demonstration within one year (1976) of the biological activity and structure of PGX, named Prostacyclin or PGI_2, an explosion of research ensued during the following five years (1977–1981) which has only now begun to subside. In the following pages, the biochemistry, pharmacology and possible roles of the prostacyclin pathway will be reviewed. The following review articles are recommended; refs. 147–154, and 295.

2. *Nomenclature*

The formal naming of products in the prostaglandin family is based on the prostanoic acid skeleton. The prostacyclins are no exception. Thus the bicyclic product now known as Prostacyclin was referred to initially as 6(9)oxy-11,15-dihydroxy prosta-5,13-dienoic acid [4] and subsequently when the stereochemical assignment of the double bonds was established as 9-deoxy-6,9α-epoxy-11,15-dihydroxy-prosta-5Z,13E-dienoic acid [15]. The trivial name Prostacyclin is generally referred to the product derived from arachidonic acid and consistent with the alphabetic naming of prostaglandins this product has been assigned the abbreviated form PGI_2.

While prostaglandins are derived from all *cis* essential fatty acids having 3, 4 and 5 double bonds, a *cis* double bond at carbon 5 of the fatty acid is essential for prostacyclin synthesis from the precursor endoperoxide. Accordingly, 8,11,14-eicosatrienoic acid, the precursor of PGE_1 and $PGF_{1\alpha}$ cannot form PGI_1. Such a product however, can be derived chemically from PGI_2 through catalytic hydrogenation [19]. PGI_3 is derived from all-*cis* 5,8,11,14,17-eicosapentaenoic acid [20,23] and PGI_2 from 5,8,11,14-eicosatetraenoic acid [4,15]. Since the biologically occurring PGIs have a vinyl ether, they are short-lived at physiological or acidic pH [15,19–21], hydrolysing in aqueous medium to products named on the basis of the primary PGs, i.e. PGI_2 hydrolyses into 6-keto $PGF_{1\alpha}$ while PGI_3 hydrolyses into Δ^{17}-6-keto $PGF_{1\alpha}$ [4,15,19,21,23]. Similarly, a proposed metabolite of 6-keto $PGF_{1\alpha}$ and PGI_2 resulting from the action of 9-hydroxydehydrogenase is 6-keto PGE_1 [23], while that which would be derived from PGI_3 would be named Δ^{17}-6-keto PGE_1.

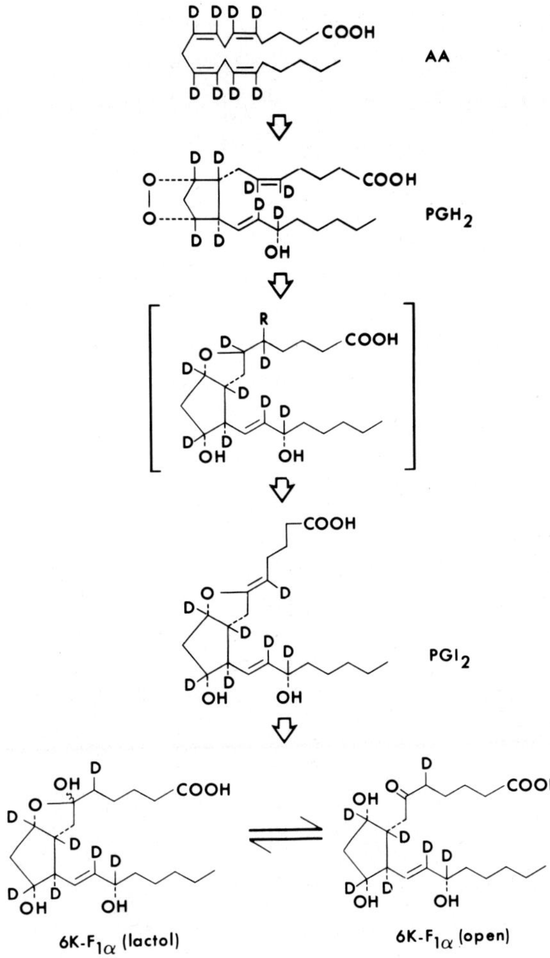

Fig. 1. Pathway showing the conversion of octadeuterated arachidonic acid into the heptadeuterated PGI_2 and 6-keto $PGF_{1\alpha}$.

3. *Biochemistry*

(a) Biosynthesis

As is the case with the classical prostaglandins and thromboxanes (see Chapters 1 and 2) products in the prostacyclin pathway were discovered using radiolabelled arachidonic acid [1–13] and the mechanism of biosynthesis was followed through use of radiolabelled prostaglandin endoperoxides [9–11] when these became available [24,25].

In 1971, Pace-Asciak and Wolfe proposed a mechanism for the conversion of arachidonic acid into the bicyclic ether now referred to as prostacyclin [4]. The

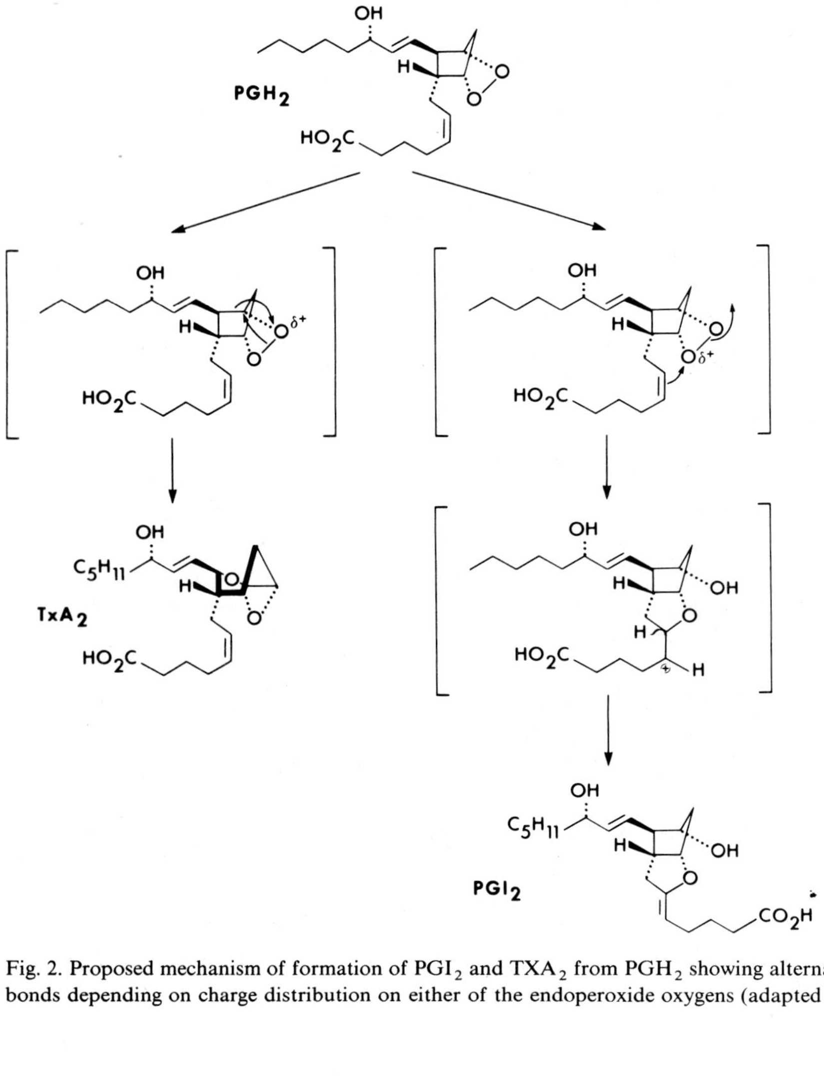

Fig. 2. Proposed mechanism of formation of PGI_2 and TXA_2 from PGH_2 showing alternative cleavage of bonds depending on charge distribution on either of the endoperoxide oxygens (adapted from ref. 29).

structural similarity of the backbone (carbons 13 to 20) of the bicyclic ether with that of PGE_2 and $PGF_{2\alpha}$ suggested a pathway in their biosynthesis not dissimilar from that proposed by Samuelsson [25] for the prostaglandins i.e. involving as intermediates the proposed endoperoxides to be isolated independently a few years later by Hamberg and Samuelsson [24] and Nugteren and Hazelhoff [25] (Fig. 1). This mechanism was confirmed in 1976 when Pace-Asciak used deuterated and tritiated arachidonic acid as well as purified octadeuterated and octatritiated endoperoxides and showed them to be converted by a rat stomach preparation into heptalabelled 6-keto $PGF_{1\alpha}$ [9–11,27]. Because prostacyclin is acid labile hydrolysing to 6-keto $PGF_{1\alpha}$ it was obvious that isolation of 6-keto $PGF_{1\alpha}$ in these studies indicated that PGI_2 had been formed. This was clearly shown in subsequent experiments where PGI_2 formed by the rat stomach was detected through bioassay on the rat blood pressure and its conversion into 6-keto $PGF_{1\alpha}$ was followed through loss of its biological activity during purification [28].

The endoperoxide, PGH_2, is the most proximal biosynthetic substrate known for PGI_2 [10,14,15,23]. Mechanistically, however, very little is known regarding the actual cleavage of the 9,11-endoperoxide group of PGH_2 with subsequent bridging (cyclisation) of the oxygen at carbon 9 with carbon 6 to form PGI_2. Fried and Just [29] have proposed a common mechanism to explain PGI_2 and TXA_2 synthesis whereby a carbonium ion is first formed on either of the endoperoxide oxygens followed by opening of the endoperoxide through participation of Δ^5 to form PGI_2 or with C11–12 cleavage to form TXA_2 (Fig. 2). It is still unclear though whether a mechanism involving free radicals or oxonium ions ensues and whether it is concerted or involves additional intermediates still to be described. Another unclear point relates to the generation of the double bond at Δ^5 (Z configuration). How is this formed? Is the initial cyclised product bound to protein possibly covalently with a sulfoprotein at position 5 [27] (Fig. 1).

(b) Tissue distribution

Although the early studies on the Prostacyclin or 6-keto $PGF_{1\alpha}$ pathway were carried out with preparations of the rat stomach in which this is the major pathway [2–13], rat brain [12,13] and liver [12] and sheep seminal vesicles [3,5] were also shown to transform arachidonic acid or prostaglandin endoperoxide into 6-keto $PGF_{1\alpha}$. Using bovine aortic rings incubated with endoperoxide Moncada et al. could demonstrate the formation of PGI_2 directly through its inhibition of platelet aggregation [14,30]. Subsequent studies have also shown that this pathway is present in an abundance of tissues representing the major pathway of arachidonic acid metabolism in vascular tissue from fetal [31–34] and adult animals [30,35–39,155], cultured endothelial [40,41], smooth muscle [42,43] and transformed cells [45], rat granuloma cells [46] fibroblasts [47] and heart [48,49]. PGI_2 has been shown to be released from isolated perfused guinea pig lungs [50] and lungs in vivo [51–53]. Through measurements of 6-keto $PGF_{1\alpha}$ in arterial vs venous blood, PGI_2 is believed to be released by human lungs in vivo [52]. Homogenates of a variety of tissues are capable of forming 6-keto

$PGF_{1\alpha}$ [54] a capacity which is not restricted to adult animals as organs and blood vessels from fetal and neonatal animals have also been shown to produce 6-keto $PGF_{1\alpha}$ [55].

The enzyme which carries out the unique cleavage of the endoperoxides with subsequent oxycyclisation of carbons 6 and 9 has been named in terms of the actual mechanism involved i.e. 6(9)oxy cyclase [27] or in terms of the product formed i.e. prostacyclin synthase [15]. This enzyme appears to be distributed unequally throughout a particular organ or tissue. In blood vessels, it was initially reported to be more abundant on the intimal surface of the vascular endothelium rather than in the smooth muscle cells [56] although cultured smooth-muscle cells are capable of forming PGI_2 [42,43]. Through use of monoclonal antibodies and immunoradiometric assay Smith et al. [64] have recently shown that the 6(9)oxy cyclase is evenly distributed in the endothelial cells and smooth muscle cells while PGH_2 synthase is enriched in the endothelial cells. Consequently, although prostacyclin may be formed by both cell types in different layers of the vasculature, each layer might utilise a different substrate. For example platelet endoperoxide or endothelial cell endoperoxide may be the substrate for PGI_2 synthesis by endothelial cells in the intimal layer while smooth muscle cells deep in the blood vessel might make use of arachidonic acid released from vascular phospholipids. Indeed the role for the two prostacyclins of different origin might be different, on the one hand endothelial prostacyclin might be involved in the 'unstickiness' of the intimal surface of the vascular endothelium to platelets due to prostacyclin's ability to prevent platelets from aggregating or adhering to its surface while prostacyclin of smooth muscle origin might, possibly in concert with PGE_2 which is also formed by vascular tissue, play a role in the regulation of the tonus of the vessel.

The 6(9)oxy cyclase is also present in the kidney [54,57] where it appears to be unevenly distributed in this organ as well. Unlike PGE_2 and $PGF_{2\alpha}$ which are mainly formed by the papilla [58], PGI_2 formation is mostly concentrated in the vasculature of the cortex or outer medulla [57,59–62]. Monoclonal antibodies to the purified enzyme have recently been reported [62] and preliminary data through immunocytofluorescent studies suggest that the 6(9)oxy cyclase is found in a previously unrecognised site of PGI_2 synthesis in the medulla, in a specialised type of medullary interstitial cell associated with capillary bundles [144]. PGI_2 synthesis within these cells appears to be restricted to the endoplasmic reticulum similar to PGH_2 synthesis. Although the function of PGI_2 within these cells is unknown, it is possible that due to the close proximity of these cells to elements of the medullary vasculature, PGI_2 formed by these cells could be involved in modulating blood flow within or to the medulla [144].

Brain contains detectable 6(9)oxy cyclase activity [13,65–67]. It is most abundant in cerebral blood vessels and capillaries [65,67–71], although a report by Gerritsen and Printz [70] has demonstrated that microvessels from the rat cerebral cortex synthesise principally PGD_2. PGI_2 is also formed by the choroid plexus [65,71] suggesting that 6-keto $PGF_{1\alpha}$ might enter the cerebrospinal fluid (see Section 4 on Levels in biological fluids). Although levels of PGs in brain are normally very low or undetectable, a transient occlusion of both common carotid arteries in the gerbil followed by reperfusion of the brain has shown rapid accumulation of PGs including 6-keto $PGF_{1\alpha}$ in the cerebral hemispheres which reach maximum level within 5 minutes of reperfusion [66]. The largest accumulation however appeared in PGD_2, a major PG found in cerebral cortex and capillaries [67,71]. These experiments suggest that formation of prostaglandins in brain is regio-selective and that their synthesis appears to be influenced by ischaemia (see Section 4 on Levels in biological fluids).

A variety of other organs and tissues have been shown to produce prostacyclin or 6-keto $PGF_{1\alpha}$; these include seminal vesicles [2,4,72–74], testes [75], gastric mucosa [76–78], lung [51], umbilical artery [79], uterus [80,81] and placenta [82]. Interestingly, while aorta of most species produces PGI_2 avidly, chicken aorta is devoid of this activity making instead PGE_2 [83]. Also in this species PGI_2 is devoid of effect as a platelet antiaggregating substance [83,84]. Another tissue devoid of PGI_2 synthetic capacity is the platelet which forms mostly thromboxane (see Chapter 2) and the lipoxygenase product 12-hydroperoxyeicosatetraenoic acid (12-HPETE).

Cofactors do not seem to be required for the conversion of endoperoxides into PGI_2. In fact this pathway was probably missed by many investigators who used arachidonic acid as substrate during measurement of PGE_2 biosynthesis because optimal conditions for PGE_2 formation require the addition of reduced gluthathione as cofactor (see Chapter 6). Thus it is quite fortuitous that the initial discovery of the 6(9)oxy bicyclic products was made in the rat stomach which has much gluthathione oxidase activity without which the radiolabelled arachidonic acid would probably have been shunted into PGE_2 [2–13]. In the absence of glutathione or other cofactors Cottee et al. could demonstrate that the seminal vesicles, a tissue capable of making PGE_2 primarily, now converted arachidonic acid mainly into 6-keto $PGF_{1\alpha}$ [72].

(c) Enzyme properties

Like other PG synthetic enzymes, the enzyme which transforms PGH_2 into PGI_2 is a particulate enzyme associated with the microsomal fraction of a tissue homogenate [72]. This enzyme, 6(9)oxy cyclase, has been solubilised from microsomes of pig and rabbit aorta with 0.5% Triton X-100 and partially purified on DEAE-cellulose chromatography [145,146]. This preparation converted PGH_2 into PGI_2 but as expected PGH_1 was not converted into a PGI_1. Instead PGH_1 was converted into the corresponding $C_{17:2}$ fatty acid (HHD) probably non-enzymatically [145]. In a recent report the 6(9)oxy cyclase from bovine aorta was purified to homogeneity through use of monoclonal antibodies and immunoaffinity chromatography on Affigel [63]. The purified enzyme exhibits a single protein band (50000 MW) on SDS polyacrylamide gel and has a reported specific activity of 570 μmoles PGI_2/min/mg of protein representing a 50 fold purification over the solubilised microsomes [143].

(d) Inhibitors

The first inhibitor discovered of the 6(9)oxy cyclase was 15-hydroperoxy arachidonic acid (15-HPETE) [85]. Since then other fatty acid hydroperoxides have been shown to inhibit this enzyme which seems to be sensitive to lipid peroxides in general [86]. Thus factors which affect lipid peroxidation are suspected to alter the activity of the 6(9)oxy cyclase. Such is believed to be the case in experimental Vitamin E deficiency which results in a decrease in vascular prostacyclin production through increased peroxidation of lipids [75,87,88]. Vitamin E supplementation restores the capacity to normal [87,88] probably through its antioxidant effects. Another example of an induced deficiency in aortic prostacyclin production is during the onset of atherosclerosis [89] and in diabetes mellitus [90–92] although essential hypertension is accompanied by an increase in vascular synthesis of PGI_2 [93–95]. In vitro, catecholamines in large quantities (10^{-5} M) also lead to an increase in PGI_2 synthesis probably through an antioxidant effect [6] as the antioxidant propyl gallate also behaves in a similar fashion [75].

Tranylcypromine, a monoamine oxidase inhibitor also inhibits prostacyclin synthetase in vitro ($IC_{50} = 160$ μg/ml) [96]. This is much weaker than the inhibition induced by the fatty acid hydroperoxides ($IC_{50} = 0.5$ μg/ml) [85]. Fortunately, the latter products are not active when administered in vivo due to active peroxidases which reduce the hydroperoxides to the inactive hydroxides. Other inhibitors of prostacyclin synthesis are the endoperoxide analogs (9,11-diaza and 9,11-epoxyimino-prosta-5,13-dienoic acid) [97] and an indole hydroperoxide [98].

(e) Catabolism

A factor with biological properties similar to PGI_2 is spontaneously released by the lungs [51]. This release can be enhanced by Angiotensin I and II [99,100] but not by norepinephrine or vasopressin. Since the release can be blocked by the converting enzyme inhibitor, captopril [101,102] or the receptor antagonist saralasin, 'prostacyclin' release is likely mediated via activation of an angiotensin II receptor.

Prostacyclin entering the circulation does not appear to be rapidly degraded as measured by the rate of disappearance of its biological activity [103–105]. Indeed, unlike other prostaglandins, prostacyclin is equally effective in reducing arterial blood pressure when administered intravenously as it is intraarterially [104,105]. Consequently it appears to survive pulmonary transit and therefore the pulmonary catabolic enzyme, 15-hydroxydehydrogenase, at least within the time frame of several passes through the lungs [106]. Whether this is due to poor transport of prostacyclin across the pulmonary endothelium due to its binding with albumin in the circulation is not known. It is, however, eventually catabolised by this enzyme as clearly shown by the studies of Sun et al. [107–109] and McGuire and Sun [108] who evaluated the profile of products appearing in the urine of the primate and the rat after intravenous infusion of 11β-[^{3}H]PGI_2 as well as the studies of Pace-Asciak et al. [106] who evaluated the rate of appearance of 9β-[^{3}H]PGI_2 metabolites in the

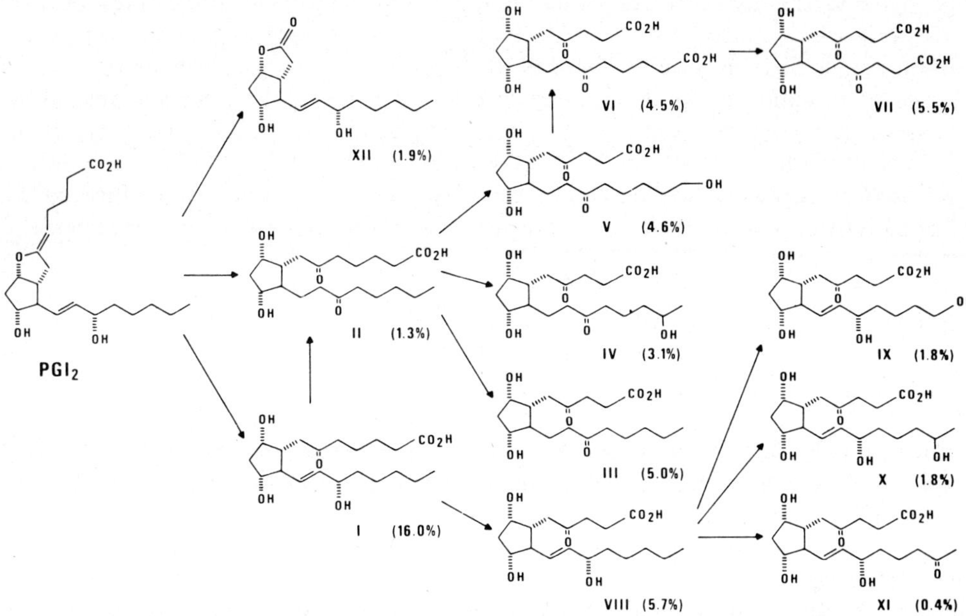

Fig. 3. Overall scheme of urinary catabolites of PGI_2 and 6-keto $PGF_{1\alpha}$ (reproduced from ref. 107 with permission).

circulation of the rat. These studies showed that PGI_2 is metabolised via 15-hydroxydehydrogenase, 13,14-reductase and β and ω-oxidation (Fig. 3). Comparison of the profile of urinary products observed after infusion of PGI_2 with the simpler pattern of products observed during infusion of 6-keto $PGF_{1\alpha}$ [110,111] in the rat indicated that while 6-keto $PGF_{1\alpha}$ is not a good substrate for 15-hydroxydehydrogenase, PGI_2 is a better substrate since in the latter experiments products were observed in blood and urine which contained a 15-keto group [109,111]. It appears that the existence of 6-keto $PGF_{1\alpha}$ in the lactol form in aqueous medium interferes with its uptake across the pulmonary endothelium hence becoming inaccessible to the dehydrogenase [112]. This concept is supported by the finding that 6-keto $PGF_{1\alpha}$ is avidly metabolised in vitro via soluble 15-hydroxydehydrogenase e.g. tissue homogenate [113]. An NADP-linked prostacyclin 15-hydroxydehydrogenase from rabbit kidney has recently been purified; $K_m PGI_2 = 278$ μM; $K_m NADP^+ = 13.4$ μM; molecular weight = 62000 [114].

When 9β-[^{3}H]PGI_2 is incubated with rat platelets, a loss of tritium takes place as a function of time [115]. This loss of tritium from the 9β-position results from the action of a 9-hydroxyprostaglandin dehydrogenase, first reported in the rat kidney [116]. Interestingly PGI_2 is reported to be a better substrate for this enzyme than 6-keto $PGF_{1\alpha}$ [114]. The product of this enzyme activity could be either 6-keto PGE_1 or its 15-keto and 15-keto-13,14-dihydro metabolites. Wong et al. first suggested that PGI_2 is converted into 6-keto PGE_1 by platelets [115] as well as after passage through the isolated perfused rabbit lung and liver although the kidney did not possess much capacity for this transformation [117–119]. It is worthwhile to mention that 6-keto PGE_1 suggested to be derived from PGI_2, possesses similar though not as potent an ability to oppose platelet aggregation as PGI_2 [120]. Since 6-keto PGE_1 is chemically more stable than PGI_2, it is possible to some extent that some of the biological effects of PGI_2 in vivo can be attributed to 6-keto PGE_1, if indeed a precursor-product relationship exists between these two products. Unfortunately, direct proof of this interaction must await further and unambiguous experiments.

4. Levels in biological fluids

(a) Plasma

While it is uncertain to what extent PGI_2 is released intact (as PGI_2) under physiological conditions or as the inactive products 6-keto $PGF_{1\alpha}$, the 15-keto 13,14-dihydro metabolite, or as the β-oxidised and ω-oxidised products, recent attempts to measure the amounts of some of these metabolites in blood and urine have been made in order to derive an estimate of the daily output of these products via the 6(9)oxy pathway of the arachidonate cascade. The findings are summarised in Table I. It is generally felt that plasma concentrations of PGI_2 are around 100 pg/ml although it has recently been reported with a highly specific and sensitive technique of negative ion chemical ionization mass spectrometry that plasma levels of 6-keto $PGF_{1\alpha}$ are less than 2 pg/ml [134]. These low levels suggest against an antiaggregatory role for PGI_2 in vivo as a circulating hormone, although the possibility must still be left open that measurements of 6-keto $PGF_{1\alpha}$ might not necessarily reflect the true concentration of endogenously produced prostacyclin. Other metabolites must inevitably be measured, preferably all, including 6-keto PGE_1 and its metabolites, if the transformation of PGI_2 into these products is indeed a prominent pathway in vivo. Estimation of all these products must be taken into account in ascertaining a true measure of PGI_2 production in the body. Such measurements will certainly become available in the near future.

With regards to the possible participation of PGI_2 as a circulating hormone with systemic antihypertensive properties, suffice it to say that arterial blood pressure of both normotensive and spontaneously hypertensive rats was unaffected by infusion of antibodies that bind PGI_2 [296]. An important observation in these experiments was the demonstration of the rate of entry of PGI_2 into the circulation since newly released PGI_2 is sequestered by the antibodies and prevented from elimination from the circulation during the time course of the experiment [297]. A rate of synthesis of 38 pg/min could be calculated from these studies [297].

There are some conflicting reports regarding plasma levels of 6-keto $PGF_{1\alpha}$ during gestation. Mitchell et al. [121] report through radioimmunological techniques that plasma levels of 6-keto $PGF_{1\alpha}$ in sheep generally tend to rise in both maternal and fetal plasma at the time of delivery. In contrast Ylikorkala and Viinikka [122] report no differences in 6-keto $PGF_{1\alpha}$ plasma levels in women during pregnancy or from the non-pregnant controls. These investigators found no correlation between the concentrations of 6-keto $PGF_{1\alpha}$ in plasma and pregnancy week, maternal age, parity or lactation, while Bolton et al. [123] report increased concentrations of 6-keto $PGF_{1\alpha}$ during the second trimester. It is unfortunate that only one product, 6-keto $PGF_{1\alpha}$, was measured in these studies. Much more consistent information would be obtained if all metabolites were profiled as this would give a more meaningful interpretation of differences in metabolic as well as synthetic capacities since PGI_2 and 6-keto $PGF_{1\alpha}$ might be handled differently during the above conditions.

Plasma concentrations of 6-keto $PGF_{1\alpha}$ have been found to be significantly reduced in the diabetic state [90,91]. Again, however, the significance of measurement of only one product in a biological fluid is quite dubious since its concentration depends on its rate of formation from PGI_2 vs its rate of catabolism and/or excretion. Should the diabetic state be associated with a greater degree of metabolism and/or excretion of either PGI_2 or 6-keto $PGF_{1\alpha}$ but not of synthesis of PGI_2, then the above interpretations of reduced PGI_2 synthesis in the diabetic or any other pathological or drug induced state are open to serious question.

(b) Urine

Although urinary products of prostacyclin and 6-keto $PGF_{1\alpha}$ have been determined after infusion of these products in experimental animals and man [107–111], actual measurements of metabolites of endogenous prostacyclin are mostly lacking. The only study available is that of Fitzgerald et al. [124] who measured through mass fragmentography two proposed urinary metabolites i.e. 2,3-dinor-6-keto $PGF_{1\alpha}$, a metabolite of 6-keto $PGF_{1\alpha}$, and 6,15-diketo-13,14-dihydro $PGF_{1\alpha}$, a proposed metabolite of PGI_2. As shown in Table 1, the amounts of these products excreted in man are approx. 80 and 100 pg/kg/min respectively. These estimates also indicate that endogenous PGI_2 is unlikely to act as a circulating anti-platelet agent in healthy man [124]. These values are in sharp contrast to those of Oliw et al. [60] who measured the excretion of 6-keto $PGF_{1\alpha}$ in the urine of rabbit. Levels of 6-keto $PGF_{1\alpha}$ in the order of 12 μg/day were found which corresponds to approx. 4 ng/kg/min. If urinary 6-keto $PGF_{1\alpha}$ reflected not only renal synthesis but also levels of PGI_2 or 6-keto $PGF_{1\alpha}$ which entered the circulation, certainly the rates shown above at 4 ng/kg/min would indeed provide for PGI_2 a significant biological function. It is important to establish now the origin of the 6-keto $PGF_{1\alpha}$ found in urine to determine whether a role for PGI_2 as a circulating hormone is still plausible at least in rabbits.

(c) Amniotic fluid

It is not unexpected that PGI_2 or 6-keto $PGF_{1\alpha}$ should be present in amniotic fluid since uteroplacental tissues are capable of synthesising these products. In a recent report Ylikorkala et al. [125] and Bodzenta et al. [126] measured the concentrations

TABLE 1
Reported levels of PGI_2 or 6-keto $PGF_{1\alpha}$ and some metabolites in biological fluids

	Level	Sex	Species	Method	Comment	Ref.
1. Blood	pg/ml					
PGI_2	21 ± 3	(M)	Rabbit	$[^3H]$cAMP		130
6-keto $PGF_{1\alpha}$	2161 ± 335	(M)	Man	RIA	Long distance runners	135
	4462 ±2405	(M)	Man	RIA		
	1630 ± 300	(M, F)	Rabbit	RIA	endotoxin	136
	740 ± 302	(F)	Man	RIA	mid-gestation – fetal blood	143
	122 ± 51	(F)	Man	RIA	term gestation – fetal blood	143
	94 ± 29	(F)	Man	RIA	mid-gestation – maternal blood	143
	115 ± 24	(F)	Man	RIA		137
	65 ± 19	(F)	Monkey	RIA		137
	25 ± 7	(F)	Sheep	RIA		137
	22 ± 3	(M)	Man	RIA		141
	255	(F)	Man	RIA	Preg. and non-preg.	122
	189 ± 9	(M)	Man	GC-MS		133
	131 ± 13	(F)	Man	GC-MS		52
	117 ± 24	(F)	Man	RIA		132
	111 ± 22	(M)	Man	RIA		132
	98	(M)	Man	GC-MS	Diabetic	90
	59 ± 5	(M, F)	Cat	RIA		131
	approx 100	(F)	Sheep	RIA		121
	> 2	(M)	Man	NICI-GC-MS		134
6-15-diketo-13,14--dihydro $PGF_{1\alpha}$	151 ± 18	(M, F)	Cat	RIA		131
2,3-dinor-6-keto $PGF_{1\alpha}$	80 ± 20	(M)	Man	GC-MS		124
15-keto-13,14-dihydro-2,3-dinor 6-keto $PGF_{1\alpha}$	100 ± 30	(M)	Man	GC-MS		124
2. Urine	pg/kg/min					
6-keto $PGF_{1\alpha}$	4097 ± 763	(F)	Rabbit	GC-MS		60
	333 ± 70	(F)	Man	RIA		142
	1282 ± 283	(F)	Man	RIA	Bartters syndrome	142
2,3-dinor 6-keto $PGF_{1\alpha}$	3.2 ± 0.50	(M)	Man	GC-MS		124
15-keto-13,14-dihydro-2,3-dinor-6-keto $PGF_{1\alpha}$	1.9 ± 0.5	(M)	Man	GC-MS		124
3. Amniotic fluid	pg/ml					
6-keto $PGF_{1\alpha}$	171 ± 9		Man	RIA	normal	125
	134 ± 9		Man	RIA	severe pre-eclampsia	125
	8800 ±1200		Man	RIA	normal	126
	2400 ±1030		Man	RIA	pre-eclampsia	126
	5.6 ± 1.1		Rat	RIA, GC-MS	normal	127

TABLE 1. Continued.

	Level	Sex	Species	Method	Comment	Ref.
4. Cerebrospinal fluid	pg/mi					
6-keto-$PGF_{1\alpha}$	120 –3600	(F)	Man	GC-MS	normal cerebral trauma, epilepsy, meningo-encephalitis, stroke, subarachnoid hemorrhage	128
	15300		Man	GC-MS	essential hypertension	128

(M) male; (F) female.

of 6-keto $PGF_{1\alpha}$ in amniotic fluid collected at amniocentesis from women at late normal pregnancy or during certain types of complicated pregnancies. The concentration of 6-keto $PGF_{1\alpha}$ reported by both groups differ. Levels of 6-keto $PGF_{1\alpha}$ around 170 pg/ml [125] and 8800 pg/ml [126] were reported in normal pregnancies. These levels did not differ in mild preeclampsia although they varied significantly in severe preeclampsia (see Table 1). Levels in diabetic pregnancies, rhesus-immunised pregnancies or intrauterine fetal growth retardation were not greatly different than normals [125,126]. 6-Keto $PGF_{1\alpha}$ has also been found in rat amniotic fluid [127]. Thus it is felt that PGI_2 may play a role in parturition.

(d) Cerebrospinal fluid

The cerebrospinal fluid acts as a sink into which prostaglandins formed within the brain enter prior to their clearance into the general circulation by transport across the blood-cerebrospinal fluid and blood-brain barriers. Thus CSF should reflect the type(s) of PGs formed by brain. Indeed all the primary PGs that have been detected in brain [13,63,65–67] have been reported in CSF [128]. The principal sites of synthesis of PGI_2 are the cerebral blood vessels and capillaries [63,66,67,129] although the origin of PGI_2 (6-keto $PGF_{1\alpha}$) in CSF seems to be the choroid plexus [63,67]. Levels of 6-keto $PGF_{1\alpha}$ in normal human CSF appear to be in the range of 100 pg/ml. Although concentrations of other prostaglandins appear to change in neurological conditions as cerebral trauma, epilepsy, meningoencephalitis, stroke and subarachnoid hemorrhage [138–140], 6-keto $PGF_{1\alpha}$ concentrations appear to be greatly increased in one patient with essential hypertension [128] (see Table 1).

5. Problems encountered with measurements of PGI_2 and 6-keto $PGF_{1\alpha}$

Although PGI_2 is unstable in physiological media it is profoundly active in vitro when assayed on smooth muscle strips (bovine coronary artery, rat stomach, chick rectum) or in inhibiting the aggregation of platelets in platelet rich plasma [298]. In fact, the demonstration of the presence of the 6(9) oxycyclase activity in bovine aorta by Moncada et al. [14] was based on these biological properties of PGI_2. While several reports have suggested that PGI_2 is present in the circulation or is released from the lungs through such bioassay techniques [51,308,309] a word of caution is needed regarding the specificity of such techniques and the interpretation of data from such experiments. Recently, using similar bioassay techniques Masotti et al reported detection of PGI_2-like activity in the circulation of man [299]. They noted that circulating levels of this PGI_2-like substance decreased with increasing age or during cigarette smoking, but increased during cold stimulation. The product they observed showed spasmogenic activity similar to PGI_2 although its concentration was estimated to be around 5 ng/ml in 60-year-old subjects and around 17–24 ng/ml in 20-year-old subjects. The potential errors in such measurements are immediately apparent. Infusion of authentic PGI_2 to achieve such high concentrations in the circulation would have profound cardiovascular effects which cannot be tolerated [160]. Consequently the true significance of the measurements reported above [299] must await further validation by more definitive techniques to show what has actually been measured.

Prostacyclin is more easily assayed as its 'stable' hydration product, 6-keto $PGF_{1\alpha}$ by radioimmunoassay [137,300–303], or by GC-MS through isotope dilution [31,134,304,305]. But this product is also subject to problems. For example, Mitchell et al. have reported that authentic 6-keto $PGF_{1\alpha}$ is transformed during TLC chromatography and subsequent extraction into as many as five unidentified products all of which cross react to a different extent with the 6-keto $PGF_{1\alpha}$ antibody [306]. Hutton and Chow have recently confirmed that plasma assays of 6-keto $PGF_{1\alpha}$ can be inaccurate due to an artefact introduced during plasma extraction [307]. Morris et al. made a careful study of variables associated with the radioimmunoassay of plasma samples showing considerable non-specificity in this assay [141]. The most specific method for the assay of 6-keto $PGF_{1\alpha}$ and other prostaglandins seems to be GC-MS in the mass fragmentography mode in which endogenous compound is diluted early in the workup by deuterium labelled product. A ratio of endogenous product to deuterium labelled product is established and this ratio will persist during sample purification until final analysis by GC-MS. This method has the benefit of normalising losses through recovery or decomposition of product and more important provides unequivocal data on the identity of the product being measured. The only limiting factor with this technique is sensitivity although in a recent report by Blair et al. using a negative ion chemical ionisation technique, a limit of detection of 0.5 pg was reached [134]. More data with this technique will surely be forthcoming.

6. *Pharmacology*

Two well-recognized pharmacological properties of PGI_2 are suppression of platelet activation [14,30] and active dilation of blood vessels [39,156,157]. Recently, fibrinolytic activity of PGI_2 has also been reported [158,159]. Because of the longevity of therapeutic effects of PGI_2 in arteriosclerosis obliterans [160,161], an additional assumption had to be put forward that PGI_2 would promote the development of collateral circulation or protect ischaemic tissue from damage, although no experimental evidence is available to support this first assumption. PGI_2 shares with other PGs a cytoprotective action on gastric mucosa [162] and an inhibitory action on secretion of gastric acid [163]. PGI_2 shares with PGE_2 [164,165] and with 6-keto PGE_1 [166] their stimulatory effect on the release of renin from the kidney. In this respect PGI_2 seems to be a proper prostanoid agonist for macula densa [166,167]. Unlike PGE_2, PGI_2 when administered by inhalation is neither a bronchodilator nor does it prevent bronchial allergic obstruction [168], although at the same time it produces profound cardiovascular effects [169]. In contrast to other PGs, PGI_2 inhibits intestinal movements and enteropooling in laboratory animals [162]. PGI_2 does not affect secretion of glucagon and insulin from the isolated perfused rat pancreas [170]; however, intravenous infusions of PGI_2 to patients with vascular disease may modify pancreatic secretion of insulin in response to the glucose pulse [171].

In summary, it appears that platelet and vascular effects of PGI_2 play the most important role in its pharmacological action.

(a) Effects on platelets in vitro

PGI_2 is a most potent inhibitor of platelet aggregation in platelet-rich plasma (PRP) of humans, dogs, rats, rabbits, sheep and horses, with IC_{50} ranging from 0.5 to 4.0 ng/ml as measured against ADP-induced aggregation [14,172]. PGI_2 inhibits aggregation induced by ADP, collagen, thrombin, arachidonic acid, TXA_2 and platelet-activating factor (PAF) [173]. The first wave of ristocetin-induced aggregation seems to be fairly resistant to the inhibitory action of PGI_2 [174]. Like PGD_2 and PGE_1, which also inhibit platelet aggregation, PGI_2 elevates cAMP levels [175,176] with a persistence of almost 300 s that is in contrast to a much shorter effect of PGE_1 and PGD_2. In human PRP antiaggregatory effect of PGI_2 is 20 times more potent than that of PGD_2 and 40 times stronger than that of PGE_1 while 6-keto-$PGF_{1\alpha}$ has less than 1/500 of the potency of PGI_2 [172]. On the other hand, 6-keto-PGE_1 [115,118,177] is only 20 times less potent than PGI_2 when tested against ADP-induced platelet aggregation in human PRP [120].

PGI_2 seems to act on the same platelet receptor site as PGE_1 and on a different receptor site than that for PGD_2. Evidence comes from the studies with compound N-0164, sodium-*p*-benzyl-4-(1-oxo-2-(4-chlorobenzyl)-3-phenylpropyl)phenyl phosphonate, which selectively antagonizes inhibition of platelet aggregation induced by PGD_2 but does not affect antiaggregatory action of PGI_2 or PGE_1 [172,178]. Indirect evidence comes from the fact that the relative potency of PGE_1 and PGI_2 is similar in PRP of several species. It varies greatly with species in the case of PGD_2, e.g. rat platelets are insensitive to antiaggregatory action of PGD_2 although they are highly susceptible to the inhibitory action of both PGI_2 and PGE_1 [172]. Furthermore, subthreshold concentrations of PGI_2 or PGE_1 desensitize platelets to the antiaggregatory action of pharmacologically effective concentrations of PGI_2 or PGE_1 but not PGD_2, whereas subthreshold concentrations of PGD_2 will only desensitize platelets to high concentrations of PGD_2 but not to PGI_2 or PGE_1 [179]. The most conclusive evidence comes from binding studies which have shown that PGE_1, PGE_2 or PGI_2, but not PGD_2, can displace $[^3H]PGI_2$ from human platelet membranes [180].

In platelet microsomes PGI_2 was shown to stimulate adenylate cyclase directly [176,181] and, therefore, platelet receptor sites for PGI_2, PGE_1 and PGD_2 are likely to be associated with the regulatory subunit of this enzyme. Phosphodiesterase inhibitors were shown to potentiate, and dibutyryl cAMP to mimic [182] the effects of PGI_2 on platelets. PGI_2 via cAMP not only inhibits platelet aggregation in vitro but also reduces platelet spreading on type III collagen fibres [183], inhibits shape change and procoagulant action of activated platelets [174,184], reduces accessibility of platelet binding sites for fibrinogen [185], seals the stomata of the open canalicular system on platelet membranes [186], inhibits adhesion of platelets to thrombin-treated cultured endothelial cells [187] to rabbit subendothelium [188–190] and to type III collagen [182]. PGI_2 inhibits the release of 5-hydroxytryptamine and ADP from dense bodies and β-thromboglobulin from α-granules [182]. The effect of PGI_2 on the platelet release reaction does not seem to be closely associated with its effect on platelet adhesion. Reduction of platelet adherence by PGI_2 may occur without inhibition of 5-hydroxytryptamine release from adherent platelets [191] whereas in other experimental conditions PGI_2 inhibits the release reaction more strongly than the adhesion of platelets to collagen [182]. Thus the experiments in vitro have shown that PGI_2 is able to suppress all forms of platelet activation such as spreading, adhesion, aggregation, mobilisation of platelet membrane binding sites for fibrinogen, the release reaction from dense bodies and α-granules as well as the release of procoagulant factors; most likely all these activities of PGI_2 are mediated by cAMP. The relative potency of PGI_2 in performing all these duties is disputable and depends largely on the choice of experimental model.

(b) Antithrombotic effect in laboratory animals

PGI_2 affects platelet function in vivo. When infused intravenously into healthy volunteers [157,192,193] or into patients with arteriosclerosis obliterans [156], PGI_2 reduces platelet sensitivity to ADP-induced platelet aggregation in PRP. It also dissipates circulating platelet aggregates and prolongs template bleeding time. When topically applied, PGI_2 prevents ADP-induced formation of platelet thrombi in arterioles and venules of the hamster cheek pouch [194]. Injected intravenously to rabbits, PGI_2 prevents electrically induced formation of thrombi in the carotid artery [195]. Laboratory animals can be protected against death resulting from disseminated thrombosis following intravenous injection of arachidonic acid [196]. Topical or intravenous administration of PGI_2 to open-chest dogs inhibits platelet thrombi formation in the partially-occluded coronary artery [197,198]. PGI_2 not only prevents platelets from clumping but also dissipates platelet thrombi that have been formed in an extracorporeal system where blood of animals [199] or humans [200,201] is perfused over collagen strips. This disaggregatory action of PGI_2 [199] allows the detection of endogenous PGI_2 that is released into the circulation by angiotensin II, bradykinin [202,203], chemoreceptor stimulants [204], nicotinic acid derivatives [205], choline esters [200] and thromboxane synthetase inhibitors [205]. In this last case the efficacy of a thromboxane synthetase inhibitor ((E)-2-methyl-3-[4-(3-pyridinylmethyl))phenyl]-2-propenoic acid, MPPA) for preventing cyclic decline in blood flow in a partially obstructed coronary artery is similar to the effect of intravenously administered PGI_2 [206].

There is no agreement concerning the mechanism of cyclic reductions of coronary blood flow which follow partial obstruction of the circumflex coronary artery. Neither is the mechanism of the beneficial action of PGI_2 clear. It was originally suggested by Folts et al. [207] that the cyclic decline in blood flow was due to platelet adhesion and aggregation in the narrowed lumen. This assumption is confirmed by Aiken et al. [206] while Uchida et al. [208] believe that the spasm of distal coronary vascular bed and not platelet aggregates or thrombi are responsible for cyclic reduction of blood pressure in the partially constricted artery. Interestingly, both American [197,198,206,209] and Japanese [210,211] authors found that intravenous infusions of PGI_2 or any of its stable analogs [209] effectively interrupt cyclic declines in blood flow in the partially occluded coronary or carotid arteries. The first group of investigators pointed to the antiaggregatory action of PGI_2 while the second group stressed the vasodilatory action of PGI_2. A similar recurring reduction in cerebral blood flow in dogs was observed after partial occlusion of the common carotid artery, and again PGI_2 and thromboxane synthetase inhibitors (OKY 046 and OKY 1580) stabilized blood flow at the highest possible level [211]. Therefore, it seems that there exists a common pathological mechanism that is set in motion when a big artery becomes partially occluded. Cyclic reduction of blood flow in distal arterial bed occurs as a symptom of PGI_2/TXA_2 imbalance.

The effectiveness of thromboxane synthetase inhibitors in interrupting this dangerous recurrence of phenomena may be explained in several ways. Thromboxane synthetase inhibitors may eliminate vasospasm evoked by TXA_2 released from platelet aggregates at the site of the occlusion [211]. In the absence of platelet thromboxane production the antiaggregatory potency of PGI_2 is enhanced 30-fold [206] and, therefore, endogenous PGI_2 may prevent the formation of platelet clumps at the site of occlusion. It is feasible that platelet endoperoxides are transferred to endothelial cells and stimulate the release of endogenous PGI_2 into the circulation [205]. Indeed, a hypothesis that the vessel wall can synthetize PGI_2 from endoperoxides provided by platelets was put forward at the time of the discovery of PGI_2 [30,39]. This concept was criticized [212,213] and supported [214–216] on the basis of data which had been obtained in various experimental models in vitro. An interaction between platelet endoperoxides and endothelial cells occurs when the number of platelets approaches that of normal blood. When the platelet count increases over this number a platelet-platelet interaction occurs resulting in an inhibition of the platelet-endothelium interaction [216]. Another concept has been put forward suggesting that vascular damage is required before endoperoxides can be utilized by prostacyclin synthetase [217]. Needleman et al. [213] observed that platelet endoperoxides are available to vessel walls only after treatment with a thromboxane synthetase inhibitor whereas Marcus et al. [216] noted enhanced production of PGI_2 in a platelet-endothelial cell monolayer mixture treated with a thromboxane synthetase inhibitor. It is highly probable that when a major artery is partially occluded in vivo [206,209,210,211] the resulting damage to the intima facilitates platelet adhesion and aggregation. At the site of constriction endothelial cells and platelets remain in close proximity. Under those conditions the pharmacological blockade of thromboxane synthetase could make platelet endoperoxides available for endothelial prostacyclin synthetase.

In summary, there is ample evidence for both antiaggregatory and disaggregatory effects of PGI_2 in vivo which may result in an overall antithrombotic action. Exogenous PGI_2 can be substituted by drugs which release endogenous PGI_2 into the circulation. Thromboxane synthetase inhibitors have a complex mechanism of action in vivo, including stimulation of the release of PGI_2 into the circulation.

(c) Cardiovascular effects

Unlike $PGF_{2\alpha}$, PGI_2 relaxes superfused strips of celiac and mesenteric arteries of rabbits and in contrast to PGE_2 it does not contract rat colon [14,30,39]. Bovine coronary strips are selectively relaxed by PGI_2 [218] making this vascular preparation most suitable for the bioassay of PGI_2. In vitro PGI_2 relaxes most vascular strips, e.g. human and baboon cerebral arteries [219], lamb ductus arteriosus [220] and canine renal artery [221]. The human umbilical artery strip is relaxed by low and contracted by high concentrations of PGI_2 [222]. In contrast, rabbit aortic strips [14,20,29] as well as human and rat venous strips are not relaxed by PGI_2 [223]. In isolated Langendorff-perfused hearts of the dog, guinea pig, rat and rabbit, PGI_2 is not only a potent vasodilator but it is also a predominant metabolite of arachidonic acid [224–226]. PGI_2 is also released from other isolated perfused vascular preparations where it exerts a strong vasodilatory action [227].

In anaesthetized or conscious dogs single bolus i.v. injection (1–3 μg/kg) or infusion (0.02–1.0 μg/kg/min) of PGI_2 results in a decrease in systemic and pulmonary blood pressure as well as in a decrease in peripheral resistance [228,229]. This last effect is greatest in renal and cerebral areas [228]. In contrast to a vasoconstrictor action of $PGF_{2\alpha}$, PGD_2, PGE_2 and arachidonic acid, PGI_2 produces a vasodilatory response in the canine and feline pulmonary vascular beds [230,231]. The pulmonary vasodilatory response to PGI_2 is enhanced when the pressure in the lobar artery is doubled by a constant infusion of an $11\alpha,9\alpha$ epoxymethano analog of PGH_2 [231]. Indeed, PGI_2 effectively lowers pulmonary vascular resistance in patients with primary and secondary pulmonary hypertension [232]. Among bisenoic PGs, only PGI_2 seems to have a vasodilatory action on pulmonary circulation. However, in the conscious newborn lamb both PGI_2 and PGE_2 increase pulmonary blood flow [232]. Otherwise, systemic hypotensive responses to PGI_2 are more or less similar to those of PGE_2. PGI_2 is equipotent as a vasodilator when given either intravenously or intraarterially [105,234,235] whereas PGE_2 is much less active when administered intravenously. This is due to inactivation of PGE_2 but not of PGI_2 through the circulation. Perhaps the lungs of anaesthetized animals remove PGE_2 from the circulation even more effectively since in conscious rats PGE_2 at doses of 0.1–5.6 μg/kg/min i.v. shows no hypotensive action whereas PGI_2 at doses of 0.1–1.0 μg/kg/min i.v. is a potent hypotensive agent [228]. The pulmonary circulation of the anaesthetized intact Rhesus monkey is resistant to the vasodilatory action of PGI_2 and PGE_2 (0.05–3.0 μg/kg into the pulmonary artery) and, at the same time, systemic cardiovascular effects of these PGs are well expressed [236]. In humans [156] and in monkeys [236] the effect of PGI_2 on diastolic blood pressure is stronger than its effect on systolic blood pressure.

A modest increase in heart rate in humans [156,157,193], monkeys [236] and cats [237] has been reported. Bradycardia accompanying PGI_2-induced hypotension was observed in anaesthetized dogs [238,239] and in healthy volunteers when high doses of PGI_2 (> 20 ng/kg/min, i.v.) were used [156,157]. This is probably due to the activation of vagal reflexes. In humans an increase in heart rate is reflected by an increase in cardiac output. However, stroke volume is not changed by PGI_2 and thus it may be concluded that in humans PGI_2 does not affect cardiac contractility [156,157]. In the intact heart of open-chest dogs PGI_2 (50–500 ng) when injected into the coronary artery increases coronary blood flow without any effect on systemic blood pressure [239,240]. Topical application of PGI_2 (20–100 μg) onto epicardium results in a prolonged coronary vasodilation and this effect is potentiated by the pretreatment with cyclo-oxygenase inhibitors [239,241]. However, it can hardly be assumed that the vasodilatory effect of PGI_2 on coronary arteries will contribute to its usefulness in acute myocardial ischemia. Administered systemically to dogs PGI_2 does not increase coronary blood flow [241,242]. Therefore, protective action of PGI_2 on myocardial ischaemia both in laboratory animals [243] and in humans [244] must seek other explanations.

The effects of PGI_2 on microcirculation, local redistribution of blood and on arterial anastomoses also have to be taken into account, in addition to the anti-platelet, fibrinolytic [158], cytoprotective [243,245] and oxygen-sparing [246] actions of PGI_2. All these effects may contribute to the beneficial effects of PGI_2 in myocardial ischaemia [243,244] as well as in ischaemia associated with arteriosclerosis obliterans [160,247], Raynaud's syndrome [248], retinal vein occlusion [249], white stroke [250], endotoxic [251,252] and traumatic [253,254] shocks.

PGI_2 reduces peripheral vascular resistance in humans [156] and in animals [240]. In the rat cremaster muscle [255] and in the hamster cheek pouch [256] preparations, PGI_2 causes a dose-dependent dilatation of arterioles whereas the postcapillary venules remain insensitive to PGI_2 [255]. The results of these simple experiments fit very well the proposed effects of PGI_2 on microcirculation in humans [156,257]. In the human, resistance vessels highly susceptible to the dilatory action of PGI_2 are those of the head, neck and palms. Erythema and a feeling of warmth in these regions were reported to occur in patients in whom PGI_2 had been administered intravenously. One of the most important papers on the effect of PGI_2 on microcirculation comes from Hallenbeck and Furlow [258]. These authors have shown that PGI_2 (30–180 μg/kg/min i.v.) increases nutrient perfusion in cortex and white matter of dog brain in the post-ischaemic period. Interestingly, indomethacin (1.5–4.0 mg/kg, i.v.) elicits a similar effect and a combination of both drugs constitutes a most effective treatment. A dramatic improvement followed PGI_2 administration to patients with hemiplegia and sensoro-motoric aphasia caused by cerebral ischaemia resulting from a thrombus in the left internal carotid artery [250]. An explanation for this may be found in the laboratory data concerning the stimulatory effect of PGI_2 on cerebral microcirculation [258] and the inhibitory effect of PGI_2 on recurring reduction of the cerebral blood flow during partial obstruction of the carotid artery [211].

In summary, PGI_2 relaxes most of arterial strips and acts as a vasodilator in perfused isolated organs. In vivo intravenous administration of PGI_2 is associated with systemic hypotension, a moderate fall in pulmonary blood pressure, decrease in peripheral vascular resistance, blunted tachycardia and a slight increase in cardiac output. Given intracoronary or epicardially PGI_2 increases blood flow through the coronary circulation. Administered systemically PGI_2 hardly influences coronary blood flow [241,242], although several authors will not agree with this statement [259,260]. Nonetheless, PGI_2 rescues heart, brain, liver and other organs from ischaemic damage. Therefore, cytoprotective and oxygen-sparing properties were ascribed to PGI_2. Another possibility is that PGI_2 redistributes blood flow in the microcirculation. Cerebral and renal microcirculation seem to be most susceptible to this action of PGI_2.

(d) Clinical trials

In the clinic PGI_2 was first used in the treatment of advanced arteriosclerosis obliterans of lower extremities [160]. PGI_2 was administered in continuous intravenous or intraarterial infusion at an average rate of 7 ng/kg/min for about 72 h. The observation period following the therapy with PGI_2 varied from 4 to 21 months [161]. The most persistent and impressive effect of the PGI_2 therapy was relief of the rest pain. Sustained elongation of the walking distance and healing of ischaemic ulcers were observed in about 40% out of 65 treated patients [161,257]. PGI_2 has also been found effective in thrombangitis obliterans [257] and in Raynaud's syndrome [248]. Indeed, the latter and another similar trial have been recently reported by Prentice et al. [247,248] as the first double blind studies on the effectiveness of PGI_2 in treatment of peripheral vascular disease. Controlled clinical trials are essential since efficacy of the therapy with PGI_2 in open clinical trials depends critically on the selection of patients [257]. Patients with spontaneous platelet aggregation [261] or with proximal localization of atheromata in the arterial tree as well as patients with gangrene [257] will not respond to the treatment with PGI_2. The duration of the PGI_2 infusion may be of importance. Initial suppression of platelet activity [257,262] is followed by a paradoxical enhancement of platelet activity that appears towards the end of a prolonged infusion of PGI_2 into patients with peripheral vascular disease [263,264]. Also the initial activation by PGI_2 of the fibrinolytic system is observed to disappear [158]. Paradoxical behaviour of platelets is probably caused by desensitization of platelet adenylate cyclase subsequently to its protracted exposure to the action of pharmacological concentrations of PGI_2 [265].

The mechanism of beneficial therapeutic action of PGI_2 in ischaemia resulting from vascular diseases is not clear. Our hypothesis [268–271] that atherosclerosis is a disease associated with a deficiency of PGI_2 constitutes a rationale for clinical trials of PGI_2 in vascular diseases associated with atherosclerosis and its thrombotic complications. PGI_2 deficiency can result from intoxication of endothelial PGI_2 synthetase by lipid peroxides [30] which most likely abide in low-density lipoproteins (LDL) of subjects with hyperlipoproteinemia [271]. Indeed, a diminished generation of PGI_2 has been observed not only in arteries of animals with experimental atherosclerosis [268–271] but also in human atherosclerotic arteries [272]. Administered into rabbits which are fed an atherogenic diet, PGI_2 prevents the development of atherosclerosis [273]. We consider the infusions of PGI_2 into patients with atherosclerosis as a substitution therapy, even though the precise mechanism of PGI_2 effectiveness remains unknown. PGE_1 is also effective in the treatment of patients with peripheral vascular disease [274].

The therapeutic potency of PGI_2 in ischaemic heart disease has not as yet been well assessed. On the basis of open clinical trials it appears that in patients with exercise angina pectoris PGI_2 is ineffective in preventing pain and ischaemic changes in ECG which occur during atrial pacing. However, in 5 out of 11 patients with spontaneous angina (including Printzmetal angina) intravenous infusion of PGI_2 reduced a daily nitroglycerine intake [244,257]. In another trial PGI_2 was ineffective in two patients with spontaneous angina [275].

Central retinal vein occlusion is another vascular disease which has been treated with PGI_2. PGI_2 (5 ng/kg/min, i.v. 72 h of continuous infusion) was administered at first to 3 patients [249] and then to another 8 patients [276] with central retinal vein occlusion. Given 24–72 h after a sudden loss of vision, PGI_2 ameliorated visual acuity, caused disappearance of hemorrhages, resorption of edema of fundus, and straightened up the tortuosity of retinal blood vessels (7 patients). Administered at a later stage of the disease PGI_2 had little effect on its natural development. The observation period after the treatment with PGI_2 was 3–12 months. During this time no secondary complications (glaucoma, maculopathia) were observed in 7 responders to the PGI_2 therapy. Another group of 10 patients with central retinal vein occlusion were treated in a typical way (anti-inflammatory drugs, vasodilators, vitamins). In only one of 10 patients the therapeutic effect was comparable to that observed in 7 out of 11 patients who had been treated with PGI_2 [276].

Most challenging is the study of effectiveness of PGI_2 in patients with acute cerebral ischaemia due to thrombotic occlusion of the internal carotid artery that shows up as hemiplegia [250]. In this study the dosage of PGI_2 was reduced to 2.5 ng/kg/min i.v. and the time of infusion was shortened to 6 hours divided into 5–8 courses of treatment. The results of the clinical trial of 10 patients will be soon published.

In patients with secondary pulmonary hypertension PGI_2 in doses of 2.5–10.0 ng/kg/min i.v. for 30 min was found to reduce significantly pulmonary wedge resistance and total pulmonary resistance. The duration of this effect was limited to the period of infusion [232,257]. A similar pharmacological effect in patients with secondary pulmonary hypertension was reported for PGE_1 [277]. PGI_2 or PGE_1 were also successfully used in children with idiopathic pulmonary artery stenosis or vasoconstriction [278,279]. Pharmacological manipulations of neonatal circulation with PGI_2, PGE_1 and PGE_2 as well as with cyclo-oxygenase inhibitors were recently reviewed by Coceani [280].

Intravenous infusions of PGI_2 were also tried in a few patients with hemolytic uremic syndrome [281], with thrombotic thrombocytopenia purpura [282] and with preeclamptic toxemia [283]. The experience of these few patients suggests that the controlled evaluation of PGI_2 in the treatment of those diseases is warranted.

Leithner et al. [284] have recently treated with PGI_2 (5 ng/kg/min i.v. for 5 days) 8 patients with chronic kidney transplant rejection. In the majority of cases this treatment improves the function of the transplant. In presensitized dogs PGI_2 suppressed the hyperacute allograft rejection [285] and in rats PGI_2 had a definite beneficial effect in prolonging survival of cardiac allografts [286]. The mechanism of this action is not clear but inhibition of the platelet release reaction and suppression of platelet clumping in the microcirculation of the grafts is likely to be of importance.

In a series of clinical trials with PGI_2 in the cardiopulmonary bypass in man, it has been shown [287–289] that PGI_2 significantly preserves platelet count and function and it potentiates the anticoagulant action of heparin when extracorporeal circulation is being maintained. These two effects of PGI_2 may well lead to reduction of postoperative blood loss and to prevention of formation of microemboli. The cardiovascular effects of PGI_2 are easily managed during surgery. The way to these clinical trials was paved by an experimental use of PGI_2 during hemodialysis [290] and cardiopulmonary bypass [291] in dogs. Similarly, laboratory data on the effect of PGI_2 on the formation of platelet aggregates and on the improvement of hemocompatibility during charcoal hemoperfusion [292] enabled the use of PGI_2 in humans in the course of treatment of fulminant hepatic failure with charcoal hemoperfusion [293].

Headache is one of the most common side effects which may occur during intravenous infusion of PGI_2. It usually appears at doses higher than 5 ng/kg/min. Headache disappears if the infusion rate is reduced. Some patients can tolerate PGI_2 at a dose of 10 ng/kg/min without headache. The most consistent but less annoying side effect is facial flush which occurs practically in all patients treated with PGI_2 along intravenous, intraarterial or inhalatory routes. Flushing of palms and feeling of warmth are also quite common. Restlessness, uneasiness and drowsiness are experienced by some patients. Typical cardiovascular effects of PGI_2 consist of a modest hypotension and blunted tachycardia. Overdosage of PGI_2 may result in a sudden drop of arterial blood pressure associated with bradycardia and fainting. We have never seen this type of side effect in our 167 patients who were treated for various reasons with PGI_2 at a dose range of 2–10 ng/kg/min i.v. A paradoxical rise in arterial blood pressure was observed in 6 out of 167 patients receiving PGI_2. Three of these subjects had a history of untreated severe arterial hypertension. In patients with a history of myocardial ischaemic disease infusions of PGI_2 may cause chest pain, and ectopic beats may appear in their ECG. Cardiac side effects of PGI_2 were relatively rare and appeared in 9 of our patients. In patients with ischaemic ulceration pain may occur during the period of infusion of PGI_2, yet finally, PGI_2 will relieve patients of rest pain.

Another local pain which is quite frequently evoked by PGI_2 is the jaw articular pain that is aggravated by chewing. The hyperglycemic effect of PGI_2 should be anticipated in patients with diabetes. The effect of PGI_2 on carbohydrate metabolism is readily reversible after termination of the infusion of PGI_2. We hardly observed in our patients any gastrointestinal disturbances during intravenous infusions of PGI_2, apart from a rare occurrence of nausea. The highest rate of intravenous infusion of PGI_2 that is presently being used in our studies is 7.5 ng/kg/min, although most frequently doses of 2.5–5.0 ng/kg/min are sufficient to obtain a therapeutic effect. In a vast majority of patients the above described side effects of PGI_2, if they appear, are readily tempered by adjustment of the rate of the drug infusion.

The above discussed side effects which may occur during the course of administration of PGI_2 to man are listed on the basis of our published [156,157,161,169,192,195,257] and unpublished clinical observations as well as those of the Wellcome group [139,294].

In conclusion, open clinical trials have led to double blind studies with PGI_2 in the treatment of peripheral vascular diseases including arteriosclerosis obliterans, thrombangitis obliterans and Raynaud's syndrome, unstable angina pectoris including Prinzmetal angina, ischaemic stroke, retinal vein occlusion and renal transplants. The usefulness of therapy with PGI_2 deserves to be evaluated in hemolytic uremic syndrome, thrombotic thrombocytopenia purpura and preeclamptic toxemia. Heparin-sparing effect of PGI_2 in extracorporeal circulation is well established.

Side effects of therapy with PGI_2 do not constitute serious clinical problems, although experienced and highly qualified staff is required to run these clinical trials.

Looking to the future one may say that the pioneer clinical trials with PGI_2 have opened the door of the clinic to stable analogs of PGI_2, to drugs which release endogenous PGI_2 and to thromboxane synthetase inhibitors.

Acknowledgements

This review was supported in part by a grant from the Medical Research Council of Canada (MT 4181).

References

1 Granström, E., Lands, W.E.M. and Samuelsson, B. (1968) J. Biol. Chem. 243, 4104–4108.
2 Pace-Asciak, C. and Wolfe, L.S. (1970) J. Chem. Soc. Chem. Commun., 1234.
3 Pace-Asciak, C. and Wolfe, L.S. (1970) J. Chem. Soc. Chem. Commun. 1235.
4 Pace-Asciak, C. and Wolfe, L.S. (1971) Biochemistry 10, 3657–3663.
5 Pace-Asciak, C. (1971) Biochemistry 10, 3664–3669.
6 Pace-Asciak, C. (1972) Biochim. Biophys. Acta, 280, 161–171.
7 Pace-Asciak, C. (1972) Adv. Biosci., 9, 29–33.
8 Pace-Asciak, C. and Nashat, M. (1976) Biochim. Biophys. Acta 424, 323–325.
9 Pace-Asciak, C. (1976) Presented at the Winter Conference on Prostaglandins, Vail, Colorado, January 24–27.
10 Pace-Asciak, C. (1976) J. Am. Chem. Soc. 98, 2348–2349.
11 Pace-Asciak, C. (1976) Experientia 32, 291–292.
12 Pace-Asciak, C. and Nashat, M. (1976) Proc. Can. Fed. Biol. Soc. 19, 268.
13 Pace-Asciak, C. and Nashat, M. (1976) J. Neurochem. 27, 551–556.
14 Moncada, S., Gryglewski, R.J., Bunting, S. and Vane, J.R. (1976) Nature 263, 663–665.
15 Johnson, R.A., Morton, D.R., Kinner, J.H., Gorman, R.R., McGuire, J.C., Sun, F.F., Whittaker, N., Bunting, S., Salmon, J., Moncada, S. and Vane, J.R. (1976) Prostaglandins 12, 915–928.
16 Sih, C. and Huang, F-C. (1978) J. Am. Chem. Soc. 100, 643–645.
17 Sih, J. and Graber, J. (1978) J. Org. Chem. 43, 3798–3800.
18 Gorman, R.R., Bunting, S. and Miller, O.V. (1977) Prostaglandins 13, 377–388.
19 Johnson, R.A., Lincoln, F.H., Nidy, E.G., Schneider, W.P., Thompson, J.L. and Axen, U. (1978) J. Am. Chem. Soc. 100, 7690–7705.
20 Chiang, Y., Kresge, A.J. and Cho, M.J. (1979) J. Chem. Soc. Chem. Commun. 129–130.
21 Pace-Asciak, C.R. and Carrara, M.C. (1979) in Prostacyclin (Vane, J.R. and Bergstrom, S., eds.) pp. 103–112, Raven Press, New York.
22 Needleman, P., Raz, A., Minkes, M.S., Ferrendelli, J.A. and Sprecher, H. (1979) Proc. Natl. Acad. Sci. USA 76, 944–948.
23 Wong, P.Y-K., Lee, W.H., Chao, P.H-W., Reiss, R.F. and McGiff, J.C. (1980) J. Biol. Chem. 255, 9021–9024.
24 Hamberg, M. and Samuelsson, B. (1973) Proc. Natl. Acad. Sci. USA 70, 899–903.
25 Nugteren, D.H. and Hazelhof, E. (1973) Biochim. Biophys. Acta 326, 448–461.
26 Samuelsson, B. (1965) J. Am. Chem. Soc. 87, 3011–3013.
27 Pace-Asciak, C. and Nashat, M. (1977) Biochim. Biophys. Acta 487, 495–507.
28 Pace-Asciak, C. and Carrara, M.C. (1978) Prostaglandins 16, 397–410.
29 Fried, G and Just, G. Discussion published in Prostaglandins (1976) 11, 433.
30 Gryglewski, R.J., Bunting, S., Moncada, S., Flower, R.J. and Vane, J.R. (1976) Prostaglandins 12, 685–714.
31 Pace-Asciak, C. and Rangaraj, G. (1977) Biochim. Biophys. Acta 486, 583–585.
32 Powell, W. and Solomon, S. (1977) Biochem. Biophys. Res. Commun. 75, 815–822.
33 Sun, F.F. and McGuire, J.C. (1978) in Adv. Prostagl. Thromb. Res. Vol. 4 (Coceani, F. and Olley, P.M., eds.) pp. 75–85, Raven Press, New York.
34 Terragno, N.A., Terragno, A., McGiff, J.C. and Rodriguez, D.J. (1977) Prostaglandins 14, 721–727.
35 Terragno, N.A., McGiff, A. and McGiff, J.C. (1978) Clin. Res. 26, 545A.

36 Skidgel, R.A. and Printz, M.P. (1978) Prostaglandins 16, 1–16.
37 Wolfe, L.S., Rostworoski, K. and Manku, M. (1979) in Prostacyclin (Vane, J.R. and Bergstrom, S., eds.) pp. 113–118, Raven Press, New York.
38 Villa, S. and de Gaetano, G. (1977) Prostaglandins 14, 1117–1124.
39 Bunting, S., Gryglewski, R.J., Moncada, S. and Vane, J.R. (1976) Prostaglandins 12, 897–913.
40 MacIntyre, D.E., Pearson, J.D. and Gordon, J.L. (1978) Nature 271, 549–551.
41 Weksler, B.B., Marcus, A.J. and Jaffe, E.A. (1977) Proc. Natl. Acad. Sci. USA 74, 3922–3926.
42 Christofinis, G.J., Moncada, S., Bunting, S. and Vane, J.R. (1979) in Prostacyclin (Vane, J.R. and Bergstrom, S., eds.) pp. 77–84, Raven Press, New York.
43 Tansik, R.L., Namm, D.H. and White, H.L. (1978) Prostaglandins 15, 399–408.
44 Silberbauer, K., Sinzinger, H. and Winter, M. (1978) Lancet i, 1356–1357.
45 Fitzpatrick, F.A., Stringfellow, D.A., Maclouf, J. and Rigaud, M. (1979) in Prostacyclin (Vane, J.R. and Bergstrom, S., eds.) pp. 55–64, Raven Press, New York.
46 Chang, W-C., Murota, S., Matsuko, M. and Tsurufuji, S. (1976) Biochem. Biophys. Res. Commun. 72, 1259–1264.
47 Baezinger, N.L., Dillander, M.J. and Majerus, P.W. (1977) Biochem. Biophys. Res. Commun. 78, 294–301.
48 Raz, A., Isakson, P.C., Minkes, M.S. and Needleman, P. (1977) J. Biol. Chem. 252, 1123–1126.
49 De Deckere, E.A.M., Nugteren, D.H. and Ten Hoor, F. (1977) Nature 268, 160–162.
50 Dawson, W., Boot, J., Cockerill, A., Mallen, D. and Osborne, D. (1976) Nature 262, 699–702.
51 Gryglewski, R.J., Korbut, R. and Ocetkiewicz, A. (1978) Nature 273, 765–767.
52 Hensby, C.N., Barnes, P.J., Dollery, C.T. and Dargie, H. (1979) Lancet, 1162–1163.
53 Edlund, A., Bomfim, W., Kaijser, L., Olin, C., Patrono, C., Pinca, E. and Wennmalm, A. (1981) Prostaglandins 22, 323–332.
54 Pace-Asciak, C.R. and Rangaraj, G. (1978) Biochim. Biophys. Acta 486, 579–582.
55 Pace-Asciak, C.R. and Rangaraj, G. (1978) Biochim. Biophys. Acta. 529, 13–20
56 Moncada, S., Herman, A.G., Higgs, E.A. and Vane, J.R. (1977) Thromb. Res. 11, 323–344.
57 Whorton, A.R., Smigel, M., Oates, J.A. and Frolich, J.C. (1978) Biochim. Biophys. Acta 529, 176–180.
58 Larsson, C. and Anggard, E. (1973) Eur. J. Pharmacol. 21, 30–36.
59 Hassid, A. and Dunn, M.J. (1980) J. Biol. Chem. 255, 2472–2475.
60 Oliw, E., Lunden, I., Sjoquist, B. and Anggard, E. (1979) Acta Physiol. Scand. 105, 359–366.
61 Sraer, J., Siess, W., Moulonguet-Doleris, L., Oudinet, J-P., Dray, F. and Andaillou, R. (1982) Biochim. Biophys. Acta 710, 45–52.
62 Terragno, N.A., Terragno, A., Early, J.A., Roberts, M.A. and McGiff, J.C. (1978) Clin. Sci. Mol. Med. 55, 199s–202s.
63 DeWitt, D.L. and Smith, W.L. (1983) J. Biol. Chem., in press.
64 Smith, W.L., DeWitt, D.L. and Day, J.S. (1983) In Prostagl. Thrombox. Leukotr. Res. Vol. 11 (Samuelsson, B. and Paoletti, R., eds) Raven Press, New York, pp. 87–92.
65 Goehlert, U.G., Ng Ying Kin, N.M.K. and Wolfe, L.S. (1981) J. Neurochem. 36, 1192–1201.
66 Gaudet, R.J., Alam, I. and Levine, L. (1980) J. Neurochem. 35, 653–658.
67 Abdel-Halim, M.S., Lunden, I., Cseh, G. and Anggard, E. (1980) Prostaglandins 19, 249–258.
68 Hagin, A.A., White, R.P. and Robertson, J.T. (1979) Stroke 10, 306–309.
69 Maurer, P., Moskowitz, M.A., Levine, L. and Melomed, E. (1980) Prostaglandins Med. 4, 153–161.
70 Gerritsen, M.E. and Printz, M.P. (1981) Prostaglandins 22, 553–566.
71 Abdel-Halim, M.S., von Holst, H., Meyerson, B., Sachs, C. and Anggard, E. (1980) J. Neurochem. 34, 1331–1333.
72 Cottee, F., Flower, R.J., Moncada, S., Salmon, J.A. and Vane, J.R. (1977) Prostaglandins 14, 413–423.
73 Salmon, J.A., Smith, D.R., Flower, R.J., Moncada, S. and Vane, J.R. (1978) Biochim. Biophys. Acta 523, 250–262.
74 Chang, W.C. and Murota, S. (1977) Biochim. Biophys. Acta 486, 136–144.
75 Carpenter, M. (1981) Fed. Proc. 40, 189–194.

76 Moncada, S., Salmon, J.A., Vane, J.R. and Whittle, B. (1977) J. Physiol. 275, 4–5P.
77 Peskar, B.M., Seyberth, H.W. and Peskar, B.A. (1980) Adv. Prostagl. Thrombox. Res. Vol. 8 (Samuelsson, B., Ramwell, P.W. and Paoletti, R., eds.) pp. 1511–1514, Raven Press, New York.
78 LeDuc, L.E. and Needleman, P. (1980) Adv. Prostagl. Thrombox. Res. Vol. 8 (Samuelsson, B., Ramwell, P.W. and Paoletti, R., eds.) pp. 1515–1517, Raven Press, New York.
79 Hamberg, M., Tuvemo, T., Svensson, J. and Jonsson, C-E. (1979) Acta Physiol. Scand. 106, 289–292.
80 Fenwick, L., Jones, R.L., Naylor, B., Poyser, N.L. and Wilson, N.H. (1977) Br. J. Pharmacol. 59, 191–199.
81 Mitchell, M.D., Ellwood, D.A., Anderson, A.B.M. and Turnbull, A.C. (1978) Prostaglandins Med. 1, 265–266.
82 Zamecnik, J., Kennedy, T.G. and Armstrong, D.T. (1980) Adv. Prostagl. Thrombox. Res. Vol. 8 (Samuelsson, B., Ramwell, P.W. and Paoletti, R., eds.) pp. 1423–1429, Raven Press, New York.
83 Bult, H., Wechsung, E., Houvenaghel, A. and Herman, A.G. (1981) Prostaglandins 21, 1045–1058.
84 Claeys, M., Wechsung, E., Herman, A. and Nugteren, D.H. (1981) Prostaglandins 21, 739–749.
85 Moncada, S., Gryglewski, R.J., Bunting, S. and Vane, J.R. (1976) Prostaglandins 12, 715–734.
86 Salmon, J.A., Smith, D.R., Flower, R.J. Moncada, S. and Vane, J.R. (1978) Biochim. Biophys. Acta 523, 250–252.
87 Okuma, M., Takayama, H. and Uchino, H. (1980) Prostaglandins 19, 527–536.
88 Chan, A.C. and Leith, M.K. (1981) Am. J. Clin. Nutr. 34, 2341–2347.
89 Gryglewski, R.J., Dembinska-Kiec, A., Zmuda, A. and Gryglewska, T. (1978) Atherosclerosis 31, 385–394.
90 Dollery, C.T., Friedman, L.A., Hensby, C.N., Kohner, E., Lewis, P.J., Porta, M. and Webster, J. (1979) Lancet ii, 1365.
91 Stuart, M.J., Sunderji, S.G. and Allen, J.B. (1981) J. Lab. Clin. Med. 98, 412–416.
92 Johnson, M., Harrison, H.E., Raftery, A.T. and Elder, J.B. (1979) Lancet i, 325.
93 Pace-Asciak, C.R., Carrara, M.C., Rangaraj, G. and Nicolaou, K.C. (1978) Prostaglandins 15, 1005–1012.
94 Pace-Asciak, C.R. and Carrara, M.C. (1978) Biochim. Biophys. Acta 574, 177–181.
95 Okuma, M., Takayama, H. and Uchino, H. (1981) Prostaglandins 19, 527–536.
96 Gryglewski, R.J., Bunting, S., Moncada, S., Flower, R.J. and Vane, J.R. (1976) Prostaglandins 12, 685–713.
97 Fitzpatrick, F.A., Bundy, G.L., Gorman, R.R. and Honohan, T. (1978) Nature 275, 764–766.
98 Terashita, Z., Nishikawa, K., Terao, S., Nakagawa, M. and Hino, T. (1979) Biochem. Biophys. Res. Commun. 91, 72–78.
99 Needleman, P., Bronson, S.D., Wyche, A., Sivakoff, M. and Nicolaou, K.C. (1978) J. Clin. Invest. 61, 839–849.
100 Dusting, G.J. (1981) J. Cardiovasc. Pharmacol. 3, 197–206.
101 Dusting, G.J. and Mullins, E.M. (1980) Clin. Exp. Pharmac. Physiol. 7, 545–550.
102 Mullane, K.M. and Moncada, S. (1980) Eur. J. Pharmacol. 66, 355–365.
103 Dusting, G.J., Moncada, S. and Vane, J.R. (1978) Br. J. Pharmacol. 64, 315–320.
104 Armstrong, J.M., Lattimer, N., Moncada, S. and Vane, J.R. (1978) Br. J. Pharmacol. 62, 125–130.
105 Pace-Asciak, C.R., Carrara, M.C. and Nicolaou, K.C. (1978) Prostaglandins 15, 999–1004.
106 Pace-Asciak, C.R., Rosenthal, A. and Domazet, Z. (1979) Biochim. Biophys. Acta 574, 182–186.
107 Sun, F.F. and Taylor, B.M. (1981) Prostaglandins 21, 307–314.
108 McGuire, J.C. and Sun, F.F. (1978) Arch. Biochem. Biophys. 189, 92–96.
109 Sun, F.F. and Taylor, B.M. (1978) Biochemistry 19, 4096–4101.
110 Sun, F.F., Taylor, B.M., Sutter, D.M. and Weeks, J.R. (1979) Prostaglandins 17, 753–759.
111 Pace-Asciak, C.R., Carrara, M.C. and Domazet, Z. (1977) Biochem. Biophys. Res. Commun. 78, 115–121.
112 Hawkins, H.J., Smith, J.B., Nicolaou, K.C. and Eling, T. (1978) Prostaglandins 16, 871–884.
113 Pace-Asciak, C.R., Domazet, Z. and Carrara, Z. (1977) Biochim. Biophys. Acta 487, 400–404.
114 Korff, J.M. and Jarabak, J. (1981) Prostaglandins 21, 719–725.
115 Wong, P.Y-K., Lee, W.H., Chao, P.H-W., Reiss, R.F. and McGiff, J.C. (1980) J. Biol. Chem. 255, 9021–9024.

116 Pace-Asciak, C. (1975) J. Biol. Chem. 250, 2789–2794.
117 Wong, P.Y-K., McGiff, J.C., Sun, F.F. and Malik, K.U. (1978) Biochem. Biophys. Res. Commun. 83, 731–738.
118 Wong, P.Y-K., Malik, K.U., Desiderio, D.M., McGiff, J.C. and Sun, F.F. (1980) Biochem. Biophys. Res. Commun. 93, 486–494.
119 Yuan, B., Tai, C.L. and Tai, H.H. (1980) J. Biol. Chem. 255, 7439–7443.
120 Miller, O.V., Aiken, J.W., Shebuski, R.J. and Gorman, R.R. (1980) Prostaglandins 20, 391–400.
121 Mitchell, M.D., Anderson, A.B.M., Brunt, J.D., Clover, L., Ellwood, D.A., Robinson, J.S. and Turnbull, A.C. (1979) J. Endocr. 83, 141–148.
122 Ylikorkala, O. and Viinikka, L. (1981) Prostaglandins and Medicine 7, 95–99.
123 Bolton, P.J., Jogee, M. and Myatt, L. (1981) Br. J. Obstet. Gynaecol. 88, 1101–1103.
124 Fitzgerald, G.A., Brash, A.R., Falardeau, P. and Oates, J.A. (1981) J. Clin. Invest. 68, 1272–1276.
125 Ylikorkala, O., Makila, U-M. and Viinikka, L. (1981) Amer. J. Obstet. Gynecol. 141, 487–490.
126 Bodzenta, A., Thomson, J.M. and Poller, L. (1980) Lancet, 650.
127 Zamecnik, J., Kennedy, T.G. and Armstrong, D.T. (1980 in Adv. Prostagl. Thrombox. Res. (Samuelsson, B., Ramwell, P.W. and Paoletti, R. eds) Vol. 8, pp. 1423–1429, Raven Press, New York.
128 Abdel-Halim, M.S., Ekstedt, J. and Anggard, E. (1979) Prostaglandins 17, 405–409.
129 Maurer, P., Moskowitz, M.A., Levine, L. and Melamed, E. (1980) Prostaglandins Med. 4, 153–161.
130 Haslam, R.J. and McClenaghan, M.D. (1981) Nature 292, 364–366.
131 Machleidt, C., Foerstermann, U., Anhut, H. and Hertting, G. (1981) Eur. J. Pharmacol. 74, 19–26.
132 Roy, A.C. and Karim, S.M.M. (1981) IRCS Med. Sci. 9, 616–617.
133 Hensby, C.N., Fitzgerald, G.A., Friedman, L.A., Lewis, P.J. and Dollery, C.T. (1979) Prostaglandins 18, 731–736.
134 Blair, I.A., Barrow, S.E., Waddell, K.A., Lewis, P.J. and Dollery, C.T. (1982) Prostaglandins, 23, 579–589.
135 Demers, L.M., Harrison, T.S., Halbert, D.R. and Santen, R.J. (1981) Prostaglandins Med. 6, 413–418.
136 Bult, H., Beetens, J. and Herman, A.G. (1980) Eur. J. Pharmacol. 63, 47–56.
137 Mitchell, M.D. (1978) Prostaglandins Med. 1, 13–21.
138 LaTorre, E., Patrono, C., Fortuna, A. and Grossi-Belloni, D. (1974) J. Neurosurg. 41, 293–299.
139 Wolfe, L.S. and Mamer, O. (1975) Prostaglandins 9, 183–192.
140 Egg, D., Herold, M., Rumpl, E. and Günther, R. (1980) J. Neurol. 222, 239–248.
141 Morris, H.G., Sherman, N.A. and Shepperdson, F.T. (1981) Prostaglandins 21, 771–788.
142 Gullner, H-G., Bryan Smith, J. and Bartter, F.C. (1980) in Adv. Prostagl. Thrombox. Res. Vol. 7 (Samuelsson, B., Ramwell, P.W. and Paoletti, R., eds) pp. 1185–1187, Raven Press, New York.
143 MacKenzie, I.Z., MacLean, D.A. and Mitchell, M.D. (1980) Prostaglandins 20, 649–654.
144 Smith, W.L., Grenier, F.C., DeWitt, D.L., Garcia-Perez, A. and Bell, T.G. (1982) in Prostaglandins and the Kidney; Biochemistry, Pharmacology and Clinical Applications (Dunn, M.J., Patrono, C. and Cinotti, G., eds) pp. 27–39, Plenum Press, New York.
145 Wlodawer, P. and Hammarstrom, S. (1980) Prostaglandins 19, 969–976.
146 Watanabe, K., Yamamoto, S. and Hayaishi, O. (1979) Biochem. Biophys. Res. Commun. 87, 192–199.
147 Moncada, S. and Vane, J.R. (1979) Agents Actions (Suppl.) 38, 66–71.
148 Gryglewski, R.J. (1980) AAS 7, 247–251.
149 Marcus, A.J., Broekman, M.J., Weksler, B.B., Jaffe, E.A., Safier, L.B., Ullman, H.L. and Tack-Goldman, K. (1981) Phil. Trans, R. Soc. Lond. Ser. B. 294, 343–353.
150 Szczeklik, A. (1981) in Prostaglandins, Platelets, Lipids: New Dev. Atheroscler. (Conn, H.L. Jr., De Felice, E. and Kuo, P.T., eds.) pp. 119–130, Spectrum Publ.
151 Moncada, S. and Vane, J.R. (1981) Phil. Trans. R. Soc. Lond. Ser. B. 294, 305–329.
152 Neri-Serneri, G.G., Masotti, G., Grensini, G.F., Abbate, R., Poggesi, L., Galanti, G. and Favilla, S. (1981) Atheroscler. Rev. 8, 139–157.
153 Needleman, P. (1979) Nature 279, 14–15.

154 Hornstra, G., Haddeman, E. and Don, J.A. (1979) Nature 279, 66–68.
155 Sinzinger, H., Clopath, P., Silberbauer, K. and Winter, M. (1980) Experientia 36, 321–323.
156 Szczeklik, A. and Gryglewski, R.J. (1979) in Prostacyclin (Vane, J.R. and Bergström, S., eds.) pp. 393–407, Raven Press, New York.
157 Szczeklik, A., Gryglewski, R.J., Nizankowski, R., Musial, J., Pieton, R. and Mruk, J. (1978) Pharmacol. Res. Commun. 10, 545–556.
158 Dembinska-Kiec, A., Kostka-Trabka, E. and Gryglewski, R.J. (1982) Thromb. Haemost. 47, 190.
159 Utsunomiya, T., Krausz, M.M., Valeri, C.R., Shepro, D. and Hechtman, H.B. (1980) Surgery 88, 25–30.
160 Szczeklik, A., Nizankowski, R., Skawinski, S., Gluszko, P. and Gryglewski, R.J. (1979) Lancet i, 1111–1114.
161 Szczeklik, A. and Gryglewski, R.J. (1981) in Clinical Pharmacology of Prostacyclin (Lewis, P.J. and O'Grady, J., eds.) pp. 159–167, Raven Press, New York.
162 Robert, A. (1980) in Adv. Prostaglandin Thromboxane Res. Vol. 8 (Samuelsson, B., Ramwell, P.W. and Paoletti, R., eds.) pp. 1533–1541, Raven Press, New York.
163 Whittle, B.J.R., Boughton-Smith, N.K., Moncada, S. and Vane, J.R. (1978) Prostaglandins 15, 955–967.
164 Whorton, A.R., Lazar, J.D., Smigel, M.D., and Oates, J.A. (1980) in Adv. Prostaglandin Thromboxane Res. Vol. 7 (Samuelsson, B., Ramwell, P.W. and Paoletti, R., eds.) pp. 1123–1129, Raven Press, New York.
165 Olson, R.D., Skoglund, M.L., Nies, A.S. and Gerber, J.G. (1980) in Adv. Prostaglandin Thromboxane Res. Vol. 7 (Samuelsson, B., Ramwell, P.W. and Paoletti, R., eds.) pp. 1135–1137, Raven Press, New York.
166 Schwertschlag, U., Stahl, T. and Hackenthal, E. (1982) Prostaglandins 23, 129–138.
167 Whorton, A.R., Lazar, J.D., Smigel, M.D. and Oates, J.A. (1981) Prostaglandins 22, 455–468.
168 Pasargiklian, M. and Bianco, S. (1980) in Adv. Prostaglandin Thromboxane Res. Vol. 7 (Samuelsson, B., Ramwell, P.W. and Paoletti, R., eds.) pp. 943–951, Raven Press, New York.
169 Szczeklik, A., Gryglewski, R.J., Nizankowska, E., Nizankowski, R. and Musial, J. (1978) Prostaglandins 16, 651–660.
170 Pek, S., Lands, W.E.M., Akpan, J. and Hurley, M. (1980) in Adv. Prostaglandin Thromboxane Res. Vol. 8 (Samuelsson, B., Ramwell, P.W. and Paoletti, R., eds.) pp. 1295–1302, Raven Press, New York.
171 Szczeklik, A., Pieton, R., Sieradzki, J. and Nizankowski, R. (1980) Prostaglandins 19, 959–968.
172 Whittle, B.J.R., Moncada, S. and Vane, J.R. (1978) Prostaglandins 16, 373–388.
173 Bussolino, F. and Camussi, G. (1980) Prostaglandins 20, 781–791.
174 Harsfalvi, J., Muszbek, L., Stadler, I. and Fesüs, L. (1980) Prostaglandins 20, 935–945.
175 Tateson, J.R., Moncada, S. and Vane, J.R. (1977) Prostaglandins 13, 389–397.
176 Gorman, R.R., Bunting, S. and Miller, O.V. (1977) Prostaglandins 13, 377–388.
177 Quilley, C.P., McGiff, J.C., Lee, W.H., Sun, F.F. and Wong, P.Y-K. (1980) Hypertension 2, 524–528.
178 MacIntyre, D.E. and Gordon, J.L. (1977) Thromb. Res. 11, 705.
179 Miller, O.V. and Gorman, R.R. (1979) J. Pharmacol. Exp. Ther. 210, 134–140.
180 Siegl, A.M., Smith, J.B. and Silver, M.J. (1979) J. Clin. Invest. 63, 215–220.
181 Best, L.C., Martin, T.J., Russell, R.G.G. and Preston, F.E. (1977) Nature 267, 850–852.
182 Karniguian, A., Legrand, Y.J. and Caen, J.P. (1982) Prostaglandins 23, 437–457.
183 Repin, A. (1982) in Abstracts of the IXth International Congress of Cardiology in Moscow, June 1982.
184 Ehrman, M.L. and Jaffe, E.A. (1980) Prostaglandins 20, 1103–1116.
185 Hawiger, J., Parkinson, S. and Timmons, S. (1980) Nature 283, 195–198.
186 Weber, G., Bianciardi, G., Toti, P. and Sinzinger, H. (1981) Prostaglandins 22, 789–793.
187 Fry, G.L., Czervionke, R.L., Hoak, J.C., Smith, J.B. and Haycraft, P.L. (1980) Blood 55, 271–275.
188 Higgs, E.A., Moncada, S., Vane, J.R., Caen, J.P., Michel, H .and Tobelem, J. (1978) Prostaglandins 16, 17–22.

189 Tschopp, T.B. and Baumgartner, H.R. (1979) Agents and Actions (Suppl.) 4, 156–162.
190 Weiss, H.J. and Turitto, V.T. (1979) Blood 53, 244–250.
191 Cazenave, J.P., Dejana, E., Kinlough-Rathbone, R.L., Richardson, M., Packham, M.A. and Mustard, J.F. (1979) Thromb. Res. 15, 273–279.
192 Gryglewski, R.J., Szczeklik, A. and Nizankowski, R. (1978) Thromb. Res. 13, 153–163.
193 O'Grady, J., Warrington, S., Moti, J., Bunting, S., Flower, R., Fowle, A.S.E., Higgs, E.A. and Moncada, S. (1980) Prostaglandins 19, 319–332.
194 Higgs, E.A., Higgs, G.A., Moncada, S. and Vane, J.R. (1978) Br. J. Pharmacol. 63, 535–539.
195 Ubatuba, F.B., Moncada, S. and Vane, J.R. (1979) Thromb. Diath. Haemorrh. 41, 425–434.
196 Bayer, B.L., Blass, K.E. and Förster, W. (1979) Br. J. Pharmacol. 66, 10–12.
197 Aiken, J.W., Gorman, R.R. and Shebuski, R.J. (1979) Prostaglandins 17, 483–494.
198 Aiken, J.W., Shebuski, R.J. and Gorman, R.R. (1980) in Adv. Prostaglandin Thromboxane Res. Vol. 7 (Samuelsson, B., Ramwell, P.W. and Paoletti, R., eds.) pp. 635–639, Raven Press, New York.
199 Gryglewski, R.J., Korbut, R. and Ocetkiewicz, A. (1978) Nature 273, 765–767.
200 Brandt, R., Dembinska-Kiec, A., Korbut, R., Gryglewski, R.J., Nowak, J. (1982) J. Acta Physiol. Scand. in press.
201 Nowak, J., Radomski, M., Kaijser, L. and Gryglewski, R.J. (1981) Acta Physiol. Scand. 112, 405–411.
202 Gryglewski, R.J., Splawinski, J. and Korbut, R. (1980) in Adv. Prostaglandin Thromboxane Res. Vol. 7 (Samuelsson, B., Ramwell, P.W. and Paoletti, R., eds.) pp. 777–787, Raven Press, New York.
203 Dusting, G.J., Mullins, E.M. and Doyle, A.E. (1980) in Adv. Prostagl. Thromb. Res. Vol. 7 (Samuelsson, B., Ramwell, P.W. and Paoletti, R., eds.) pp. 815–819, Raven Press, New York.
204 Gryglewski, R.J. (1980) Ann. Anest. Frans. 6, 613–619.
205 Gryglewski, R.J., Szczeklik, A., Kostka-Trabka, E. and Zygulska-Mach, H. (1982) in Abstract Book of Vth International Conference on Prostaglandins in Florence, May 1982, p. 593.
206 Aiken, J.W., Shebuski, R.J., Miller, O.V. and Gorman, R. (1981) J. Pharmacol. Exp. Ther. 219, 299–308.
207 Folts, J.D., Crowell, E.P. and Rowe, G.G. (1976) Circulation 54, 365–370.
208 Uchida, Y., Yoshimoto, N. and Murao, S. (1980) Jpn. Circ. J. 44, 163–171.
209 Aiken, J.W. and Shebuski, R.J. (1980) Prostaglandins 19, 629–643.
210 Uchida, Y. and Murao, S. (1979) Jpn. Circ. J. 43, 645–652.
211 Uchida, Y. and Murao, S. (1981) Stroke 12, 786–792.
212 Hornstra, G., Haddeman, E. and Don, J.A. (1979) Nature 279, 66–68.
213 Needleman, P., Wyche, A. and Raz, A. (1979) J. Clin. Invest. 63, 345–349.
214 Nordoy, A., Svensson, B. and Hoak, J.C. (1978) Thromb. Res. 12, 597–608.
215 Tansik, R.L., Namm, D.H and White, H.L. (1978) Prostaglandins 15, 399–408.
216 Marcus, A.J., Broekman, M.J., Weksler, B.B., Jafffe, E.A., Safier, L.B., Ullman, H.L. and Tack-Goldman, K. (1982) in Cardiovascular Pharmacology of Prostaglandins (Herman, A.G. et al., eds.) pp. 125–135, Raven Press, New York.
217 Needleman, P., Brouson, S.D. and Wyche, A. (1978) J. Clin. Invest. 61, 839–849.
218 Dusting, G.J., Moncada, S. and Vane, J.R. (1977) Prostaglandins 13, 3–15.
219 Boullin, D.J., Bunting, S., Blaso, W.P., Hunt, T.M. and Moncada, S. (1979) Br. J. Clin. Pharmacol. 7, 139–147.
220 Coceani, F., Bishai, I., White, E., Bodach, E. and Olley, P.M. (1978) Am. J. Physiol. 234, 1117–1122.
221 Sintetos, A.L., Bogler, P.M. and Ramwell, P.W. (1979) in Prostacyclin (Vane, J.R. and Bergström, S., eds.) pp. 269–274, Raven Press, New York.
222 Pomerantz, K., Sintetos, A. and Ramwell, P.W. (1978) Prostaglandins 15, 1035–1044.
223 Levy, J.V. (1978) Prostaglandins 16, 93–97.
224 Raz, A., Isakson, P.C., Minkes, M.S. and Needleman, P. (1977) J. Biol. Chem. 252, 1123–1126.
225 Schrör, K., Moncada, S., Ubatuba, F.B. and Vane, J.R. (1978) Eur. J. Pharmacol. 47, 103–114.
226 De Deckere, E.A.M., Nugteren, D.H. and Ten Hoor, F. (1977) Nature 268, 160–163.
227 Grodzinska, L. and Gryglewski, R.J. (1980) Pharmacol. Res. Commun. 12, 339–347.
228 Weeks, J.R. and DuCharme, S. (1978) in Abstracts of Ist Soviet Union Conference, Prostaglandins in Experimental and Clinical Medicine Moscow, April 1978, pp. 76.

229 Armstrong, J.M., Chapple, D.J., Dusting, G.J., Hughes, R., Moncada, S. and Vane, J.R. (1978) Br. J. Pharmacol. 61, 136P.

230 Kadowitz, P.J., Chapnick, B.M., Feigen, L.P., Hyman, A.L., Nelson, P.K. and Spannhake, E.W. (1978) J. Appl. Physiol. 45, 408–413.

231 Kadowitz, P.J., She, S.S., McNamara, D.B., Spannhake, E.W. and Hyman, A.L. (1982) in Cardiovascular Pharmacology of Prostaglandins (Herman A.G. et al., eds.) pp. 287–302, Raven Press, New York.

232 Szczeklik, J., Szczeklik, A. and Nizankowski, R. (1980) Lancet ii, 1076.

233 Lock, J.E., Coceani, F. and Olley, P.M. (1980) in Adv. Prostaglandins and Thromboxane Res. Vol. 7 (Samuelsson, B., Ramwell, P.W. and Paoletti, R., eds). pp. 751–753, Raven Press, New York.

234 Armstrong, J.M., Lattimer, N., Moncada, S. and Vane, J.R. (1978) Br. J. Pharmacol. 62, 125–130.

235 Dusting, G.J., Moncada, S. and Vane, J.R. (1978) Br. J. Pharmacol. 64, 315–320.

236 Fletcher, J.R. and Ramwell, P.W. (1979) in Prostacyclin (Vane, J.R. and Bergström, S., eds.) pp. 259–267, Raven Press, New York.

237 Lefer, A.M., Ogletree, M.L., Smith, J.B., Silver, M.J., Nicolaou, K.C., Barnette, W.E. and Gasic, G.P. (1978) Science 200, 52–54.

238 Hintze, T., Kaley, G., Martin, E.G. and Messina, E.J. (1978) Prostaglandins 15, 712.

239 Dusting, G.J., Chapple, D.J., Hughes, R., Moncada, S. and Vane, J.R. (1978) Cardiovasc. Res. 12, 720–730.

240 Armstrong, J.M., Chapple, D.J., Dusting, G.J., Hughes, R., Moncada, S. and Vane, J.R. (1977) Br. J. Pharmacol. 61, 136P.

241 Fiedler, V.R. (1982) in Abstract Book of Vth International Conference on Prostaglandins, Florence, May 1982, pp. 273.

242 Jentzer, J.H., Sonnenblick, E.H. and Kirk, E.S. (1979) in Prostacyclin (Vane, J.R. and Bergström, S., eds.) pp. 323–338, Raven Press, New York.

243 Lefer, A.M. and Smith III, E.F. (1979) in Prostacyclin (Vane, J.R. and Bergström, S., eds.) pp. 339–447, Raven Press, New York.

244 Szczeklik, A., Szczeklik, J., Nizankowski, R. and Gluszko, P. (1980) New Engl. J. Med. 303, 881.

245 Araki, H. and Lefer, A.M. (1980) Am. J. Physiol. 238, H176–H181.

246 Giessen, W.J. and Verdouw, P.D. (1982) in Abstract Book of Vth International conference on Prostaglandins, Florence, May 1982, pp. 274.

247 Belch, J.J.F., McKay, A.J., Lowe, C.D.O., McLaren, M., Leiberman, D.P., Pollock, J.G., Forbes, C.D. and Prentice, C.R.M. (1982) in Abstract Book of Vth Int. Conf. Prostagl. Florence, May 1982, pp. 292.

248 Belch, J.J.F., Newman, P., Drury, J.K., Capell, H., Leiberman, P., Forbes, C.D. and Prentice, C.R.M. (1982) in Abstract Book of Vth International Conference on Prostaglandins, Florence, May 1982, pp. 291.

249 Zygulska-Mach, H., Kostka-Trabka, E., Niton, A. and Gryglewski, R.J. (1980) Lancet ii, 1075.

250 Gryglewski, R.J., Nowak, S., Kostka-Trabka, E., Bieron, K., Dembinska-Kiec, A., Btaszczyk, B., Kusmiderski, J., Markowska, E. and Szmatata, S. (1982) Pharmacol. Res. Commun. 14, 879–908.

251 Lefer, A.M., Tabas, J. and Smith, E.F. (1980) Pharmacology 21, 206–212.

252 Krausz, M.M., Utsunomiya, T., Feurstein, G., Shepro, D. and Hechtman, H.B. (1980) Surg. Forum 31, 37–39.

253 Lefer, A.M., Sollott, S.L. and Galvin, M.J. (1979) Prostaglandins 17, 761–767.

254 Bult, H. and Herman, A.G. (1982) in Cardiovasc. Pharmacol. Prostagl. (Herman, A.G. et al., eds.) pp. 327–345, Raven Press, New York.

255 Messina, E.J. and Kaley, G. (1980) in Adv. Prostaglandin Thromboxane Res. Vol. 7 (Samuelsson, B., Ramwell, P.W. and Paoletti, R., eds.) pp. 719–722, Raven Press, New York.

256 Higgs, G.A. (1982) in Cardiovascular Pharmacology of Prostaglandins (Herman, A.G. et al., eds.) pp. 315–325, Raven Press, New York.

257 Szczeklik, A. and Gryglewski, R.J. (1982) in Cardiovascular Pharmacology of Prostaglandins (Herman, A.G. et al., eds.) pp. 347–359, Raven Press, New York.

258 Hallenbeck, J.M. and Furlow, T.W.Jr. (1979) in Prostacyclin (Vane, J.R. and Bergström, S., eds.) pp. 299–310, Raven Press, New York.
259 Smirnov, I.E., Mentz, P.R. and Markov, C.M. (1980) in Adv. Prostaglandin Thromboxane Res. Vol. 7 (Samuelsson, B., Ramwell, P.W. and Paoletti, R., eds.) pp. 631–634, Raven Press, New York.
260 Ito, T., Ogawa, K., Enomoto, J., Hashimoto, H., Kai, J. and Satake, T. (1980) in Adv. Prostaglandin Thromboxane Res. Vol. 7 (Samuelsson, B., Ramwell, P.W. and Paoletti, R., eds.) pp. 641–646, Raven Press, New York.
261 Machin, S.J., Defreyn, S.G., Chamone, D.A.F. and Vermylen, J. (1981) in Clinical Pharmacology of Prostacyclin (Lewis, P.J. and O'Grady, J., eds.) pp. 173, Raven Press, New York.
262 Fitzgerald, G.A., Haviger, J., Oates, J.A. and Roberts, L.J. (1982) in Abstract Book of Vth International Conference on Prostaglandins, Florence, May 1982, p. 308.
263 Sinzinger, H., Silberbauer, K., Horsch, A.K. and Gall, A. (1981) Prostaglandins 21, 49–51.
264 Dembinska-Kiec, A., Zmuda, A., Grodzinska, L., Bieron, K., Basista, M., Kedzior, A., Kostka-Trabka, E., Telesz, E. and Zelazny, T. (1981) Prostaglandins 21, 827–832.
265 Miller, O.V., Brown, W.P., Lund, J.E. and Gorman, R.R. (1982) in Abstract Book of Vth International Conference on Prostaglandins, Florence, May 1982, p. 307.
266 Carlson, L.A. and Eriksson, J. (1973) Lancet i, 155.
267 Carlsson, L.A. and Olsson, A. (1976) Lanct ii, 810.
268 Dembinska-Kiec, A., Gryglewska, T., Zmuda, A. and Gryglewski, R.J. (1977) Prostaglandins 14, 1025–1034.
269 Gryglewski, R.J., Dembinska-Kiec, A., Zmuda, A., Chytkowski, A. and Gryglewska, T. (1978) Atherosclerosis 31, 385–394.
270 Gryglewski, R.J. (1980) CRC Series Biochem. 7, 291–338.
271 Gryglewski, R.J. and Szczeklik, A. (1982) in Cardiovascular Pharmacology Prostaglandins (Herman, A.G. et al., eds.) pp. 215–223, Raven Press, New York.
272 Sinzinger, H., Silberbauer, K. and Feigl, W. (1979) Lancet i, 469–470.
273 Makary, A., Pataki, M., Lusztig, G., Stadler, J. and Virag, S. (1982) in Abstract Book of Vth International Conference on Prostaglandins, Florence, May 1982, p. 224.
274 Carlsson, L.A. (1982) in Abstract Book of Vth International Conference on Prostaglandins, Florence, May 1982, p. 592.
275 Dargie, H.J. and Lewis, P.J. (1981) in Clinical Pharmacology of Prostacyclin (Lewis, P.J. and O'Grady, J., eds.) pp. 177–180, Raven Press, New York.
276 Zygulska-Mach, H., Kostka-Trabka, E. and Gryglewski, R.J. (1982) unpublished observations.
277 Szczeklik, J., Dubiel, J.S., Mysik, M., Krol, R. and Horzela, T. (1978) Br. Heart J. 40, 1397–1401.
278 Lock, J.E., Olley, P.M., Coceani, F., Swyer, P.R. and Rowe, R.D. (1979) Lancet i, 1343.
279 Watkins, W.D., Peterson, M.P., Brone, R.K., Shannon, D.C. and Levin, L. (1980) Lancet i, 1083.
280 Coceani, F. and Olley, P.M. (1982) in Cardiovascular Pharmacology on Prostaglandins (Herman, A.G. et al., eds.) pp. 303–314, Raven Press, New York.
281 Webster, J., Borysiewicz, L.K., Rees, A.J. and Lewis, P.J. (1981) in Clinical Pharmacology of Prostacyclin (Lewis, P.J. and O'Grady, J., eds.) pp. 77–80, Raven Press, New York.
282 Fitzgerald, G.A., Roberts, L.J., Maas, D., Brash, A.R. and Oates, J.A. (1981) in Clinical Pharmacology of Prostacyclin (Lewis, P.J. and O'Grady, J., eds) p. 81, Raven Press, New York.
283 Fidler, J., Ellis, C., Bennett, M.J., deSwiet, M. and Lewis, P.J. (1981) in Clinical Pharmacology of Prostacyclin (Lewis, P.J. and O'Grady, J., eds.) pp. 141–143, Raven Press, New York.
284 Leithner, C., Sinzinger, H. and Schwartz, M. (1981) Prostaglandins 22, 783–788.
285 Mundy, A.R., Bewick, M., Moncada, S. and Vane, J.R. (1980) Prostaglandins 19, 595–604.
286 Shaw, J.F.L. (1982) in Abstract Book of Vth International Conference on Prostaglandins, Florence, May 1982, p. 637.
287 Bunting, S., O'Grady, J., Fabiani, J.N., Terrier, E., Moncada, S., Vane, J.R. and Dubost, Ch. (1981) in Clinical Pharmacology of Prostacyclin (Lewis, P.J. and O'Grady, J., eds.) pp. 181–193, Raven Press, New York.
288 Walker, J.D., Davidson, J.F., Faichney, A., Wheatley, D. and Davidson, K. (1981) in Clinical Pharmacology of Prostacyclin (Lewis, P.J. and O'Grady, J., eds) pp. 195–199, Raven Press, New York.

289 Bennett, J.G., Longmore, D.B. and O'Grady, J. (1981) in Clinical Pharmacology of Prostacyclin (Lewis, P.J. and O'Grady, J., eds.) pp. 201–208, Raven Press, New York.
290 Woods, H.F., Ash, G., Weston, M.J., Bunting, S., Moncada, S. and Vane, J.R. (1978) Lancet ii, 1075.
291 Longmore, D.B., Bennett, G., Gueirrara, D., Smith, M., Bunting, S., Reed, P., Moncada, S., Read, N.G. and Vane, J.R. (1979) Lancet i, 1002.
292 Bunting, S., Moncada, S., Vane, J.R., Woods, H.F. and Weston, M.T. (1979) in Prostacyclin (Vane, J.R. and Bergström, S., eds.) pp. 361–369, Raven Press, New York.
293 Gimson, A.E.S., Canalese, J., Hughes, R.D., Langley, P.G. Mellon, P.J. and Williams, R. (1981) in Clinical Pharmacology of Prostacyclin (Lewis, P.J. and O'Grady, J., eds.) pp. 211–218, Raven Press, New York.
294 O'Grady, J., Warrington, J., Moti, M.J., Bunting, S., Flower, R., Fowle, A.S.E., Higgs, E.A. and Moncada, S. (1979) in Prostacyclin (Vane, J.R. and Bergström, S., eds.) pp. 409–417, Raven Press, New York.
295 Nelson, N.A., Kelly, R.C. and Johnson, R.A. (1982) Chem. Eng. News, Aug 16, 30–44.
296 Pace-Asciak, C.R., Carrara, M.C., Levine, L. and Nicolaou, K.C. (1980) Prostaglandins 20, 1053–1060.
297 Pace-Asciak, C.R., Carrara, M.C. and Levine, L. (1980) Biochim. Biophys. Acta 620, 186–192.
298 Moncada, S., Ferreira, S.H. and Vane, J.R. (1978) in Adv. in Prostaglandin and Thromboxane Research, Vol. 5 (Frolich, J.C., ed.) pp. 211–236, Raven Press, New York.
299 Masotti, G., Poggesi, L., Galanti, G., Trotta, F. and Neri-Serneri, G. (1981) in Clinical Pharmacology of Prostacyclin (Lewis, P.J. and O'Grady, J., eds.) pp. 9–20, Raven Press, New York.
300 Salmon, J.A. (1978) Prostaglandins 15, 383–397.
301 Dighe, K.K., Jones, R.L. and Poyser, N.L. (1978) Proc. Br. Pharmacol. Soc. 406P.
302 Levine, L. and Alam, I. (1979) Prostaglandin Med. 3, 295–304.
303 Dray, F., Gerozissis, K., Kouznetzova, B., Mamas, S., Pradelles, P. and Trugnan, G. (1980) in Adv. Prostaglandin & Thromboxane Research, Vol. 6 (Samuelsson, B., Ramwell, P.W. and Paoletti, R., eds.) pp. 167–180, Raven Press, New York.
304 Pace-Asciak, C.R. (1977) Anal. Biochem. 81, 251–255.
305 Falardeau, P., Oates, J.A. and Brash, A.R. (1981) Anal. Biochem. 115, 359–367.
306 Mitchell, M.D., Brunt, J.D. and Webb, R. (1981) Prostaglandin Med. 6, 437–440.
307 Hutton, R.A. and Chow, F.P.R. (1982) Br. J. Hematol. 51, 327.
308 Moncada, S., Korbut, R., Bunting, S., and Vane, J.R. (1978) Nature 273, 767–769.
309 Neri-Serneri, G.G., Masotti, G., Poggesi, L. and Galanti, G. (1980) Thromb. Res. 17, 197–208.

CHAPTER 4

The leukotrienes and other lipoxygenase products

GÖRAN HANSSON *, CURT MALMSTEN and OLOF RÅDMARK

Department of Physiological Chemistry, Karolinska Institutet, S-104 01 Stockholm, (Present address AB Hässle, S-431 83, Mölndal) Sweden*

1. Introduction

The importance of arachidonic acid as a precursor of regulators and mediators of various cell functions is well recognized [1,2]. Although research was initially focused upon the cyclooxygenase pathway with formation of the prostaglandin endoperoxides (PGG_2, PGH_2), prostaglandin E_2, $F_{2\alpha}$ and D_2, prostacyclin (PGI_2) and thromboxane (TXA_2), an alternate metabolic pathway via a lipoxygenase-catalyzed reaction has recently been demonstrated [3,4]. Thus, lipoxygenase products of arachidonic acid in platelets are known to induce directed movement of leukocytes [5], and the carrageenan-induced leukocyte migration in vivo is stimulated by inhibition of the cyclooxygenase pathway [6].

A major step in the understanding of lipoxygenase metabolism of arachidonic acid and its pathophysiological importance was the discovery of new arachidonate derived metabolites – the leukotrienes and also various hydroxy- and hydroperoxy derivatives (for reviews, see refs. 7–11). In these studies the chemical structure of the slow reacting substance of anaphylaxis (SRS-A) was elucidated [3] and a new understanding of the biochemical mechanisms underlying hypersensitivity reactions and inflammation arrived at. Unlike the prostaglandins and thromboxanes, some of which play important roles as biological regulators, the actions of the lipoxygenase products of arachidonic acid, so far demonstrated, appear to be exclusively of a pathophysiological nature [12].

2. Leukotrienes: classification and nomenclature

The leukotrienes constitute a group of fatty acid derivatives, formed predominantly in various inflammatory cells. Most of the leukotrienes described to date are derived

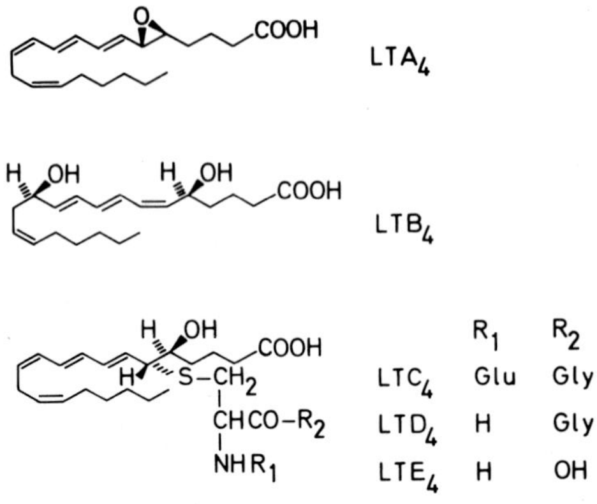

Fig. 1. Structures of the leukotrienes.

from arachidonic acid (5,8,11,14-eicosatetraenoic acid). In this section, the structures of the various leukotrienes are presented, and the nomenclature explained.

The term leukotriene (LT) was introduced for compounds which are non-cyclicized C_{20} carboxylic acid, with one or two oxygen substituents, and three conjugated double bonds. Structurally different leukotrienes are distinguished by capital letters A, B, C, etc. [13]. A subscript denotes the number of double bonds in the structures [14]. More recently another criterion has been added. To be regarded as a leukotriene, the biosynthesis leading to the compound shall involve an allylic epoxide intermediate of the LTA-type [15]. In Fig. 1 the structures of LTA_4, LTB_4, LTC_4, LTD_4 and LTE_4 are given.

To permit denotation of isomerism of leukotrienes, regarding positions of substituents and configurations of double bonds, prefixes are used. As examples; the structures of an isomer of LTA_4 (i.e. 14,15-LTA_4), an isomer of LTB_4 (i.e. 8(S),15(S)-LTB_4), and an isomer of LTE_4 (i.e. 11-trans-LTE_4) are shown in Fig. 2.

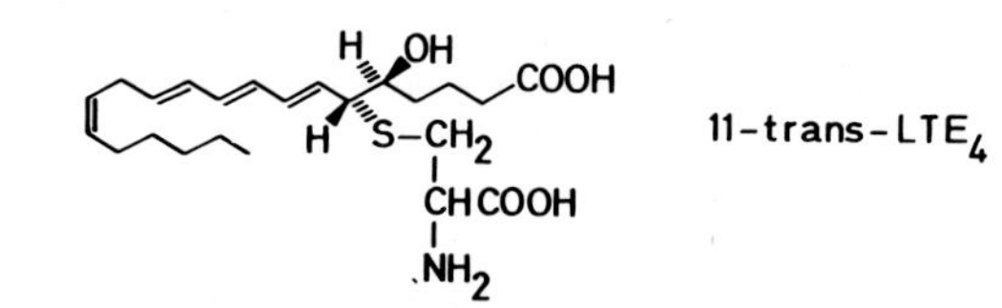

Fig. 2. Structures of some leukotriene isomers.

3. *Biosynthesis of leukotrienes*

In this section, papers concerning the structures and biosynthesis of leukotrienes are reviewed. Initially leukotrienes of the A and B types (oxygen substituents only) are described, while the latter part deals with the leukotrienes of C, D and E types (i.e. amino acid containing compounds with SRS properties).

(a) Leukotrienes of types A and B

The first enzymatic transformation in the biosynthesis of leukotrienes is an oxygenation of the fatty acid substrate, by a lipoxygenase, giving a hydroperoxide. Thus, arachidonic acid can be converted to 5-hydroperoxyeicosatetraenoic acid (5-HPETE)

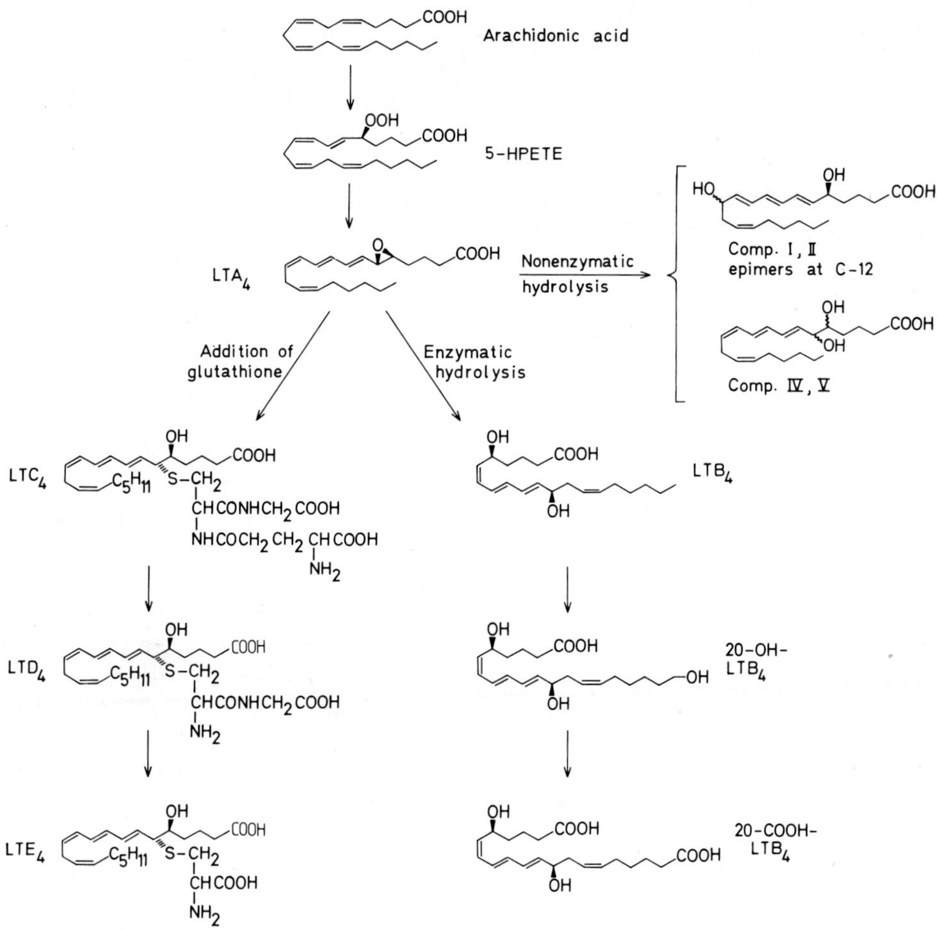

Fig. 3. Leukotriene biosynthesis originating with oxygenation at C-5 of arachidonic acid.

when incubated with rabbit polymorphonuclear leukocytes (PMNL) [16] or human PMNL [17], as demonstrated by the isolation of the corresponding hydroxyacid (5-HETE) from these incubations. The hydroperoxy- and hydroxyacids are discussed further in Section 4. Alternatively to reduction, the hydroperoxy acid can be dehydrated in a reaction (presumably enzymatic), in which one of the hydrogens at C-10 of 5-HPETE is abstracted and the allylic epoxide 5(S)-*trans*-oxido-7,9-*trans*-11,14-cis-eicosatetraenoic acid (LTA_4) is formed (Fig. 3). This is the second transformation in leukotriene biosynthesis. The LTA_4 structure was first described in ref. 18. In this study it was shown that LTA_4 is an unstable compound with a half-life of 2 minutes in a living cell preparation. In a water/acetone mixture of pH 7.4, the half-life increases to 4–5 minutes, whereas the compound is very short-lived under acidic conditions [18]. The detailed structure of LTA_4 was determined by stereochemically controlled organic synthesis of the correct isomer of LTA_4 [19], which is accepted by an enzyme and is converted further to LTB_4 (see below) [20]. LTA_4 can be isolated from cellular incubations as the methyl ester [21], showing that it exists in the cell as a free entity.

The isolation and handling of LTA_4 requires special precautions, since the compound is very sensitive to acid, radicals and oxygen [22]. Thus, it cannot be isolated by acidic extraction to an organic phase, and when chromatographed, stationary and mobile phases should be slightly alkaline [19,21]. LTA_4 exhibits a triplet in the UV spectrum with maxima (in methanol) at 269, 278 and 289 nm. The molar extinction coefficient is 40000 at 278 nm [19]. LTA_4 formation has been demonstrated as such in human PMNL [21] and as methanol-trapping products in rabbit PMNL [13] and in rat basophilic leukemia cells [23]. Additional synthetic approaches leading to LTA_4 and isomers are presented in refs. 22, and 24–30.

From LTA_4, the biosynthetic scheme of the leukotrienes diverges, i.e. LTA_4 can undergo various reactions. When LTA_4 reacts with water, five different compounds arise [18,20,31,32]. One of these results from enzymatic hydrolysis, while the other four are products of non-enzymatic hydrolysis of LTA_4. The product of enzymatic hydrolysis is referred to as LTB_4 with the structure 5(S),12(R)-dihydroxy-6-*cis*-8,10-*trans*-14-*cis*-eicosatetraenoic acid. The covalent structure and the configurations at C-5 and C-12 were determined in ref. 32. The configurations of the double bonds were shown by comparison of native LTB_4 with a synthetic product of known stereochemistry [33]. Parallel to the enzymatic hydrolysis, LTA_4 is also subjected to nonenzymatic hydrolysis in the cell. This gives two additional 5,12-dihydroxy acids, epimeric at C-12 (5(S),12-dihydroxy-6,8,10-*trans*-14-*cis*-eicosatetraenoic acids), and also in lesser amounts, two diastereo-isomeric 5,6-dihydroxy-7,9,11,14-eicosatetraenoic acids [31]. When these four compounds are discussed in conjunction with LTB_4, they are often referred to as compounds (or isomers) I, II, IV and V, respectively, (the original compound/isomer III is LTB_4) [31]. Compounds I and II have also been denoted as the epimers at C-12 of 6-*trans*-LTB_4 [34]. LTB_4 and the compounds I, II, IV and V are stable compounds, so traditional techniques for isolation and purification of fatty acid derivatives can be utilized. For separation of LTB_4, I, II, IV and V, HPLC (reverse or straight phase) is necessary [31]. They all

TABLE 1
Reports on formation of LTB_4
In the references underlined, the identification was based on GC-MS.

Rabbit	Human	Rat	Guinea pig
Neutrophils	Neutrophils	Peritoneal PMNL	Peritoneal PMNL
(32, 36)	(17, 35, 37, 38)	(36, 37)	(45)
	Eosinophils	Peritoneal macrophages	
	(39)	(42)	
	Synovial fluid from RA patients	Neutrophils	
	(40)	(43)	
		Basophilic leukemia cells	
		(44)	

exhibit typical triplets in the UV-spectra with maxima around 260, 270 and 280 nm [31–34]. For LTB_4 the maxima are at 260, 270.5 and 280 nm with molar extinction coefficients of 38 000, 50 000 and 39 000, respectively [33].

LTB_4 was originally isolated from incubations of rabbit PMNL with arachidonic acid [32], but human PMNL also have the capacity to synthesize LTB_4. An interesting feature in these cells is that the calcium ionophore A23187 greatly enhances the biosynthesis [17]. Opsonized zymosan, a phagocytic stimulus, also induces formation of LTB_4 [35]. LTB_4 formation has been demonstrated in leukocytes from several species (see Table 1). Organic syntheses leading to LTB_4 and isomers of LTB_4 are described in refs. 33, 34, 46 and 47.

In this context it may be helpful to mention the finding of another isomer of LTB_4. This is 5(S),12(S)-dihydroxy-6-*trans*,8-*cis*,10-*trans*,14-*cis*-eicosatetraenoic acid, that is not formed via the leukotriene-pathway. It will therefore be discussed in Section 4.

A biosynthetic pathway in which leukotrienes are formed with oxygen substituents at C-14 and C-15, or at C-8 and C-15 of arachidonic acid has been demonstrated [48–50]. The first reaction in this pathway is oxygenation of arachidonic acid at C-15 rather than at C-5, giving 15-hydroperoxy-eicosatetraenoic acid (15-HPETE). 15-HPETE can subsequently be converted into an allylic epoxide with the structure of 14,15-oxido-5,8,10,12-eicosatetraenoic acid, referred to as 14,15-LTA_4. The 14,15-LTA_4 can be hydrolyzed into two isomers of 14,15-dihydroxy-5,8,10,12-eicosatetraenoic acid (14,15-LTB_4), and also two isomers of 8,15-dihydroxy-5,9,11,13-eicosatetraenoic acid (8,15-LTB_4) [48,50]. This pathway has been demonstrated in human [48,49] and in porcine leukocytes [50]. 14,15-LTA_4 has been prepared chemically [51].

(b) Leukotrienes of types C, D and E (slow reacting substances SRS)

The elucidation of the chemistry of the biologically highly potent principle SRS has attracted the interest of many laboratories for several years. Recently, when the various compounds comprising SRS were structurally determined and found to be members of the leukotriene group, they were named according to the LT nomenclature. Previously, however, they were referred to as SRS, classified depending on cellular origin and the stimulus for the biosynthesis. The SRS nomenclature is now used in parallel with the LT nomenclature.

The term slow reacting substance (SRS) was originally introduced by Feldberg and Kellaway [52]. In 1938 they described a factor in perfusates from guinea pig and cat lungs formed upon treatment with cobra venom. The factor induced a prolonged contraction with slow onset of the guinea pig jejunum. Two years later Kellaway and Trethewie described a similar substance released from sensitized guinea pig lung during anaphylaxis [53]. Using the guinea pig ileum bioassay, Brocklehurst showed that the factor was a pharmacological entity distinct from histamine and other contractile agents, and introduced the term slow reacting substance of anaphylaxis (SRS-A) for immunologically released SRS [54]. The early pharmacology and chemistry of SRS-A was reviewed in 1962, and it was shown that lung segments from human asthmatics have the capacity to produce SRS-A [55]. Subsequent work has suggested that SRS-A plays an important role as a mediator in asthma and other types of immediate type hypersensitivity reactions [56].

The elucidation of the structures of the SRS compounds has been complicated. Difficulties in purification and problems of identifying small amounts of biologically active components without destroying the chemical structure hampered many attempts. In order to achieve more material for structural analysis, systems other than lung tissue with SRS-producing capacity have been used, such as rat peritoneal cavity cells [57–61], rat basophilic leukemia cells [62,63], mouse mastocytoma cells [64], the perfused cat paw [65] and human peripheral polymorphonuclear leukocytes [66]. The immunologically formed SRS-A and non-immunological SRS from different cells and species were found to have similar, although not identical, biological and chromatographic properties [67–74]. Thus, the more productive "non-immunological" sources could be used to generate enough material for structural elucidation. The ionophore A23187 was found to be a potent stimulus for SRS-formation in rat peripheral cells [59] and has been used extensively in many other systems. The purification of SRS from the various sources has been made possible through use of HPLC [67,75].

The connection between fatty acid metabolism and SRS formation was made when it was discovered that an intact lipoxygenase reaction was essential for SRS formation [76–81]. Conversely, inhibition of lipoxygenase prevented SRS formation as determined by prevention of anaphylactic bronchoconstriction [82,83]. Further evidence for lipoxygenase involvement is provided by the enhanced antigen-induced tracheal contraction demonstrated during cyclooxygenase inhibition [84–86] as well as the finding of clinical cases with aspirin-induced asthma [87]. The observations that 5-HPETE potentiates SRS formation [88,89] and is incorporated in the biologically active compound [90], and that also labelled arachidonic acid is incorporated [62,91,92], showed that SRS is a fatty acid derivative.

Sulphur was found through spark source mass spectrometry to be abundant in SRS-A [93]. Also, incorporation of ^{35}S into SRS has been reported [64,94–96]. The observation that several thiols enhance SRS formation in different systems [97–100] and that arylsulfatase (an enzyme that cleaves sulfate monoesters of phenolic and other unsaturated hydroxylated systems) inactivates SRS-A [101,102] opened the view that a thiol is a constituent of the active compound. However, it has recently been shown that the SRS-inactivating action of commercially available arylsulfatase is not due to sulfate ester cleavage, but to a dipeptidase contaminant [103,104]. The destruction of different SRS compounds by lipoxygenase [67,105,106] shows that SRS contains a *cis,cis*-1,4-pentadiene structure, since this is a prerequisite for a lipoxygenase substrate [107]. For a review of the earlier structural work on SRS, see ref. 108.

One of the important observations that linked SRS with the leukotrienes was the UV spectrum of SRS-A [67] which indicated a conjugated triene in the SRS molecule. This and other similarities were noted during the initial studies on the leukotrienes in leukocytes. Subsequently, this proved to be very fruitful when the observations from the work on leukotrienes were applied to the structural determination of SRS.

Thus, the first complete structure of an SRS-compound was described as 5(S)-hydroxy-7,9-*trans*-11,14-*cis*-eicosatetraenoic acid with a glutathionyl substituent at C-6 (R-configuration) [64,109,110]. This compound was originally isolated from murine mastocytoma cells, and it is named leukotriene C_4 (LTC_4). The structural analysis of LTC_4 is reviewed in refs. 7 and 12.

LTC_4 is enzymatically formed from LTA_4 [23,111] by addition of glutathione to the epoxide-function of LTA_4, catalyzed by a glutathione-*S*-transferase (Fig. 3). LTC_4 has now been isolated in SRS derived from different cells and species, such as human peripheral polymorphonuclear leukocytes [112], rat basophilic leukemia cells [113–115], rat peritoneal mononuclear cells [116], anaphylactic rat peritoneal cavity [117], guinea pig lung [117,118] and mouse peritoneal macrophages [119–121]. Also the stereo-isomeric 11-*trans* LTC_4 has been demonstrated as a naturally occurring SRS compound [122].

LTC_4 is enzymatically transformed by a γ-glutamyltranspeptidase into LTD_4 (5S-hydroxy-6S-cysteinylglycyl-7,9,11,14-eicosatetraenoic acid) [123,124] (Fig. 1). This compound has been reported as a component of SRS formed in rat basophilic leukemia cells [113,114,123], rat peritoneal mononuclear cells [125], anaphylactic rat peritoneal cavity [117], cat paw perfused with histamine releasing compound 48/80 [126] and in anaphylactic human and guinea pig lung [117,118,125] and in sputum from patients with cystic fibrosis [41]. The 11-*trans* isomer of LTD_4 is described in ref. 127.

Finally, LTD_4 is enzymatically transformed to LTE_4 (5S-hydroxy-6S-cysteinyl-7,9,11,14-eicosatetraenoic acid) by removal of the glycine residue [114,124,126–130].

This compound is also a naturally occurring part of native SRS, and the 11-*trans* isomer of LTE_4 has been described [127].

The ratio of LTC_4, LTD_4, LTE_4 and the 11-*trans* isomers thus varies in SRS from different sources and possibly also with other parameters (e.g. stimulus, time, substrates, cofactors). Since the different leukotrienes have a biological profile which differs both quantitatively and qualitatively [117,131–135] (see below), it seems appropriate to use the chemical characterization to describe the defined compounds, and to use SRS nomenclature only to design biological materials where the relative amounts of the different leukotrienes are unknown.

LTC_4, LTD_4 and LTE_4 exhibit triplets in the UV spectra with maxima at 270, 280 and 290 nm [19,64,123,127,136]. The molar extinction coefficients at 280 nm are 40 000 [19,127,136]. The origin of the 11-*trans* isomers of these leukotrienes is unclear, and several alternative explanations are given [122,137]. The UV spectra of the 11-*trans* isomers are shifted to 2 nm lower values [122,127]. The first organic synthesis of LTC_4 that was instrumental for the elucidation of the exact stereochemistry is described in ref. 19. Syntheses of LTC_4, LTD_4, LTE_4 and isomers of these compounds are also described in refs. 22, 26, 51, 122, 127, 136, 138 and 139.

(c) Some characteristics of leukotriene producing systems

The leukotrienes described above in Sections 3(a) and 3(b) are all derived from arachidonic acid. Other substrates, for example 5,8,11-eicosatrienoic acid and 5,8,11,14,17-eicosapentaenoic acid, are converted to leukotrienes of the 3- and 5-series, respectively, i.e. LTC_3 [140] and LTC_5 [141,142]. The essential structure required for a fatty acid to be converted to leukotrienes in rat basophilic leukemia cells appears to be a $\Delta^{5,8,11}$-unsaturation [143]. Fatty acids with this feature give LTB-like compounds and SRS activity in $10\,000 \times g$ supernatants from rat basophilic leukemia (RBL) cell homogenates [143]. However, 8,11,14-eicosatrienoic acid, the precursor of the prostaglandins and thromboxanes of the 1 series, can also be converted into a leukotriene i.e. 8,9-LTC_3, but in low yield [144]. The production of SRS activity in the RBL supernatant is dependent on glutathione [145], and biosynthesis of 5-HETE, 5,12-DHETE (LTB_4) and SRS activity is stimulated by calcium [44,145]. The enzyme thought to depend on calcium in the RBL cell is the lipoxygenase [44], which is also thought to discriminate towards the substrate structure [143].

4. Other lipoxygenase products

This section reviews the formation of fatty acid derivatives not belonging to the leukotriene group formed by lipoxygenases in some mammalian cells. The much larger literature on lipoxygenases and their products of the plant world is reviewed in refs. 146–149. This knowledge is of interest since many features of lipoxygenases from different sources are similar.

(a) Lipoxygenase products

A variety of oxygenated derivatives is formed during the reaction of lipoxygenases with fatty acid substrates. The biosynthesis of the monohydroxy and dihydroxy acids proceeds via the corresponding hydroperoxy acids, as is the case in the plant systems. The immediate product of the lipoxygenase thus is a hydroperoxy acid. This product is reduced to the corresponding hydroxy acid, presumably both enzymatically by peroxidases and through non-enzymatic decomposition. However, the hydroperoxy acid can also be converted to a ketone or to an epoxy-hydroxy acid that can hydrolyze into a trihydroxy acid (see below).

The criterion required of a compound to serve as a plant lipoxygenase substrate, i.e. a *cis,cis*-1,4-pentadiene structure [146], seems to be valid also for the mammalian lipoxygenases. All reports so far fit with this concept, and arachidonic acid (all *cis*-5,8,11-14-eicosatetraenoic acid) is by far the substrate most studied. Oxygen can be introduced at various positions of arachidonic acid (Fig. 4), and in Table 2 the different monohydroxy-eicosatetraenoic acids (HETE) obtained from arachidonic acid in different cells are summarized.

When a lipoxygenase acts on the same fatty acid substrate molecule twice, and the hydroperoxide groups are reduced, a dihydroxy acid results. The formation of such a compound, isomeric with LTB_4, has been reported in suspensions of human PMNL. The structure of this compound is 5(S),12(S)-dihydroxy-6,8,10,14-eicosatetraenoic acid, and most probably the double bonds have the *trans,cis-trans,cis* configuration, respectively (Fig. 4) [15,228]. Another dihydroxy acid formed by

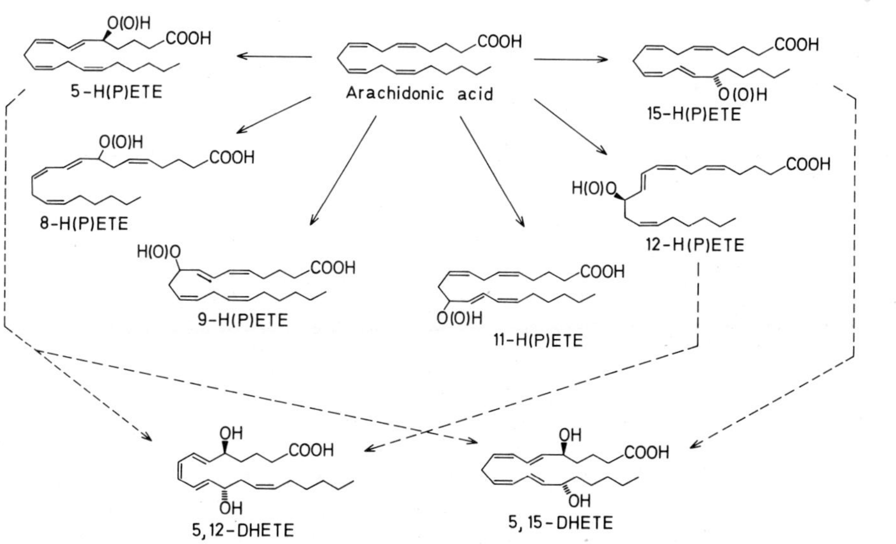

Fig. 4. Mono- and dihydroxylated derivatives of arachidonic acid, formed by single or double dioxygenation followed by reduction.

TABLE 2
Formation of monohydroxylated derivatives of arachidonic acid in various cells and tissues
References in parentheses.

5-HETE	8-HETE	9-HETE	11-HETE	12-HETE	15-HETE
Rabbit PMNL (16, 36)	Human PMNL (151)	Human PMNL (151)	Human PMNL (150, 151)	Human PMNL (151)	Human PMNL (17)
Human PMNL (17, 38, 150–152)	Mouse peritoneal monocytes (157)	Mouse peritoneal monocytes (157)	Guinea pig lung (158)	Mouse peritoneal macrophages (155, 162,163)	Human lung (175)
RBL-cells (44, 88)	Mouse peritoneal macrophages (155)	Mouse peritoneal macrophages (155)	Cyclooxygenase (159, 160)	Human lymphocytes (154)	Guinea pig lung (158)
Rabbit alveolar macrophages (153)		Pig liver macrophages (156)	Rabbit alveolar macrophages (153)	Platelets, human bovine (164, 165)	Rat peritoneal macrophages (42)
Rat peritoneal macrophages (42)			Rat neutrophils (161)	Guinea pig lung and spleen (158, 166)	Cyclooxygenase (160, 176)
Human lymphocytes (154)			Human eosino-phils (39)	Normal and psoriatic epi-	Rat neutrophils (161)

fluid (40)	monocytes (157)	(169)	monocytes (157)
Rat neutrophils (43)	Mouse peritoneal macrophages (155)	Rat serosal mast cells (170)	Mouse peritoneal macrophages (155)
Human eosinophils (39)	Pig liver microsomes (156)	Rat peritoneal macrophages (42)	Rabbit peritoneal tissues (177)
Guinea pig PMNL (45)		Human eosinophils (39)	Pig liver micro-somes (156)
Mouse peritoneal macrophages (155)		Rabbit pericardium, pleura, peritoneum (171)	
Pig liver micro-somes (156)		Rat brain cortex (172)	
		Human colonic tissue (173)	
		Perfused dog lung (174)	
		Pig liver microsomes (156)	
		Rat lung (416)	

double deoxygenation of arachidonic acid is 5,15-dihydroxy-6,8,11,13-eicosatetraenoic acid, isolated from rat mononuclear cells [178]. Further oxygenated metabolites of dihydroxy acids, i.e. trihydroxy acids, have been described [15,179].

Another series of trihydroxyacids has been described in platelets and lung. In this case, the hydroperoxy acid is first converted to an epoxy-hydroxy acid. From 12-HPETE, 10-hydroxy-11,12-epoxy-eicosa-5,8,14-trienoic acid and 8-hydroxy-11,12-epoxy-eicosa-5,9,14-trienoic acid can be formed. The former compound has been isolated as such [180]. The hydrolysis products of the latter allylic epoxide are two isomeric trihydroxy acids. Formation of such trihydroxy acids was reported in platelets [181–183] and lung [415–417]. These conversions of the hydroperoxy acid seem to be favoured when the reducing capacity of the peroxidases present is insufficient [184] and diminished when peroxidase activity is augmented [185].

(b) Some properties of lipoxygenases

Regarding the characteristics and properties of various mammalian lipoxygenases, most data have been accumulated for the enzyme in platelets, which was the first mammalian lipoxygenase described. Some data have also been presented concerning lipoxygenases in inflammatory cells. In human platelets, however, arachidonic acid is converted to 12(L)-hydroxy-eicosatetraenoic acid (12-HETE), via the corresponding hydroperoxy acid [164,165]. 12-HPETE has been isolated as such from platelets in which the peroxidase-activity was inhibited [186]. Platelets from many other species were shown to have the same capacity [165] and the substrate specificity of the bovine lipoxygenase was determined [165]. Two *cis* double bonds at position 8 and 11 (*n*-6, *n*-12) are required of eicosapolyenoic acids for them to be converted efficiently. The specificity seemed to be related more to the distance between the diene and the methyl end group than to the carboxyl group.

The lipoxygenase in bovine platelets was recovered in the $100\,000 \times g$ supernatant of the platelet homogenate [165]. A conflicting report on the enzyme localization in human platelets stated that the lipoxygenase is found in the microsomal fraction, the explanation for this could be a species difference or methodological discrepancy [187]. In a third study on the platelet lipoxygenase, however, presence of enzyme activity was found both in the $100\,000 \times g$ supernatant and in the particulate fraction [188]. The cytosolic enzyme could be separated into two active fractions, one of which also contained peroxidase activity. Data regarding pH optimum, molecular weights, and inhibitory effects of drugs are given in ref. 188. The preparation of platelet lipoxygenase as an acetone-pentane powder is described in ref. 189. pH optimum, heat stability and solubility data have also been reported. Also, several divalent cations have been tested as inhibitors for the enzyme, and Michaelis constants for three fatty acids are presented.

In a mechanistic study using [10L-^{3}H,3-^{14}C]arachidonic acid as substrate for the platelet lipoxygenase, it was found that stereospecific removal of the "L"-hydrogen from C-10 of arachidonic acid is probably the initial step in conversion to 12-HPETE [190]. This study also describes the activation of lipoxygenase by endoperoxides, in accordance with earlier reports [186,191] concerning activation of lipoxygenase activity by its product, 12-HPETE. 15-HPETE, on the other hand, inhibits metabolism of endogenous arachidonic acid in platelets. This is regarded as an effect of inhibition of platelet diglyceride lipase [192]. A high molecular weight factor present in serum from adjuvant arthritic rats has been reported to stimulate lipoxygenase activity in platelets [193].

Ferric ion is a necessary cofactor for lipoxygenase activity in platelets, and various chelators inhibit the enzyme [194,195]. The role of vitamin E in relation to platelet lipoxygenase is unclear. An inhibitory effect has been reported [196,197], whereas others have found no effect [198]. The lipoxygenase activity of human neutrophils (see below) has been reported to be enhanced by normal plasma concentrations of vitamin E, whereas higher concentrations are suppressive [199].

The lipoxygenases of various inflammatory cells have attracted an increasing interest and a number of lipoxygenase metabolites have been described (see Table 2). Some properties of the enzymes involved have also been reported. Thus, the 5-lipoxygenase in the $10\,000 \times g$ supernatant from homogenized rat basophilic leukemia (RBL) cells is stimulated by Ca^{2+}. This lipoxygenase, which catalyzes insertion of oxygen at C-5 of arachidonic acid, thus differs from the platelet lipoxygenase in calcium dependency [44]. For efficient conversion to monohydroxy acids by the RBL-lipoxygenase, an all *cis*-5,8,11-structure is required [143]. The calcium dependence of a lipoxygenase inserting oxygen at C-5 of arachidonic acid also in rat neutrophils has been implicated. These cells produce 5-HETE only when stimulated with a calcium ionophore, whereas in response to arachidonic acid they only produce 11-HETE, 15-HETE as well as prostaglandins [43,161]. The calcium dependency and other metabolic requirements of rabbit PMNL lipoxygenase have been reported [200].

In another study, a lipoxygenase from rabbit PMNL which inserts oxygen at C-15 of arachidonic acid is described. Its molecular weight is 61 000 and the effects of various inhibitors were studied [201].

An interesting lipoxygenase has been characterized in reticulocytes from rabbits [202]. The molecular weight (78 000), isoelectric point (5.5) and sugar content (5%), as well as the association of two iron atoms per enzyme molecule were reported. This lipoxygenase was found to inactivate respiratory proteins of the developing reticulocyte.

The purification and characterization of a lipoxygenase-like enzyme in rat testis has also been described. The enzyme activity could be purified from the microsomes to almost homogeneity by affinity chromatography [203,204].

(c) Alternative preparations of lipoxygenase products

The synthetic approaches leading to hydroperoxy acids have mostly consisted of indirect oxidations of arachidonic acid. Various methods have been described. Oxidation with air [205], with singlet oxygen [206,207], with H_2O_2 in presence of Cu^{2+} [208,209], give mixtures of H(P)ETE isomers that can be separated on HPLC.

Oxidation catalyzed by hemoglobin or myoglobin [210] or by xanthine oxidase [211] also give mixtures of isomers. However, specific procedures giving various isomers of HETE as pure products have also been reported. Thus, organic syntheses of 11-HETE, 12-HETE and 15-HETE are described in ref. 212, and of 5-HETE in ref. 213. Furthermore, methods for conversion of the hydroxy acids into hydroperoxy acids of opposite stereochemistry are given in these last two chapters.

5-HETE and 5-HPETE can also be produced in incubations of arachidonic acid with the lipoxygenase in potato and tomato [213,214].

5. *Metabolism of leukotrienes*

(a) Metabolism of cysteinyl-containing leukotrienes

LTC_4, LTD_4 and LTE_4, and possibly also the 11-*trans* isomers, are all components of native SRS-A. In peripheral airways, the system where SRS-A has been suggested to exert its main effect [215,216], all the cysteinyl-containing leukotrienes have been shown to be equipotent as constrictors [217,218], although they can differ in potency in contracting other smooth muscle preparations [123,124,219].

LTD_4 and LTE_4 are metabolites of LTC_4 and are formed by a successive elimination of glutamic acid and glycine from the peptide-chain of LTC_4 [123,124,129,130]. In some cell types and tissues, LTC_4 has been identified as the main SRS component, while LTD_4 is the main component in some others (see above, Section 3(b)). The varying ratios of LTC_4, LTD_4, LTE_4 and the 11-*trans* isomers reflect differences in the metabolic conditions in various cell types and tissues. Part of the differences is also due to the experimental conditions used for their isolation, e.g. incubation time and concentrations of cofactors. The sequential conversion LTC to LTD to LTE has been demonstrated in RBL cells simply by increasing the incubation time [124,129]. This has also been shown in rat peritoneal mononuclear cells [220] and in human PMNL (Hansson, G., unpublished observations). Some of the thiols, which have been used to enhance SRS formation and therefore often are included in incubations for SRS generation, have recently been found to interfere with the transformation of LTC to LTD to LTE. For example, high concentrations of glutathione prevent the conversion of LTC to LTD, and in fact they have also been shown to stimulate the reverse transformation, i.e. LTD to LTC [221]. L-Cysteine, on the other hand, inhibits the conversion of LTD to LTE [114,129] leading to an accumulation of D-type leukotrienes.

The transformation of LTC_4 to LTD_4 [123], as well as LTC_3 to LTD_3 [140] and LTC_5 to LTD_5 [141,142] is reversibly catalyzed by γ-glutamyl transpeptidase (EC 2.3.2.2), a membrane-bound enzyme of widespread occurrence [222]. The kidney possesses high concentrations of this enzyme. Inhibitors of γ-glutamyl transpeptidase, such as L-serine-borate [223], AT-125 (L-(αS,5S)-α-amino-3-chloro-4,5-dihydro-5-isoxazoleacetic acid) [129] and δ-D-glutamyl-*O*-carboxy phenylhydrazine [224], result in the accumulation of LTC_4 in RBL cells.

A dipeptidase catalyzes the transformation of LTD_3, LTD_4, LTD_5 and 11-*trans*

LTD_4 to corresponding E leukotrienes [114,130,221]. This enzyme has been partially purified from kidney [130], human plasma [128], RBL cells, guinea pig lung, and guinea pig peritoneal eosinophils [104]. In the latter preparations, the peptidase activity could be resolved from the arylsulfatase activity [104], which had earlier been suggested to be responsible for inactivation of SRS [101,102]. Inhibitors of the dipeptidase, more potent than L-cysteine, are 3-mercaptopropionic acid and D-penicillamine [114].

Very few studies on the metabolism of leukotrienes of the 4-series have been reported so far. This is mainly due to difficulties in preparing labeled leukotrienes of this series with high enough specific activity and with the label in a metabolically stable position. However, metabolism of LTC_3 has been investigated using tritium-labeled material of high specific activity and with the label in the fatty acid of the molecule [221]. Homogenates of guinea pig lung convert labeled LTC_3 into LTD_3, while liver and kidney homogenates do not catabolize LTC_3 to any appreciably extent, probably due to high tissue concentrations of glutathione [221]. When LTD_3 was added to liver and kidney homogenates, however, it was rapidly metabolized into LTE_3.

Distribution studies by whole body autoradiography have been performed in mice after intravenous injection of labeled LTC_3 [225]. The radioactivity was distributed mainly into the liver, bile and kidney, but also to lung and connective tissue in various organs. Analysis of the major radioactive metabolites present in lung, liver, bile, intestine, heart and blood of the animals, after 5, 20 and 60 min, showed compounds with chromatographic properties identical to those of LTC_3, LTD_3 and LTE_3. In the kidney, several additional unidentified metabolites were seen. The relatively large amount of unaltered LTC_3 present in liver and bile indicated a poor metabolism of LTC_3 in the liver, which agreed with the in vitro results from guinea pig liver homogenates [221].

Excretion of metabolites of LTC_3 has been followed in guinea pigs after subcutaneous injection of labeled LTC_3 [221]. Quantitative excretion of the given dose was achieved in 5 days after administration with about 60% recovered in feces and 40% in urine. Analysis of the excreted material showed that these metabolites were not identical to LTC_3, LTD_3 or LTE_3 [221]. Others have reported that LTE_4 might be one of several products found in the urine of mice after intravenous injection of LTD_4 [128].

In vivo metabolism of LTC_3 has also been investigated in the monkey [226]. After injection of tritium-labeled LTC_3 into the right atrium, the radioactivity was rapidly eliminated from the circulation with a hundred-fold decrease over a period of 15 min. After one passage through the lungs (within 15 s), 40% of the recovered radioactivity was accounted for by LTD_3 and LTE_3, and after 2 min LTE_3 predominated in the blood.

(b) Metabolism of LTB compounds

Metabolites of LTB_4 have been identified from suspensions of human PMNL [179] and rat mononuclear cells [178]. LTB_4 is metabolized in these preparations by ω-oxidation mainly to 20-hydroxy-LTB_4 (20-OH-LTB_4), but a small amount of 19-hydroxy-LTB_4 (19-OH-LTB_4) was also found. In the human PMNL preparation, 20-OH-LTB_4 is then further oxidized to the dicarboxylic acid, 20-carboxy-LTB_4 (20-COOH-LTB_4) [179]. This metabolite is the main leukotriene found when human leukocytes were stimulated by the chemotactic tripeptide formyl-methionyl-leucyl-phenylalanine (fMLP) [227]. The ω-oxidized metabolites of LTB_4 were somewhat less potent than LTB_4 as chemotactic agents [227] and in causing leukocyte adherence to postcapillary venules [179], although they were equipotent with LTB_4 in contracting the guinea pig lung parenchyma [179] (see below, Section 6). Another abundant 5,12-dihydroxy acid formed in preparations of human and porcine peripheral PMNL, 5S,12S-dihydroxy-6-*trans*,8-*cis*,10-*trans*,14-*cis*-eicosatetraenoic acid [15,228] has also been shown to be metabolized by ω-oxidation to the corresponding metabolites [15,179].

6. *Biological effects of leukotrienes and other lipoxygenase products*

A role has been proposed for cyclooxygenase products of arachidonic acid in different aspects of the inflammatory response (reviewed in refs. 229–231). Most of the evidence originates in the finding that non-steroidal anti-inflammatory drugs inhibit prostaglandin cyclooxygenase [232]. With the newly discovered lipoxygenase products a new approach has been opened for elucidating the role of arachidonic acid metabolism in inflammation as many of the effects of "the leukotriene family" are closely linked to different aspects of inflammation. Below, the effects of these compounds on various cells and tissues are reviewed.

(a) Effects of LTB compounds

i. Polymorphonuclear neutrophil leukocytes (PMNL)

The PMNL play an important role in inflammation. These cells are also of special interest since they are fairly well studied concerning the metabolism of arachidonic acid, and since the biological effects of different arachidonate metabolites have been studied in many laboratories. PMNL transform arachidonic acid to small amounts of prostaglandins [233] and thromboxanes [234] but the main products are several hydroxyacid derivatives [17,31,32,43,48,234] and leukotrienes [18,20,21,43,70,112]. The formation of these metabolites is markedly increased in the presence of calcium ionophore A23187 [17,235]. Whether this reflects Ca^{2+} dependence of the enzymatic reactions [44,145,235–237] or whether it is an effect on the release of endogenous arachidonic acid from the phospholipids [238–240], or both, is not clear. PMNL functions which have been studied with regard to arachidonate lipoxygenase metabolism are chemotaxis and chemokinesis, enzyme secretion, aggregation/adhesion and superoxide production.

Chemotaxis and chemokinesis Among cyclooxygenase products thromboxane B_2 [241] and some prostaglandins [242] exert a slight chemoattractant effect in some species but give no significant response per se in human PMNL. Lipoxygenase products from platelets (12-HETE and 12-HPETE) show some chemotactic activity [5,243].

Chemoattractants induce release of arachidonic acid from phospholipids in PMNL [244] and the arachidonate metabolism is stimulated in a manner similar to that of ionophore A23187 [235,245]. Inhibitors of arachidonate metabolism inhibit leukocyte migration [246–248]. However, with inhibition mainly of the cyclooxygenase pathway, an increase of PMNL migration is observed in vitro [150,247,249] and in vivo [6,250,251]. Formation of LTB_4 and 5-HETE is significantly increased in synovial fluid in rheumatoid arthritis [40]. These data support the concept that an endogenous lipoxygenase product is involved in the PMNL chemotactic response.

Among the monohydroxy compounds formed from PMNL [31,32,151], 5-HETE exerts the most potent chemoattractant effect upon human PMNL in vitro and is considerably more active than 8-HETE which in turn is more active than 11-HETE [150,252]. The latter compound is equally potent with 12-HETE in promoting leukocyte migration [252]. 15-HETE is virtually inactive in this respect [253].

The most effective chemotactic agent within the lipoxygenase series of products so far studied in vitro [37,247,254–257] and in vivo [258,259] is LTB_4. It is almost as active as fMLP at equimolar concentrations, and the response is stereospecific since the non-enzymatic stereoisomers of LTB_4 give much less activity [247,249,260,261]. The ω-oxidation products of LTB_4 are less active than LTB_4 itself [179], and the cysteinyl-containing leukotrienes are inactive [247,256]. At this point, it has to be stressed that the response in leukocyte migration to some extent depends upon the technique and species used [253]. It also varies considerably between individuals [262], with cell concentration [263] and with temperature [264].

The mechanism by which the arachidonate metabolites exert their chemotactic effect is still unclear. The observation that methyl esters of biologically active compounds in some cases inhibit the chemotactic response [265] indicates that a free carboxyl group is essential. This, together with the finding that chemotactic hydroxy acids are incorporated into the phospholipids [266], has given the hypothesis that membrane modulation might be important for the response. Some support for this idea is the observation that the chemotactic factor fMLP [267] as well as active arachidonate metabolites [267,268] lead to an increase in plasma membrane permeability to Ca^{2+} [269]. However, although often used as a model for physiological chemotactic peptides, it should be mentioned that fMLP might induce a cellular response diverging from that of naturally occurring compounds [270]. Positive evidence for this resemblance to physiological stimuli is that fMLP binds to and activates surface receptors [271–273].

The differentiation between chemokinesis (increase of spontaneous movement) and chemotaxis (increase of directed movement) might also be of importance [274]. Thus, dibutyryl cyclic adenosine 3′,5′-monophosphate produces divergent effects upon the two parameters of leukocyte locomotion under certain conditions [275]; consequently it would seem that leukocyte movement should include measurements of both chemokinesis and chemotaxis. It is also noteworthy that too large a concentration of a chemotaxin might cause "deactivation" and inhibition of cell movement [247,276]. This 'over-stimulation' might result from a pathological increase in activity of the hexose monophosphate shunt [277].

Finally, it should be mentioned that generation of a chemotactic lipid from arachidonic acid has been reported during exposure to a superoxide generating system [278]. Under physiological conditions products of this free radical reaction might be of importance together with the enzymatically formed compounds, since in vivo administration of scavengers of superoxide [279] or hydrogen peroxide [280] inhibit infiltration during inflammation. The structure of this directly oxygenated compound has not been established but it seems less potent that LTB_4.

Enzyme secretion In contrast to lipid mediators, which are formed after simulation of the cell, different lytic enzymes (e.g. lysozyme and β-glucuronidase) are stored in granules in the PMNL, ready to be released at stimulation. Although critical for host defence, these mediators are also responsible for a part of the tissue damage characterising inflammation [276,281,282].

The mechanisms of enzyme secretion and chemotaxis have obvious similarities. Thus, many chemotactic factors are also secretagogues for lysosomal enzyme secretion, e.g. fMLP [283,284]. Compounds causing secretion [285] and/or phagocytosis [286] increase the liberation of arachidonic acid from the phospholipids in a Ca^{2+}-dependent manner [287]. Arachidonic acid in the presence of cytochalasin B causes enzyme release from rabbit peritoneal PMNL but not from human PMNL [152,288,290]. The acetylenic analog of arachidonic acid (5,8,11,14-eicosatetraenoic acid, ETYA) and nordihydroguiaiaretic acid (NDGA), both inhibitors of lipoxygenase, inhibit enzyme secretion induced by arachidonic acid [291,292] or chemotactic peptides and the complement factor C5a [289].

These observations again focus the attention on the biological activity of different lipoxygenase products of arachidonate. Both 5-HETE and to a lesser extent 12-HETE have been reported to possess enzyme releasing potency in chemotactic concentrations [152]. In other studies no effect was observed under these conditions [252,293]. However, LTB_4 was found to be a more potent releasing agent [254,293,294], but it should be stressed that the maximal level of enzyme release was far less than that of the chemotactic fragment of C5 and formylmethionyl peptides. The cysteinyl-containing leukotrienes are not active in this respect [293].

Although less clear than in chemotaxis, there is strong evidence that lipoxygenase products of arachidonic acid are involved in enzyme secretion from PMNL. The situation is made more complex by the observation that the response in fact might be divided into two classes: one response induced by agents (fMLP, calcium ionophore A23187, and immune complexes) which provoke release of both azurophil granules (with e.g. lysozyme) and specific granules (with e.g. β-glucuronidase), and another response induced by agents (the lectin concanavalin A and phorbol myristate acetate) which provoke discharge of enzymes from specific granules only [295,296]. The enzyme release induced by 5-HETE was of the latter class [152], whereas LTB_4 also causes release of β-glucuronidase [254,293]. Whether this reflects real differences in mode of action of the two compounds, or depends on experimental conditions, is not known.

Aggregation and adherence Aggregation and adherence are two closely related characteristics of the PMNL. Although poorly understood these mechanisms seem to be of importance in the inflammatory response. Thus, adherence of leukocytes to the endothelium of microvessels and the sticking phenomena are considered initial hallmarks of an inflammatory process in vivo [297]. As in chemotaxis and degranulation these actions involve a contractile process of the cell.

Many phagocytic and/or chemotactic agents cause PMNL aggregation [289–300]. Arachidonic acid itself aggregates human [290,301,302] and rat [303] leukocytes in vitro in a manner which resembles that of the chemotactic formylpeptide and other agents [304]. The response is inhibited by the acetylenic analog of arachidonic acid, is stimulated by cytochalasin B and is dependent on divalent cations [304]. The fact that inhibitors of arachidonate metabolism also inhibit aggregation induced by agents other than the acid itself [290,301] supports the idea that lipoxygenase products might also be of importance in this case. Release of endogenous arachidonic acid by phorbol myristate acetate also induces PMNL aggregation. However, in this case the response is relatively independent of extracellular Ca^{2+} concentration, cytochalasin B and inhibitors of arachidonate metabolism [305].

Among lipoxygenase products LTB_4 is a potent inducer of aggregation of rat and human neutrophils [10,37]. Isomers of LTB_4 are less potent in this respect [260]. No significant response has been reported with monohydroxy derivatives. Also, PMNL adherence to nylon fibers is significantly increased by LTB_4 in vitro [249].

In vivo LTB_4 causes a conspicuous and reversible adhesion of leukocytes to the endothelium in post-capillary venules [135], and the metabolites 20-OH-LTB_4 and 20-COOH-LTB_4 are approximately 50 times less potent than LTB_4 itself [179]. LTC_4 and LTD_4 do not enhance leukocyte adherence in this way [135].

Superoxide production Oxygen transformed by phagocytosing leukocytes to the biologically active species (O_2^-, H_2O_2, $OH^{\cdot}$ and $^1O_2$) is suggested to be the form for killing off bacteria [284] and for participating in the tissue damaging effect during inflammation. Oxygen activation is induced by NADPH oxidase [306,307] or possibly by a direct cytochrome *b* effect [308].

Formyl-Met-Leu-Phe is involved in oxygen activation and the respiratory burst induced by this peptide is inhibited by ETYA, but not by inhibitors of cyclooxgenase [309]. The chemotactic peptide [309,310] and other superoxide generating agents [310] stimulate glucose metabolism via the hexose monophosphate shunt, although it is blocked by lipoxygenase inhibition. Similar to the enzyme secretion, superoxide production is stimulated by cytochalasin B [311], is dependent on esterase activity [312] and on extracellular Ca^{2+} [313]. Corticosteroids, which among other effects inhibit liberation of arachidonic acid from phospholipids [314], decrease superoxide production [315,316], whereas phorbol myristate acetate, which stimulates acylhydrolase activity, enhances oxygen activation [317,318].

From a physiological point of view, it is curious that some chemoattractants are capable of activating the superoxide-generating system in vitro in addition to the cell-directing effect. If this were to occur in vivo, a premature release of activated oxygen would be expected. Therefore, a more complex modulation has been proposed in the control of this mechanism [319] or alternative pathways of activation [320]. This might be a plausible explanation why neither leukotrienes nor other hydroxylated lipoxygenase products of arachidonic acid have been reported to significantly activate superoxide production per se [249], although there is some evidence that lipoxygenase products might be involved also in this aspect of PMNL function. This biological aspect might also explain why LTB_4 is considerably less active in inducing enzyme secretion than chemotaxis [254,293,294].

ii. Macrophages

In addition to phagocytosis and release of different kinds of prostaglandins and hydrolytic enzymes [321,322], macrophages have an important role in the initiation of the cell-mediated immune reaction in response to the antigen presented. The cells are activated by a variety of agents such as immune complexes, lymphokines, zymosane and C3b.

The macrophages contain large amounts of esterified arachidonic acid in their phospholipids, and up to 50% of this is released in the form of oxygenated metabolites in response to phagocytic stimuli [323]. The main metabolic products in mouse peritoneal macrophages are LTC_4 and hydroxy acids in addition to lesser amounts of prostaglandins [119,120,162,323,324]. This has led to the hypothesis that lipoxygenase products might be of pathophysiological importance in these cells [325]. Thus, the alveolar macrophage derived factor (AMCF), low molecular weight factor(s) derived from macrophages by a variety of potentially pathogenic stimuli that preferentially attract neutrophils [326] is proposed to be a lipoxygenase product [153,327], possibly similar or identical to LTB_4. Also in macrophages lysosomal enzyme secretion is increased by inhibition of cyclooxygenase or in presence of phorbol myristate acetate [328]. The association of arachidonic acid metabolism with reactive oxygen production in peritoneal macrophages is also analogous to that observed in PMNL [329].

iii. Lymphocytes

Following macrophage activation, which is considered to be the first step of cell-mediated immune response, three events involving lymphocytes occur: mitogen or antigen induced lymphocyte transformation, blastogenesis, and the cytotoxic effect of the activated lymphocyte [231].

The role of lipoxygenase in these events is still unknown. Mitogens cause release of arachidonic acid from the phospholipids [330] and generation of thromboxane B_2 and lipoxygenase products [154]. Arachidonic acid, but not other fatty acids, stimulates blast transformation and incorporation of radiolabeled thymidine and uridine [331], and this effect is inhibited by lipoxygenase inhibition [232]. Thus, it is proposed that the lipoxygenase pathway produces factor(s) that promote mitogenesis.

However, the only presented significant effect upon mitogenesis exerted by a product of arachidonic acid lipoxygenation was the opposite one, viz. inhibition.

Thus, 15-HPETE causes inhibition of RNA and DNA synthesis and blastogenesis [333] with alteration of intracellular cyclic nucleotide concentrations [334]. LTB_4 is not generated in significant amounts in rat or human lymphocytes, and LTB_4 does not change the lymphocyte response to mitogen stimulation [335]. The modulation of lymphocyte function is still more complicated when the response to neutrophil-derived factors is considered [336].

It should also be mentioned that arachidonate metabolism via lipoxygenase has been reported to be of importance for T-lymphocyte chemokinesis [337].

iv. Basophils

Basophils are active in immediate type inflammatory reactions, but they also function in important aspects of the entire inflammatory process [338]. They exert their effects by release of mediators such as histamine and large molecular weight mediators termed "basophil kallikrein-like activities" [338]. When stimulated, these cells also release SRS [92,339], now chemically characterized as mainly LTC_4 and LTD_4 [114,115,123,125]. Arachidonic acid [340] and cyclooxygenase inhibitors [341] enhance histamine release, whereas lipoxygenase inhibitors abolish the response [342]. As in secretion from other leukocytes, the phorbol ester induces histamine release [343], presumably by its arachidonic acid liberation, whereas inhibition of phospholipid methylation gives the opposite effect [344]. These observations indicate that the mechanism of histamine release may resemble or be identical to the enzyme secretion of PMNL. However, no leukotrienes or any other lipoxygenase products of arachidonic acid have been reported to induce histamine release.

v. Eosinophils

It is well known that eosinophils migrate into the site of immediate type hypersensitivity reactions. Among attractants the eosinophil chemotactic factor of anaphylaxis (ECF-A) has drawn special attention. This activity is released from sensitized human and guinea pig lung by antigen challenge [345] and in skin slices from actively sensitized guinea pigs [346]. The factor is chemically heterogeneous and consists of two components of MW 15000 and MW 70000 in addition to a low molecular weight (approximately MW 500) factor, which is independent of the complement system [345]. This last factor is also formed in PMNL after stimulation with calcium ionophore, phagocytosis of zymosan particles [346] and arachidonic acid [348]. Its formation is phospholipase and lipoxygenase dependent [349,350]. There is much evidence that ECF of low molecular weight is identical to LTB_4 or very similar. When incubated with arachidonic acid, eosinophils form 11-HETE, 9-HETE, 5-HETE and LTB_4 [39]. These monohydroxy acids are all active in inducing chemokinesis and chemotaxis, 5-HETE being the most potent compound. In accordance with PMNL migration, preliminary data indicate that LTB_4 is a considerably more potent chemotactic agent in eosinophils. No effect of LTB_4 is reported on release of eosinophilic enzymes (β-glucuronidase and arylsulfatase B) [39].

It is thus proposed that lipoxygenase products derived from the eosinophils themselves, as well as from other cells, are active in modulating eosinophil function.

(b) Effects of cysteinyl-containing leukotrienes

The immediate-type hypersensitivity reaction has many common features with the inflammatory response. In asthma, for instance, the initiation of the reaction is the interaction between antigens, such as pollen, etc., and IgE molecules bound to membrane receptors of mast cells [4,351]. This results in release of factors which influence vascular and pulmonary smooth muscles, vascular permeability and eosinophil recruitment.

i. Effects on smooth muscle
The main LTs affecting smooth muscle tone are LTC_4, LTD_4, LTE_4 and their 11-*trans* isomers in various ratios (= SRS-A) together with histamine. Since antihistamines are not effective pharmacological tools in the treatment of asthma, histamine might be less important.

The effects upon *guinea pig ileum* are interesting from the point of view that it is a classical bioassay preparation used to define the biological activity of one unit SRS in relation to histamine. The contractions of SRS compounds are selectively inhibited by FPL 55712 [352,353] but unaffected by atropine and mepyramine. LTC_4, LTD_4 and LTE_4 are all potent constrictors of guinea pig ileum. LTD_4 is in this respect more potent than LTC_4 and LTE_4 (approximately 5 to 20 fold) [117,123,134,219]. LTC_5 [142] and 11-*trans* LTC_4 [122] are less potent than LTC_4, whereas LTC_3 and LTD_3 are almost as potent as LTC_4 and LTD_4, respectively [140]. LTB_4 is virtually inactive in this respect. All active leukotrienes are considerably more potent than histamine on a molar basis (> 50 fold).

LTC_4 and LTD_4 are largely equipotent in inducing contractions of *tracheal spirals* from guinea pigs and are 30 to 100 fold more potent than histamine [131,132,134]. However, the effect differs between species, since rabbit bronchial preparations do not respond to leukotrienes, whereas human bronchi are remarkably sensitive to LTC_4 and LTD_4, 10^{-10} M being sufficient for a significant response in the latter tissue [131,354,355]. LTE_4 induces bronchoconstriction in guinea pig but not in rat after intravenous injection in vivo [219]. Also LTA_4 and LTB_4 are potent bronchoconstrictors although considerably less active than cysteinyl-containing leukotrienes [131].

Strips of *pulmonary parenchymal tissue* from man [354] and guinea pig [117,131,132,134] are still more sensitive to LTC_4 and LTD_4 (1000 fold more potent than histamine), indicating that the main effect of the leukotrienes is exerted upon peripheral airways, as earlier suggested for SRS-A [215,216] and prostaglandins [356]. Interestingly, LTB_4 is also potent as a constrictor of the parenchymal strip [357,358]. The mechanism differs from that of other leukotrienes since this effect is inhibited by indomethacin. It has been suggested that the mechanism of this contractile effect is activation of a specific LTB_4 receptor, which in turn provokes stimulation of prostaglandin and thromboxane formation [357]. However, under certain experimental conditions the contraction of guinea pig lung parenchymal strips induced by LTC_4 can be inhibited by indomethacin [224,359–361]. Indeed,

LTC_4 and LTD_4 have been shown to induce prostaglandin release in rat peritoneal macrophages [362] and thromboxane release in guinea pig lung [363], and SRS-A induces formation of 12-HETE in isolated lung [364]. Other interactions between the lipoxygenase and cyclooxygenase systems are that hydroperoxides of arachidonic acid inhibit prostaglandin [191] and prostacyclin formation [365].

A vascular effect of LTC_4 and LTD_4 when injected intradermally is a rapid *constriction of the microvasculature* [131–133]. Intravenous infusion in unanaesthetized guinea pigs causes a short phase of hypertension, peaking at 60 s, followed by transient hypotension. These observations are consistent with the findings in the hamster check pouch, where LTC_4 and LTD_4 induce a short-lived constriction of arterioles [135], whereas LTB_4 does not have this effect.

ii. Vascular permeability

The increase in lung vascular permeability by bacteria and endotoxins [366,367] is augmented by inhibition of prostaglandin synthesis [368]. Some of the increased permeability demonstrated under clinical and experimental conditions may be due to histamine release, but since H_1 antagonists only partially inhibit the increase, other factors have to be considered [369].

Among arachidonate lipoxygenase products 5-HETE and LTB_4 showed little effect upon vascular permeability, whereas a purified homogeneous SRS-A produced a clear increase [369]. Plasma exudation in this study was measured as accumulation of intravenously injected [^{131}I]albumin in guinea pig skin. Using the same technique pure LTC_4 and LTD_4 were found to be potent and largely equi-active in one study [131], whereas another group found a significant increase of vascular permeability by LTC_4 and LTD_4 only in the presence of the vasodilator prostaglandin E_2 [133]. Since this might reflect experimental differences, an in vivo model has been used in which the terminal vascular bed can be studied with regard to different vascular events, such as blood flow, vessel diameter, macromolecular permeability and blood cell-endothelium interaction, i.e. the hamster cheek pouch preparation [370]. Under these specific conditions, LTB_4 was shown to cause cell adhesion to the endothelium but not to promote plasma leakage [135], while LTC_4 and LTD_4 both caused a marked dose-dependent extravasation of macromolecules from post-capillary venules.

Reports that LTB_4 increases vascular permeability [371,372] might therefore reflect the essential recruitment of leukocytes necessary for the increase of permeability rather than a direct effect [373,374]. Evidence for this theory is that factors like histamine and bradykinin exert a direct effect upon the vessel wall, whereas the action of C5a, LTB_4 and formyl-tripeptides are dependent on PMNL [375].

LTC_4, LTD_4 and LTE_4 (possibly also the 11-*trans* isomers) fulfill two important biological criteria previously attributed to the pathophysiological agent SRS-A, i.e. the potent smooth muscle effects preferentially in peripheral human airways and the marked increase of vascular permeability in the venules.

7. Assay methods for leukotrienes and other lipoxygenase products

Methods for detection and quantitation of leukotrienes and several other related lipoxygenase products are so far predominantly based on their strong biological activities (see above, Section 4) and ultraviolet absorption in combination with chromatographic properties.

(a) Assays based on biological activity

Bioassays are particularly useful in determining the presence of unstable biologically active compounds and are often the first method of choice for detection of unknown substances. Bioassays for leukotrienes can be highly sensitive, but in contrast to most chemical and physical methods, bioassays usually have a very low specificity, and quantifications can only be approximate. The specificity can however be somewhat increased by combining different bioassay systems, by using inhibitors and antagonists, or by prior purification of the samples. The classical bioassay for determination of SRS-A in relation to histamine is the guinea pig ileum assay [56]. Strips of guinea pig ileum are either suspended in organ baths filled with Tyrode's solution or superfused with buffer containing the sample to be tested. Administration of histamine gives rise to an immediate contraction of the ileum, while SRS-A or each of the cysteinyl-containing leukotrienes (LTC, LTD and LTE) produce a slow onset of the contraction after a short latency period [56,64,123,130,376,377]. The contraction usually reaches a plateau within 1 to 3 minutes and persists for a long time. Repeated washing or administration of the antagonist FPL 55712 results in relaxation of the ileum [352]. Blockade of muscarinic and histamine receptors by atropine and mepyramine does not affect the contraction caused by the leukotrienes. The mechanism of the contraction is unknown, but is thought to involve a leukotriene receptor, which utilizes a pool of calcium channels common to all smooth muscle agonists [377]. LTC_4, LTD_4 and LTE_4 are much more potent than histamine (50–200 times) in the guinea pig ileum assay, and around 0.1 pmol (10^{-10} M) of LTD_4 is sufficient to cause a contraction of the ileum [360]. LTD_4 is more potent than LTC_4 or LTE_4, and also shows a somewhat faster onset of the contraction [123,126,134,224,378]. LTB_4 is considered to be "inactive" in this assay since much higher doses, around 1 nmol (10^{-6} M) [379], are required to obtain a contraction.

Several other smooth muscle preparations from guinea pig and man show a similar type of contraction of cysteinyl-containing leukotrienes (e.g. guinea pig trachea spirals and lung parenchymal strips, uterine strips from virgin and adult ovariectomized guinea pig, human bronchus and human lung parenchyma) [117,131,132,134,354,376], while corresponding preparations from rat and rabbit do not respond or respond only weakly to leukotrienes. This fact can be used in a differential bioassay to additionally distinguish the biological activity of SRS or cysteinyl-containing leukotrienes from that of other chemical mediators (histamine, serotonin, bradykinin, prostaglandin, etc.) [56].

Guinea pig lung parenchymal strips are still more sensitive to cysteinyl-containing leukotrienes than guinea pig ileum. In such an assay, where these substances were added to the bath fluid under conditions of no flow, the detection limit was around 0.03 pmol (3×10^{-11} M) [360]. LTC_4 LTD_4 and LTE_4 as well as the 11-*trans* isomers and the corresponding leukotrienes of the 3- and 5-series are equipotent constrictors of the lung parenchyma [217]. However, some laboratories report that even in this tissue LTD_4 is more potent than LTC_4 and LTE_4, which are more potent than their 11-*trans* isomers [117,127,132,224,378]. Part of these and several other contradictory bioassay results might be due to differences in experimental conditions [360]. One important finding to take into consideration when pulmonary parenchymal strips are used for bioassay is the fact that leukotrienes cause tachyphylaxis of the tissue, which makes it impossible to use cumulative administration of leukotrienes [217]. Leukotriene induced contraction of superfused guinea pig lung strips were inhibited by indomethacin, indicating that at least part of the response was due to the release of one or more cyclooxygenase products [224,359]. Other studies have also shown that LTC_4 and LTD_4 stimulate formation and release of TXA_2 from isolated perfused guinea pig lung [67,363]. However, in a guinea pig lung strip assay using the organ bath technique, where the bath fluid was changed intermittently, indomethacin treatment had no effect on the contraction induced by LTC_4 [217].

In a superfused guinea pig ileum assay a major part of the LTC_4-induced contraction was reported to be due to conversion of LTC_4 to LTD_4 by γ-glutamyl transpeptidase present in the ileum. This was shown by the use of δ-D-glutamyl-*O*-carboxyphenyl hydrazine, an inhibitor of γ-glutamyl transpeptidase [224]. Such a conversion does not seem to be essential for the contracting activity of LTC_3 in the lung parenchymal strip assay, using the organ bath technique with stopped flow [217]. When HPLC analysis of the bath fluid was performed at regular intervals after addition of radiolabeled LTC_3 to guinea pig lung strips, no LTD_3 could be detected after 3 minutes when half-maximal contraction was reached. After 10 minutes, 25% of the amount of LTC_3 had been converted to LTD_3.

The guinea pig lung parenchymal strip has also been used to assay LTB_4 [357,358]. With 30–1500 pmol LTB_4, a dose dependent but relatively short-lived contraction was seen, which was not antagonized by FPL 55712, but was nearly completely abolished by indomethacin. The ω-oxidized metabolites of LTB_4 give a similar type of contraction of the guinea pig lung strip [179]. 20-hydroxy-LTB_4 was somewhat more potent than LTB_4, while 20-carboxy-LTB_4 was less potent.

Among other biological effects of leukotrienes that can be used in bioassays are the ability of LTC_4 and LTD_4 to increase the vascular permeability in guinea pig and rat skin, but not in rabbit skin [131,132,224,369,380]. Intradermal injection of 0.1 pmol or more of LTC_4 or LTD_4 in guinea pig skin causes an exudation of intravenously injected dye in the presence of histamine receptor blockers. Higher doses produced dose-dependent increase in spot diameter, which were homogenous with LTD_4, but with LTC_4 showed a central blanching at the site of injection. A more sophisticated and better system for measuring macromolecular leakage in relation to other vascular events is the hamster cheek pouch preparation [135]. Leukotrienes were applied topically to an everted hamster cheek pouch and the leakage of macromolecules was studied under the microscope after intravenous injection of fluorescent dextran as a tracer.

Although LTB_4 has some spasmogenic properties, it is primarily involved in leukocyte function and more sensitive assays can be obtained by following its effect on leukocyte adherence, aggregation, enzyme secretion, chemotaxis and chemokinesis. In some assays based on these effects around 0.1 pmol of LTB_4 can be detected. In adherence assays for LTB_4, leukocyte adherence to nylon fibers [249] or to the endothelium in post-capillary venules in the hamster cheek pouch preparation [135] have been used. Aggregation of leukocytes caused by addition of LTB_4 has been assessed by nephelometry in an aggregometer [37]. In chemotaxis and chemokinesis assays for LTB_4, 5-HETE, and related compounds, different techniques have been used: the Boyden chamber technique [254], the agarose microdroplet assay [37] or studies of leukocyte migration under agarose [247].

(b) Assays based on chromatography and UV absorption

The rapid progress over the last years in research on SRS-A and the leukotrienes is to a large extent due to the introduction of HPLC combined with UV detectors for purification and analysis of these compounds. Several laboratories have now described HPLC methods (reverse phase and/or straight phase-adsorption chromatography) with UV absorbance measurements for separation and quantification of the different HETE, HPETE [17,205,381], di-HETE including LTB_4 [15,17,71] and cysteinyl-containing leukotrienes [64,71,117,127,129,382].

Before analysis by HPLC can be performed, an initial sample purification is often necessary. Various purification methods for leukotrienes have been described in the literature. Depending on the type and size of the sample, and whether a total analysis is intended or if only certain components should be analyzed, different procedures can be used. The cysteinyl-containing leukotrienes are somewhat acid labile and require mild conditions for extraction and purification. A first extraction of leukotrienes from biological samples can be achieved by adsorption to some resin, e.g. Amberlite XAD-8 or XAD-7, at slightly acid or neutral pH [64,91,112,215] or adsorption to charcoal [75,118] or to Sephadex LH-20 [69]. Mild extraction into organic solvents at low temperature has also been used for cysteinyl-containing leukotrienes [119], although this method has preferably been used at a later step in the purification procedure for these compounds [75].

The extracts are then further purified using methods such as silicic acid chromatography on a neutral silicic acid column [64,124], ion exchange chromatography [95,178] or gel filtration [73,75,92]. By these methods a group separation between the cysteinyl-containing leukotrienes and the different hydroxy acids (mono-, di- and trihydroxy acids, as well as dicarboxylic metabolites) can be achieved, which may simplify the subsequent HPLC profile.

After initial purification and group fractionation of the leukotrienes, the different fractions are usually subjected to reverse phase HPLC, using either gradient or isocratic elution systems. However, although HPLC methods usually have a high separation efficiency, several of the lipoxygenase products cannot be completely separated from each other even by reverse phase chromatography. To eliminate cochromatography and to obtain sufficient separation between all the different isomers of lipoxygenase products which can appear in biological samples, it is often necessary to use at least two different types of HPLC columns, e.g. reverse phase and straight phase adsorption columns. For example, LTB_4, prepared from human and porcine peripheral leukocyte preparations, was recently shown to be contaminated with another isomer, 5S,12S-dihydroxy-6-*trans*,8-*cis*,10-*trans*,14-*cis*-eicosatetraenoic acid, which cochromatographed on reverse phase HPLC [15,228]. This isomer had a similar UV spectrum to LTB_4 but was considerably less active on the guinea pig lung strip [228] and in a leukotactic assay [360]. The two compounds could however be well separated as methyl esters on straight phase adsorption HPLC. The early attempts to quantify LTB_4 from biological samples by the HPLC-UV method, using only reverse phase systems, must therefore be re-evaluated. It might also be necessary to confirm some data on biological activity of LTB_4 obtained from such isomeric mixtures.

UV spectrometry is the most frequently used method for detection and quantification of lipoxygenase products in HPLC assays. The leukotrienes and related compounds with three conjugated double bonds, exhibit characteristic triplets in their UV spectra [383] with maxima around 270, 280 and 290 nm for LTA_4 and the cysteinyl-containing leukotrienes [19,64,123,127,136], and around 260, 270 and 280 for LTB-like compounds [15,31–34,48]. All lipoxygenase products with conjugated double bonds possess relatively high molar extinction coefficients: 23 000–31 000 for HPETEs and HETEs at 232–236 nm [16,107,205, 213], 50 000 for LTB_4 at 270 nm [33], 40 000–56 000 at around 270 nm for related dihydroxy acids with triene structure [31,46,163], 33 500 at 243 nm for the 5,15-dihydroxy acid with a double diene structure [163], and 40 000 for LTA_4 and the cysteinyl-containing leukotrienes at 278–280 nm [19]. This makes it possible to detect about 10 pmol of these substances. For convenient UV detection of all different lipoxygenase products, it is desirable to have simultaneous detection of at least two different wavelengths (e.g. 235 nm and 270 nm or 280 nm), or the possibility to get complete UV spectra of the compounds during chromatography. In order to establish the identity and purity of a chromatographic peak, it is important to register the complete UV spectrum before reliable quantitative UV absorption measurements can be performed. Recoveries of lipoxygenase products in HPLC assays can sometimes be relatively low. In one study, only 65% of 12-HETE and 50% of arachidonic acid were recovered after chromatography on one reverse HPLC column [381]. To this should be added the inevitable losses during the initial purification of samples. Correction for losses during the purification procedure and in the HPLC systems can be made by addition of radiolabeled internal standards of high specific activity prior to purification. Since some of the leukotrienes have so far been difficult to prepare with high enough specific activity, other approaches have been made. Borgeat and Samuelsson [17] added PGB_2 as an internal reference and standard for estimation of the production of LTB_4 and the non-enzymatically formed isomers under various conditions. PGB_2 has strong UV absorption at 278 nm ($E = 26\,800$ [384]) and chromatographic properties very similar to LTB_4.

The labile epoxide intermediate, LTA_4, cannot be assayed directly with the above-mentioned procedure, since LTA_4 is very sensitive to acid, radicals and oxygen [22]. LTA_4 must therefore first be converted into a stable derivative. Analysis of the kinetics of appearance and disappearance of LTA_4 in rabbit peripheral leukocyte preparations and RBL cells have been performed after such a conversion into stable 12-*O*-methylated dihydroxy derivatives by using methanol as a trapping agent and PGB_2 as internal standard [18,23].

Another sensitive method for detection of cysteinyl-containing leukotrienes in HPLC assays is measurement of fluorescence, which has been used in combination with UV absorbance and radioactivity monitoring [119]. Post-column derivatization of compounds containing free amino groups was performed on-line with fluorescamine.

In certain well-defined in vitro systems more unspecific and simplified radiochemical assays without HPLC can be used. Such an assay has been described to follow the release of LTC_4 in macrophages after labeling of the phospholipids with $[^{14}C]$arachidonic acid [120].

(c) Gas chromatography-mass spectrometry and radioimmunoassays

Assay methods using combined gas chromatography-mass spectrometry with selected ion monitoring and addition of stable isotopes as carriers and internal standards have been published for the different HETE isomers [208,236,385]. However, so far no GC-MS-assay for LTB_4 and related dihydroxy acids or the cysteinyl-containing leukotrienes have been described. Deuterated standards of HETEs were prepared from octadeuterated arachidonic acid either by biosynthesis in mammalian tissues [236,385] or by chemical methods [208]. Preparation of internal standards by chemical methods resulted in deuterated standards with minimal contamination of unlabeled material. This resulted in assays with a detection limit of about 1 pmol for the different HETEs. A GC-MS assay without addition of deuterated internal standards has also been described for analysis of the ratio between different HETEs in the same sample [210].

Radioimmunoassays (RIA) have been developed for 12-HETE [386,387] and 15-HETE [388]. These compounds showed relatively weak immunogenic properties and the titer of the antibodies was much lower than for many cyclooxygenase products. The detection limit for these assays was around 1 pmol. A report on the development of RIA for LTC_4 and LTD_4 has also appeared [389]. The antisera for LTD_4 showed a considerable cross-reactivity with LTC_4 and LTE_4 [389]. These biologically potent compounds are most likely produced in very small amounts during physiological conditions. Since radioimmunological methods can often become extremely sensitive, a further development of RIA for leukotrienes or for their metabolites and stable degradation products will provide important tools for evaluation of their roles in hypersensitivity and inflammation.

8. *Inhibitors of lipoxygenase and leukotriene biosynthesis, SRS antagonists*

Initially inhibitors of lipoxygenase will be discussed (Section a). Inhibitors of the other enzymes involved in the pathways are discussed thereafter (Section b). Finally, the antagonists of the action of SRS (cysteinyl-containing leukotrienes) are reviewed (Section c).

(a) Lipoxygenase inhibitors

The classical soybean lipoxygenase inhibitors are the antioxidant nordihydroguaiaretic acid (NDGA) [390] and the substrate analogue 5,8,11,14-eicosatetraynoic acid (ETYA) [391,392] that also inhibits cyclooxygenase (for review see ref. 393). Lipoxygenases of plants and animals are similar in many ways, including their response to inhibitors [394]. In this review, however, only drugs that inhibit mammalian lipoxygenases are included. Most studies regard the n-8 lipoxygenase (that gives 12-HETE), mostly in platelets, but several reports deal with the lipoxygenases of inflammatory cells. Intact cells were usually studied after stimulation with arachidonic acid.

ETYA (10^{-5} M) inhibits the formation of 12(L)-HETE in intact platelets [164]. The platelet lipoxygenase is insensitive to indomethacin, aspirin and cyanide [164,165]. The 12-lipoxygenase present in guinea pig spleen homogenates is inhibited completely by 2×10^{-4} M ETYA, and to 90% by 5×10^{-4} M NDGA [166]. The particulate lipoxygenase prepared from platelet microsomes [190] is sensitive to Cu^{2+} and hydroquinone. A series of phenylhydrazones has been tested as inhibitors for platelet lipoxygenase (acetone-pentane powder preparation) and found effective with IC_{50} values in the 10^{-7}–10^{-6} M range [189]. The cations Zn^{2+} and Sn^{2+} are also inhibitory. The phenylhydrazones also inhibit soybean lipoxygenase and cyclooxygenase.

Since ferric ion is a cofactor for platelet lipoxygenase, various chelators should be inhibitory. Thus, EDTA exhibited an IC_{50} of 7×10^{-6} M [194] and toluene-3,4-dithiol an IC_{50} of 10^{-5} M [195]. High speed supernatant preparations were used in these studies. The latter study also stated cyanide as a lipoxygenase inhibitor, IC_{50} 2×10^{-3} M. The neuroleptic drug chlorpromazine is a weak inhibitor of lipoxygenase in high speed supernatants from platelets, IC_{50} at 10^{-3} M [395].

Extracts from onion and garlic inhibit arachidonic acid metabolism in platelets. The exact nature of the inhibiting factor and the mechanism is not fully understood [396,397].

Various flavonoids and related compounds have been tested as inhibitors for cyclooxygenase and lipoxygenase. Some are more effective as lipoxygenase inhibitors, and some more effective as cyclooxygenase inhibitors. Thus, 3′,4′-dihydroxyflavone and 1,5-dihydroxy-naphthalene are potent inhibitors of 12-HETE formation in rat lung and spleen homogenates. IC_{50} values are 3.3×10^{-5} M and 2×10^{-5} M, respectively [394].

There is a need for lipoxygenase inhibitors that are specific in that they do not also inhibit cyclooxygenase. Various poly-ynoic fatty acids are promising in this respect. One such study concerned 5,8,11-eicosatetraynoic acid [398] which inhibited formation of 12-HETE by intact platelets with $IC_{50} = 2.4 \times 10^{-5}$ M. In two other studies some very selective lipoxygenase inhibitors are described [399,400]. One of the most selective was 4,7,10,13-eicosatetraynoic acid. Stated IC_{50} values varied (intact platelets) from 3×10^{-7} M [400] to 7.8×10^{-6} M [399].

Two other drugs that are more efficient as lipoxygenase than as cyclooxygenase inhibitors are benoxaprofen [401] and acetone phenylhydrazone [399]. Benoxaprofen inhibits the lipoxygenases of ionophore stimulated rabbit PMNL with an IC_{50} of 6×10^{-5} M [401,402]. Acetone phenylhydrazone inhibits platelet 12-lipoxygenase, $IC_{50} = 1.6 \times 10^{-6}$ M [403].

A very interesting inhibitor of the lipoxygenases which catalyzes the synthesis of 12-HETE in rabbit and human platelets and 5-HETE in rabbit and human PMNL is 15-hydroxy-5,8,11,13-eicosatetraenoic acid (15-HETE), an endogenous arachidonate metabolite [36,404]. 15-HETE given exogenously inhibited the conversion in intact rabbit cells with IC_{50} values of 5.7×10^{-6} M for the 5-lipoxygenase and 3.4×10^{-7} M for the 12-lipoxygenase. Also, 15-HETE was found to have more than ten times lower effect towards the cyclooxygenase pathways.

Two structurally related drugs that have a common feature in that they inhibit both the cyclooxygenase and lipoxygenase pathways are phenidone and BW 755C. Thus, phenidone (1-phenyl-3-pyrazolidone) inhibits lipoxygenase in intact platelets (IC_{50} 3×10^{-4} M) and more effectively in lung [405]. The related compound called BW 755C (3-amino-1-(-m(trifluoromethyl)-phenyl)-2-pyrazoline), is a more potent lipoxygenase inhibitor. The IC_{50} for the lipoxygenase from disrupted horse platelets is 7.5×10^{-6} M [406]. Also, the biosynthesis of 5-HETE in glycogen-elicited rabbit leukocytes was inhibited by BW 755C with an IC_{50} close to 5×10^{-6} M [250], while the same conversion in human PMNL (ionophore A23187 stimulated) required a higher dose (IC_{50} $10–20 \times 10^{-6}$ M) [407]. In a study where rabbit PMNL were stimulated with ionophore A23187, the IC_{50} for 5-HETE production was found to be close to 10^{-4} M for BW 755C [402]. In this study NDGA was also tried and found to have an IC_{50} close to 3×10^{-6} M for the same conversion. The high IC_{50} value for inhibition of ionophore stimulated 5-HETE synthesis by BW 755C (approximately 10^{-4} M) was also reported for the enzyme in rat neutrophils [43].

Regarding the lipoxygenase-catalyzed 5-HETE production in leukocytes, there is some controversy about the inhibitory effect of ETYA. The observed differences have been explained as a species- and/or tissue dependency [45]. Thus, ETYA (6.5×10^{-5} M) did not inhibit the biosynthesis of 5-HETE in arachidonate-stimulated rabbit PMNL [16]. This is reconfirmed in rabbit PMNL [36] and in guinea pig PMNL [45]. Inhibition of the same pathway did occur though in human neutrophils (IC_{50} close to 10^{-5} M [152] and $3–20 \times 10^{-6}$ M [150]), in human eosinophils (10^{-5} M [39]), in rat neutrophils (IC_{50} around 3×10^{-5} M [43]), and in RBL-cells ($3–34 \times 10^{-6}$ M [88] and 6.7×10^{-5} M [145]). In human lymphocytes ETYA inhibition of 5-HETE formation was poor, but effective for 12-HETE [154].

The antioxidant NDGA has also been tested for inhibition of 5-HETE formation. It was found effective in human neutrophils (5–10 $\times 10^{-6}$ M [39]), in RBL cells (3×10^{-6} M [88]), in guinea pig peritoneal PMNL (5×10^{-6} M [45]), and in rabbit PMNL (3×10^{-6} M [403]). Poor efficiency was stated though in human lymphocytes [154].

When hydroxyacids (11-HETE and 15-HETE) are produced as byproducts of the cyclooxygenase pathway, inhibition is effected by cyclooxygenase inhibitors as indomethacin and flurbiprofen [159,160]. Indomethacin inhibits formation of thromboxane B_2 in platelets effectively at 2.8×10^{-5} M, while no inhibitory effect was seen on the formation of 12-HETE at 2.8×10^{-4} M [164]. In leukocytes, however, inhibition of lipoxygenases at an indomethacin concentration of 10^{-4} M has been reported [245].

(b) Inhibitors of other enzymes in the leukotriene pathways

The initial product resulting from the action of a lipoxygenase is a hydroperoxy acid. This is quickly followed by reduction to a hydroxyacid by peroxidase. Some common anti-inflammatory drugs have been shown to cause accumulation of 12-HPETE in platelets by inhibition of the enzymatic reduction into 12-HETE [186,188]. Among the drugs showing this effect are aspirin, indomethacin, sodium salicylate and phenylbutazone.

Some data have been presented regarding inhibition of the production of leukotrienes. A number of studies have compared the effects of various lipoxygenase inhibitors on production of 5-HETE and LTB_4, and found similar effects for the two compounds [36,43,250,401,402,407]. There are numerous observations on inhibition of SRS production by lipoxygenase inhibitors [88,223,402]. These drugs appear to inhibit the lipoxygenase and have little if any, effect on the additional enzymes involved in LTB_4 production, although the specific effect on the additional leukotriene-forming enzymes cannot be determined from these studies.

Effects of drugs on LTB_4 production have also been studied utilizing bioassay techniques. With this technique comprehensive data for many drugs studied in the same system is presented [42,245,303,408].

Inhibition of LTA_4-synthetase has been reported [45]. In this study ETYA inhibited production in guinea pig peritoneal PMNL of LTB_4 and its non-enzymatically formed isomers, while 5-HETE synthesis was augmented. This is interpreted as inhibition of the LTA_4-synthetase and a shunting of the 5-HPETE towards the peroxidase [45].

The γ-glutamyl transpeptidase which catalyzes conversion of LTC_4 to LTD_4 has been studied with regard to its inhibition by the transition state inhibitor L-serine-borate. When this complex was added to incubations of RBL cells, the amount of LTD_4 formed was decreased, while the amount of LTC_4 was increased [223].

(c) Antagonists to SRS

A compound that inhibits the contractions induced in the guinea pig ileum by SRS is FPL 55712. As a selective inhibitor of SRS-A [352] it has been used extensively in research concerning SRS compounds since its discovery in 1973. In fact one of the important criteria for SRS activity has been its inhibition by FPL 55712. The IC_{50} value against SRS-A-induced contractions of guinea pig ileum is reported to be 10 nM [352]. FPL 55712, and also related compounds, inhibits the action of SRS-A in other preparations of smooth muscle as well [353,409]. It is also active in vivo, in inhibiting antigen-induced bronchoconstriction, when given as an aerosol to guinea pigs [353]. FPL 55712 has been administered to human asthmatics although no firm conclusions from these results can be drawn [410].

Regarding selectivity of action, FPL 55712 has been shown to inhibit antigen-induced histamine release and thromboxane synthesis [411]. Hence it is claimed that used at concentrations exceeding 1 μM, FPL 55712 can act through mechanisms other than simply antagonism of SRS-A.

New drugs similar to FPL 55712 but which are more effective in inhibiting the actions of SRS and leukotrienes C and D have recently been reported [412,413]. Rotenone, a natural product used as a fish and insect poison, is also active as an SRS-A antagonist. Inhibition of SRS-A induced constriction of the guinea pig ileum was reported at IC_{50} 110 nM [414].

Acknowledgments

Part of this work was supported by grants from the Swedish Medical Research Council (project no. 03X-217), from Riksförbundet mot Reumatism, and from Konung Gustaf V:s 80-årsfond.

References

1 Samuelsson, B., Goldyne, M., Granström, E., Hamberg, M., Hammarström, S. and Malmsten, C. (1978) Annu. Rev. Biochem. 47, 997–1029.
2 Ramwell, P.W. (1981) Arch. Internal Med. 141, 275–278.
3 Austen, K.F. (1978) J. Immunol. 121, 793–805.
4 Dawson, W. (1979) Eur. J. Rheum. Inflamm. 3, 1–2.
5 Turner, S.R., Tainer, S.A. and Lynn, W.S. (1975) Nature 257, 680–681.
6 Eakins, K.E., Higgs, G.A., Moncada, S., Mugridge, K.G. and Vane, J.R. (1980) Br. J. Pharmacol. 69, 270P–271P.
7 Samuelsson, B., Hammarström, S., Murphy, R.C. and Borgeat, P. (1980) Allergy 35, 375–381.
8 Samuelsson, B., Borgeat, P., Hammarström, S. and Murphy, R.C. (1980) in Advances in Prostaglandin and Thromboxane Research (Samuelsson, B., Ramwell, P. and Paoletti, R., eds.) Vol. 6, pp. 1–18, Raven Press, New York.
9 Borgeat, P. and Sirois, P. (1981) J. Med. Chem. 24, 121–126.

10 Ford-Hutchinson, A.W., Bray, M.A. and Smith, M.J.H. (1980) Agents and Actions 10, 548–549.
11 Samuelsson, B. and Hammarström, S. (1981) Immunology Today 2, 3–6.
12 Kuehl, F.A. Jr, and Egan, R.W. (1980) Science 210, 978–934.
13 Samuelsson, B., Borgeat, P., Hammarström, S. and Murphy, R.C. (1979) Prostaglandins 17, 785–787.
14 Samuelsson, B. and Hammarström, S. (1980) Prostaglandins 19, 645–648.
15 Lindgren, J-Å., Hansson, G. and Samuelsson, B. (1981) FEBS Lett. 128, 329–335.
16 Borgeat, P., Hamberg, M. and Samuelsson, B. (1976) J. Biol. Chem. 251, 7816–7820 (see correction (1977) J. Biol. Chem. 252, 8772).
17 Borgeat, P. and Samuelsson, B. (1979) Proc. Natl. Acad. Sci. USA 76, 2148–2152.
18 Borgeat, P. and Samuelsson, B. (1979) Proc. Natl. Acad. Sci. USA 76, 3213–3217.
19 Corey, E.J., Clark, D.A., Goto, G., Marfat, A., Mioskowski, C., Samuelsson, B. and Hammarström, S. (1980) J. Am. Chem. Soc. 102, 1436–1439.
20 Rådmark, O., Malmsten, C., Samuelsson, B., Clark, D.A., Goto, G., Marfat, A. and Corey, E.J. (1980) Biochem. Biophys. Res. Commun. 92, 954–961.
21 Rådmark, O., Malmsten, C., Samuelsson, B., Goto, G., Marfat, A. and Corey, E.J. (1980) J. Biol. Chem. 255, 11828–11831.
22 Corey, E.J., Barton, A.E. and Clark, D.A. (1980) J. Am. Chem. Soc. 102, 4278–4279.
23 Hammarström, S. and Samuelsson, B. (1980) FEBS Lett. 122, 83–86.
24 Rokach, J., Young, R.N., Kakushima, M., Lau, C.-K., Seguin, R., Frenette, R. and Guindon, Y. (1981) Tetrahedron Lett. 22, 979–982.
25 Corey, E.J., Arai Y. and Mioskowski, C. (1979) J. Am. Chem. Soc. 101, 6748–6749.
26 Rosenberger, M. and Neukom, C. (1980) J. Am. Chem. Soc. 102, 5426.
27 Baker, S.R., Jamieson, U.B., McKay, S.W. Morgan, S.E., Rackham, D.M., Ross, W.J. and Shrubsall, P.R. (1980) Tetrahedron Lett. 21, 4123–4126.
28 Cohen, N., Banner, B.L. and Lopresti, R.J. (1980) Tetrahedron Lett. 21, 4163–4166.
29 Corey, E.J., Hashimoto, S. and Barton, A.E. (1981) J. Am. Chem. Soc. 103, 721–722.
30 Gleason, J.G., Bryan, D.B. and Kinzig, C.M. (1980) Tetrahedron Lett. 21, 1129–1132.
31 Borgeat, P. and Samuelsson, B. (1979) J. Biol. Chem. 254, 7865–7869.
32 Borgeat, P. and Samuelsson, B. (1979) J. Biol. Chem. 254, 2643–2646.
33 Corey, E.J., Marfat, A., Goto, G. and Brion, F. (1980) J. Am. Chem. Soc. 102, 7984–7985.
34 Corey, E.J., Marfat, A. and Hoover, D.J. (1981) Tetrahedron Lett. 22, 1587–1590.
35 Claesson, H.E., Lundberg, U. and Malmsten, C. (1981) Biochem. Biophys. Res. Commun. 98, 1230–1237.
36 Vanderhoek, J.Y., Bryant, R.W. and Bailey, J.M. (1980) J. Biol. Chem. 255, 10064–10066.
37 Ford-Hutchinson, A.W., Bray, M.A., Doig, M.V., Shipley, M.E. and Smith, M.J.H. (1980) Nature 286, 264–265.
38 Stenson, W.F. and Parker, C.W. (1979) J. Clin. Invest. 64, 1457–1465.
39 Goetzl, E.J., Weller, P.F. and Sun, F.F. (1980) J. Immunol. 124, 926–933.
40 Klickstein, L.B., Shapleigh, C. and Goetzl, E.J. (1980) J. Clin. Invest. 66, 1166–1170.
41 Cromwell, O., Morris, H.R., Hodson, M.E., Walport, M.J., Taylor, G.W., Batten, J. and Kay, A.B. (1981) Lancet ii, 164–165.
42 Doig, M.V. and Ford-Hutchinson, A.W. (1980) Prostaglandins 20, 1007–1019.
43 Siegel, M.I., McConnell, R.T., Bonser, R.W. and Cautrecasas, P. (1981) Prostaglandins 21, 123–132.
44 Jakschik, B.A., Sun, F.F., Lee, L. and Steinhoff, M.M. (1980) Biochem. Biophys. Res. Commun. 95, 103–110.
45 Bokoch, G.M. and Reed, P.W. (1981) J. Biol. Chem. 256, 4156–4159.
46 Corey, E.J., Hopkins, P.B., Munroe, J.E., Marfat, A. and Hashimoto, S. (1980) J. Am. Chem. Soc. 102, 7986–7987.
47 Corey, E.J., Marfat, A., Munroe, J., Kim, K.S., Hopkins, P.B. and Brion, F. (1981) Tetrahedron Lett. 22, 1077–1080.
48 Jubiz, W., Rådmark, O., Lindgren, J.-Å., Malmsten, C. and Samuelsson, B. (1981) Biochem. Biophys. Res. Commun. 99, 976–986.

49 Lundberg, U., Rådmark, O., Malmsten, C. and Samuelsson, B. (1981) FEBS Lett. 126, 127–132.
50 Maas, R., Brash, A. and Oates, J. (1981) Proc. Natl. Acad. Sci. USA 78, 5523–5527.
51 Corey, E.J., Marfat, A. and Goto, G. (1980) J. Am. Chem. Soc. 102, 6607–6608.
52 Feldberg, W. and Kellaway, C.H. (1938) J. Physiol. (Lond.) 94, 187–226.
53 Kellaway, C.H. and Trethewie, E.R. (1940) Q.J. Exp. Physiol. 30, 121–145.
54 Brocklehurst, W.E. (1953) J. Physiol. (Lond.) 120, 16P.
55 Brocklehurst, W.E. (1962) Progr. Allergy 6, 539–558.
56 Orange, R.P. and Austen, K.F. (1969) Adv. Immunol. 10, 104–144.
57 Bach, M.K., Brashler, J.R. and Gorman, R.R. (1977) Prostaglandins 14, 21–28.
58 Burka, J.F. and Flower, R.J. (1979) Br. J. Pharmacol. 65, 35–41.
59 Bach, M.K. and Brashler, J.R. (1974) J. Immunol. 113, 2040–2044.
60 Orange, R.P., Moore, E.G. and Geltand, E.W. (1980) J. Immunol. 124, 2264–2267.
61 Yecies, L.D., Wedner, A.J., Johnson, S.M., Jakschik, B.A. and Parker, C.W. (1979) J. Immunol. 122, 2083–2089.
62 Jakschik, B.A., Kulzycki, A., MacDonald, H.H. and Parker, C.W. (1977) J. Immunol. 119, 618–622.
63 Jakschik, B.A., Lee, L.H., Shaffer, G. and Parker, C.W. (1978) Prostaglandins 16, 733–749.
64 Murphy, R.C., Hammarström, S. and Samuelsson, B. (1979) Proc. Natl. Acad. Sci. USA 76, 4275–4279.
65 Strandberg, K. and Uvnäs, B. (1971) Acta Phys. Scand. 82, 358–374.
66 Conroy, M.C., Orange, R.P. and Lichtenstein, L.M. (1976) J. Immunol. 116, 1677–1681.
67 Morris, H.R., Piper, P.J., Taylor, G.W. and Tippins, J.R. (1979) Br. J. Pharmacol. 67, 179–184.
68 Sirois, P., Engineer, D.M., Piper, P.J. and Moore, E.G. (1979) Experientia 35, 361–363.
69 Watanabe-Kohno, S. and Parker, C.W. (1980) J. Immunol. 125, 946–955.
70 Findlay, S.R., Lichtenstein, L.M. and Grant, J.A. (1980) J. Immunol. 124, 238–242.
71 Morris, H.R., Taylor, G.W., Piper, P.J. and Tippins, J.R. (1979) Agents and Actions Suppl. 6, 27–36.
72 Sirois, P., Moore, E.G. and Orange, R.P. (1979) Agents and Actions 9, 337–343.
73 Watanabe, S. and Koda, A. (1979) Microbiol. Immunol. 23, 1009–1022.
74 Piper, P.J. and Seale, J.P. (1979) Br. J. Pharm. 67, 67–72.
75 Morris, H.R., Taylor, G.W., Piper, P.J., Sirois, P. and Tippins, J.R. (1978) FEBS Lett. 87, 203–206.
76 Piper, P.J., Tippins, J.R., Morris, H.R. and Taylor, G.W. (1980) in Advances in Prostaglandin and Thromboxane Research (Samuelsson, B., Ramwell, P. and Paoletti, R., eds.) Vol. 6, pp. 121–124, Raven Press, New York.
77 Burka, J.F. and Paterson, N.A. (1980) Prostaglandins 19, 499–515.
78 Morris, H.R., Piper, P.J., Taylor, G.W. and Tippins, J.R. (1980) Prostaglandins 19, 371–383.
79 Paterson, N.A.M. and Craig, I.D. (1981) Aust. N. Zeal. J. Med. 11, 104.
80 Piper, P.J., Tippins, J.R., Morris, A.R. and Taylor, G.W. (1979) Agents and Actions Suppl. 6, 37–48.
81 Walker, J.L. (1973) in Advances in Biosciences 9 (Bergström, S. and Bernard, S., eds.) pp. 235–239, Pergamon Press, Oxford.
82 Nijkamp, F.P. and Ramakers, A.G. (1980) Eur. J. Pharmacol. 62, 121–122.
83 Yen, S.S. and Kreutner, W. (1980) Agents and Actions 10, 274–278.
84 Burka, J.F. and Paterson, N.A. (1980) in Advances in Prostaglandin and Thromboxane Research, Vol. 8 (Samuelsson, B., Ramwell, P. and Paoletti, R., eds.) pp. 1755–1758, Raven Press, New York.
85 Hitchcock, M. (1980) Br. J. Pharmacol. 71, 65–73.
86 Laekeman, G.M. and Herman, A.G. (1979) Arch. Int. Pharmacodyn. 242, 307–309.
87 Chaud, N. and Altura, B.M. (1981) Prostaglandins Med. 6, 249–258.
88 Falkenhein, S.F., MacDonald, H., Huber, M.M., Koch, D. and Parker, C.W. (1980) J. Immunol. 125, 163–168.
89 Adcock, J.J., Garland, L.G., Moncada, S. and Salmon, J.A. (1979) Prostaglandins 16, 163–181.
90 Parker, C.W., Koch, D., Huber, M.M. and Falkenhein, S.F. (1980) Biochem. Biophys. Res. Commun. 94, 1037–1043.
91 Jakschik, B.A., Falkenhein, S. and Parker, C.W. (1977) Proc. Natl. Acad. Sci. USA 74, 4577–4581.
92 Yecies, L.D., Parker, C.W. and Watanabe, S. (1979) Life. Sci. 25, 1909–1916.
93 Orange, R.P., Murphy, R.C., Karnovsky, M.L. and Austen, K.F. (1973) J. Immunol. 110, 760–770.

94 Parker, C.W., Huber, M.T. and Falkenhein, S. (1980) Fed. Proc. 38, 1167.
95 Parker, C.W., Jakschik, B.A., Huber, M.G. and Falkenhein, S.F. (1979) Biochem. Biophys. Res. Commun. 89, 1186–1192.
96 Dawson, W., Lewis, R.L. and Tomlinson, R. (1975) J. Physiol. (Lond.) 247, 37–38P.
97 Orange, R.P. and Chang, P.-L. (1975) J. Immunol. 115, 1072–1077.
98 Orange, R. and Moore, E.G. (1976) J. Immunol. 116, 392–397.
99 Parker, C.W., Fischman, C.M. and Wedner, H.J. (1980) Proc. Natl. Acad. Sci. USA 77, 6870–6873.
100 Bach, M.K. and Brashler, J.R. (1978) Life Sci. 23, 2119–2126.
101 Orange, R.P., Murphy, R.C. and Austen, K.F. (1974) J. Immunol. 113, 316–323.
102 Wasserman, S.I., Goetzl, E.J. and Austen, K.F. (1975) J. Immunol. 114, 645–652.
103 Parker, C.W., Koch, D.A., Huber, M.M. and Falkenhein, S.F. (1980) Prostaglandins 20, 887–908.
104 Sok, D.-E., Pai, J.-K., Atrache, V., Kang, Y.-C. and Sih, C.J. (1981) Biochem. Biophys. Res. Commun. 101, 222–229.
105 Sirois, P. (1979) Prostaglandins 17, 395–404.
106 Sirois, P. (1980) in Advances in Prostaglandin and Thromboxane Research Vol. 6 (Samuelsson, B., Ramwell, P. and Paoletti, R., eds.) pp. 125–128, Raven Press, New York.
107 Hamberg, M. and Samuelsson, B. (1967) J. Biol. Chem. 242, 5329–5335.
108 Sirois, P. and Borgeat, P. (1980) Int. J. Immunopharmacol. 2, 281–294.
109 Hammarström, S., Murphy, R.C., Samuelsson, B., Clark, D.A., Mioskowski, C. and Corey, E.J. (1979) Biochem. Biophys. Res. Commun. 91, 1266–1272.
110 Hammarström, S., Samuelsson, B., Clark, D.A., Goto, G., Marfat, A., Mioskowski, C. and Corey, E.J. (1980) Biochem. Biophys. Res. Commun. 92, 946–953.
111 Rådmark, O., Malmsten, C. and Samuelsson, B. (1980) Biochim. Biophys. Res. Commun. 96, 1679–1687.
112 Hansson, G. and Rådmark, O. (1980) FEBS Lett. 122, 87–90.
113 Morris, H.R., Taylor, G.W., Piper, P.J., Samhoun, M.N. and Tippins, J.R. (1980) Prostaglandins 19, 185–201.
114 Sok, D.E., Pai, J.K., Atrache, V. and Sih, C.J. (1980) Proc. Natl. Acad. Sci. USA 77, 6481–6485.
115 Parker, C.W., Huber, M.M., Hoffman, M.K. and Falkenhein, S.R. (1979) Prostaglandins 18, 673–686.
116 Bach, M.K., Brashler, J.R., Hammarström, S. and Samuelsson, B. (1980) J. Immunol. 125, 115–117.
117 Lewis, R.A., Austen, K.F., Drazen, J.M.,, Clark, D.A., Marfat, A. and Corey, E.J. (1980) Proc. Natl. Acad. Sci. USA 77, 3710–3714.
118 Morris, H.R., Taylor, G.W., Piper, P.J. and Tippins, J.R. (1980) Nature 285, 104–106.
119 Rouzer, C.A., Scott, W.A., Cohn, Z.A., Blackburn, P. and Manning, J.M. (1980) Proc. Natl. Acad. Sci. USA 77, 4928–4932.
120 Rouzer, C.A., Scott, W.A., Hamill, A.L. and Cohn, Z.A. (1980) J. Exp. Med. 152, 1236–1247.
121 Rouzer, C.A., Scott, W.A., Griffith, O.W., Hamill, A.L. and Cohn, Z.A. (1981) Proc. Natl. Acad. Sci. USA 78, 2532–2536.
122 Clark, D.A., Goto, G., Marfat, A., Corey, E.J., Hammarström, S., and Samuelsson, B. (1980) Biochem. Biophys. Res. Commun. 94, 1133–1139.
123 Örning, L., Hammarström, S. and Samuelsson, B. (1980) Proc. Natl. Acad. Sci. USA 77, 2014–2017.
124 Parker, C.W., Falkenhein, S.F. and Huber, M.M. (1980) Prostaglandins 20, 863–886.
125 Bach, M.K., Brashler, J.R., Hammarström, S. and Samuelsson, B. (1980) Biochem. Biophys. Res. Commun. 93, 1121–1126.
126 Houglum, J., Pai, J.K., Atrache, V., Sok, D.E. and Sih, C.J. (1980) Proc. Natl. Acad. Sci. USA 77, 5688–5692.
127 Lewis, R.A., Drazen, J.M., Austen, K.F., Clark, D.A. and Corey, E.J. (1980) Biochem. Biophys. Res. Commun. 96, 271–277.
128 Parker, C.W., Koch, D., Huber, M.M. and Falkenhein, S.F. (1980) Biochem. Biophys. Res. Commun. 97, 1038–1046.
129 Örning, L., Bernström, K. and Hammarström, S. (1981) Eur. J. Biochem. 120, 41–45.
130 Bernström, K. and Hammarström, S. (1981) J. Biol. Chem. 256, 9579–9582.

131 Hedqvist, P., Dahlén, S.-E., Gustafsson, L., Hammarström, S. and Samuelsson, B. (1980) Acta Physiol. Scand. 10, 331–334.
132 Drazen, J.M., Austen, K.F., Lewis, R.A., Clark, D.A., Goto, G., Marfat, A. and Corey, E.J. (1980) Proc. Natl. Acad. Sci. USA 77, 4354–4358.
133 Peck, M.J., Piper, P.J. and Williams, T.J. (1981) Prostaglandins 21, 315–322.
134 Palmer, M.H., Piper, P.J., Samhoun, M.N. and Tippins, J.R. (1981) Br. J. Pharmacol. 73, 213P.
135 Dahlén, S.-E., Björk, J., Hedqvist, P., Arfors, K.-E., Hammarström, S., Lindgren, J.-Å. and Samuelsson, B. (1981) Proc. Natl. Acad. Sci. USA 78, 3887–3891.
136 Corey, E.J., Clark, D.A., Marfat, A. and Goto, G. (1980) Tetrahedron Lett. 2, 3143–3146.
137 Atrache, V., Sok, D.-E., Pai, J.-K. and Sih, C.J. (1981) Proc. Natl. Acad. Sci. USA 78, 1523–1526.
138 Rokach, J., Girard, Y., Guidon, Y., Atkinson, J.G., Larue, M., Young, R.N., Massaon, P. and Holme, G. (1980) Tetrahedron Lett. 21, 1485–1488.
139 Corey, E.J. and Clark, D.A. (1980) Tetrahedron Lett. 21, 3547–3548.
140 Hammarström, S. (1981) J. Biol. Chem. 256, 2275–2279.
141 Hammarström, S. (1981) Biochim. Biophys. Acta 663, 575–577.
142 Hammarström, S. (1980) J. Biol. Chem. 255, 7093–7094.
143 Jakschik, B.A., Sams, A.R., Sprecher, H. and Needleman, P. (1980) Prostaglandins 20, 401–410.
144 Hammarström, S. (1981) J. Biol. Chem. 256, 7712–7714.
145 Jakschik, B.A. and Lee, L.H. (1980) Nature 287, 51–52.
146 Axelrod, B. (1979) Adv. Chem. Ser. 136, 324–348.
147 Easkin, N.A., Grossman, S. and Pinsky, A. (1977) Crit. Rev. Food, Sci. Nutr. 9, 1.
148 Grossman, S. and Zakut, R. (1979) Methods Biochem. Anal. 25, 303–329.
149 Hamberg, M., Samuelsson, B., Björkhem, I. and Danielsson, H. (1974) in Mechanisms of Oxygen Activation (Hayaishi, O., ed.) pp. 29–85, Academic Press, New York.
150 Goetzl, E.J. (1980) Immunology 40, 709–719.
151 Goetzl, E.J. and Sun, F.F. (1979) J. Exp. Med. 150, 406–411.
152 Stenson, W.F. and Parker, C.W. (1980) J. Immunol. 124, 2100–2104.
153 Valone, F.H., Franklin, M., Sun, F.F. and Goetzl, E.J. (1980) Cell Immunol. 54, 390–401.
154 Parker, C.W., Stenson, W.F., Huber, M.G. and Kelly, J.P. (1979) J. Immunol. 122, 1572–1577.
155 Rabinovitch, H., Durand, J., Rigaud, M., Mendy, F. and Breton, J.-C. (1981) Lipids 16, 518–524.
156 Capdevila, J., Parkhill, L., Chacos, N., Ocita, R., Masters, B.S.S. and Estabrook, R.W. (1981) Biochem. Biophys. Res. Commun. 101, 1357–1363.
157 McGuire, J.C. and Sun, F.F. (1980) in Advances in Prostaglandin and Thromboxane Research vol. 8 (Samuelsson, B., Ramwell, P. and Paoletti, R., eds.) pp. 1665–1667, Raven Press, New York.
158 Hamberg, M. and Samuelsson, B. (1974) Biochem. Biophys. Res. Commun. 61, 942–949.
159 Hemler, M.E., Crawford, C.G. and Lands, W.E.M. (1978) Biochemistry 17, 1772–1779.
160 Hubbard, W.C., Hough, A.J., Brash, A.R., Watson, J.F. and Oates, J.A. (1980) Prostaglandins 20, 431–447.
161 Siegel, M.I., McConnell, R.T., Porter, N.A., Selph, J.L., Truax, J.F., Vinegar, R. and Cuatrecasas, P. (1980) Biochem. Biophys. Res. Commun. 92, 688–695.
162 Rigaud, M., Durand, J. and Breton, J.C. (1979) Biochim. Biophys. Acta 573, 408–412.
163 van Os, C.P.A., Rijke-Schilder, P.M., van Halbeck, H., Verhagen, J. and Vliegenhart, F.G. (1981) Biochim. Biophys. Acta 663, 177–193.
164 Hamberg, M. and Samuelsson, B. (1974) Proc. Natl. Acad. Sci. USA 71, 3400–3404.
165 Nugteren, D.H. (1975) Biochim. Biophys. Acta 380, 299–307.
166 Hamberg, M. (1976) Biochim. Biophys. Acta 431, 651–654.
167 Hammarström, S., Hamberg, M., Samuelsson, B., Duell, E.A., Stawiski, M. and Voorhees, J.J. (1975) Proc. Natl. Acad. Sci. USA 72, 5130–5134.
168 Hammarström, S., Lindgren, J.Å., Marcelo, C., Duell, E., Anderson, T. and Voorhees, J.J. (1979) J. Investigative Dermatology 73, 180–183.
169 Greenwald, J.E., Bianchine, J.R. and Wong, L.K. (1979) Nature 281, 588–589.
170 Robert, L.J., Lewis, R.A., Oates, J.A. and Austen, K.F. (1979) Biochim. Biophys. Acta 575, 185–192.
171 Herman, A.G., Claeys, M., Moncada, S. and Vane, J.R. (1979) Prostaglandins 18, 439–452.

172 Sautebin, L., Spagnuolo, C., Galli, C. and Galli, G. (1978) Prostaglandins 16, 985–988.
173 Bennet, A., Hensby, C.N., Sanger, G.J. and Stanford, J.F. (1981) Br. J. Pharmacol. 74, 435–444.
174 Barnes, P., Dollery, C.T. and Hensby, C.N. (1980) in Advances in Prostaglandin and Thromboxane Research, Vol. 7 (Samuelsson, B., Ramwell, P. and Paoletti, R., eds.) pp. 933–936, Raven Press, New York.
175 Hamberg, M., Hedqvist, P. and Rådegran, K. (1980) Acta Physiol. Scand. 110, 219–221.
176 Wlodawer, P. and Samuelsson, B. (1973) J. Biol. Chem. 248, 5673–5678.
177 Claeys, M., Coene, M.-C., Herman, A.G., van der Planken, M., Jouvenaz, G.H. and Nugteren, D.H. (1981) Arch. Int. Pharmacodyn. 250, 305–308.
178 Maas, R.L., Brash, A.R. and Oates, J.A. (1981) in SRS-A and Leukotrienes (Piper, P.J., ed.) pp. 151–159, John Wiley and Sons Ltd., Chichester, England.
179 Hansson, G., Lindgren, J.-Å. Dahlén, S.-E., Hedqvist, P. and Samuelsson, B. (1981) FEBS Lett. 130, 107–112.
180 Walker, I.C., Jones, R.L. and Wilson, N.H. (1980) Prostaglandins 18, 173–180.
181 Falardeau, P., Hamberg, M. and Samuelsson, B. (1976) Biochim. Biophys. Acta 441, 193–200.
182 Jones, R.L., Kerry, P.J., Poyser, N.L., Walker, I.C. and Wilson, N.H. (1978) Prostaglandins 16, 583–589.
183 Bryant, R.W. and Bailey, J.M. (1979) Prostaglandins 17, 9–18.
184 Bryant, R.W. and Bailey, J.M. (1980) Biochem. Biophys. Res. Commun. 92, 268–276.
185 Bryant, R.W. and Bailey, J.M. (1980) in Advances in Prostaglandin and Thromboxane Research, Vol. 6 (Samuelsson, B., Ramwell, P. and Paoletti, R., eds.) pp. 95–99, Raven Press, New York.
186 Siegel, M.I., McConnell, R.T. and Cuatrecasas, P. (1979) Proc. Natl. Acad. Sci. USA 76, 3774–3776.
187 Ho, P.P.K., Walter, C.P. and Sullivan, H.R. (1977) Biochem. Biophys. Res. Commun. 76, 398–405.
188 Siegel, M.I., McConnell, R.T., Porter, N.A. and Cuatrecasas, P. (1980) Proc. Natl. Acad. Sci. USA 77, 308–312.
189 Wallach, D.P. and Brown, V.R. (1981) Biochim. Biophys. Acta 663, 361–372.
190 Hamberg, M. and Hamberg, G. (1980) Biochem. Biophys. Res. Commun. 95, 1090–1097.
191 Siegel, M.I., McConnell, R.T., Abrahams, S.L., Porter, N.A. and Cuatrecasas, P. (1979) Biochem. Biophys. Res. Commun. 89, 1273–1280.
192 Lagarde, M., Vericel, E., Guichardant, M. and Dechavanne, M. (1981) Biochem. Biophys. Res. Commun. 99, 1398–1402.
193 Ahnfelt-Rønne, I. and Arrigoni-Martelli, E. (1980) Agents and Actions 10, 550–553.
194 Greenwald, J.E., Alexander, M.S., Fertel, R.H., Beach, C.A., Wong, L.K. and Bianchine, J.R. (1980) Biochem. Biophys. Res. Commun. 96, 817–822.
195 Aharony, D., Smith, J.B. and Silver, M.J. (1981) Prostaglandins Med. 6, 237–242.
196 Rao, G.H.R., Gerrard, J.M., Eaton, S.W. and White, J.G. (1978) Photochem. Photobiol. 28, 845–850.
197 Gwebu, E.T., Trewyn, R.W., Cornwell, D.G. and Panganamala, R.V. (1980) Res. Commun. Chem. Pathol. Pharmacol. 28, 361–376.
198 Butler, A.M., Gerrard, J.M., Peller, J., Stoddard, S.F., Rao, G.H.R. and White, J.G. (1979) Prostaglandins Med. 2, 203–216.
199 Goetzl, E.J. (1980) Nature 288, 183–185.
200 Walker, J.R. and Parich, H.A. (1981) Int. Arch. Allergy Appl. Immunol. 66, 83–90.
201 Naruyima, S., Salmon, J.A., Cottee, F.H., Weatherley, B.C. and Flower, R.J. (1981) J. Biol. Chem. 256, 9583–9592.
202 Rapoport, S.M., Schewe, T., Wiesner, R., Halangk, W., Ludwig, P., Janicke-Höhne, M., Tannert, C., Hiebsch, C. and Klatt, D. (1979) Eur. J. Biochem. 96, 545–561.
203 Shahin, I., Grossman, S. and Sredni, B. (1978) Biochim. Biophys. Acta 529, 300–308.
204 Grossman, S., Shalim, I. and Sredni, B. (1979) Biochim. Biophys. Acta 572, 293–297.
205 Porter, N.A., Wolf, R.A., Yaxbro, E.M. and Weenen, A. (1979) Biochem. Biophys. Res. Commun. 89, 1058–1064.
206 Porter, N.A., Logan, J. and Kontoyiannidou, V. (1979) J. Org. Chem. 44, 3177–3181.
207 Terao, J. and Matsushita, S. (1981) Agric. Biol. Chem. 45, 587–593.
208 Boeynaems, J.M., Brash, A.R., Oates, J.A. and Hubbard, W.C. (1980) Anal. Biochem. 104, 259–267.

209 Boeynaems, J.M., Oates, J.A. and Hubbard, W.C. (1980) Prostaglandins 19, 87–97.
210 Terao, J. and Matsushita, S. (1981) Agric. Biol. Chem. 45, 595–599.
211 Fridovich, S.E. and Porter, N.A. (1981) J. Biol. Chem. 256, 260–265.
212 Corey, E.J., Marfat, A., Falck, J.R. and Albright, J.O. (1980) J. Am. Chem. Soc. 102, 1433–1435.
213 Corey, E.J., Albright, J.O., Barton, A.E. and Hashimoto, S. (1980) J. Am. Chem. Soc. 102, 1435–1436.
214 Galliard, T. and Phillips, D.R. (1971) Biochemical J. 124, 431–438.
215 Drazen, J.M., Lewis, R.A., Wasserman, S.I., Orange, R.P. and Austen, K.F. (1979) J. Clin. Invest. 63, 1–5.
216 Michoud, M.C., Pare, P.J., Orange, R.P. and Hogg, J.C. (1979) Am. Rev. Respir. Dis. 119, 419–424.
217 Hedqvist, P., Dahlén, S.-E. and Björk, J. (1982) in Advances in Prostaglandin, Thromboxane and Leukotriene Research, Vol. 9 (Samuelsson, B. and Paoletti, R., eds.) pp. 187–200. Raven Press, New York.
218 Hedqvist, P., Dahlén, S.-E. and Björk, J. (1983) in: Leukotrienes and Prostacyclin (Berti, F., ed.) NATO-ASI-series, Plenum Press, New York, Vol. 4, pp. 81–107.
219 Welton, A.F., Crowley, H.J., Miller, D.A. and Yaremko, B. (1981) Prostaglandins 21, 287–296.
220 Bach, M.K., Brashler, J.R., Johnson, H.G. and Mc Nee, M.L. (1981) in SRS-A and Leukotrienes (Piper, J., ed.) pp. 161–180, John Wiley and Sons Ltd., Chichester, England.
221 Hammarström, S. (1981) J. Biol. Chem. 256, 9573–9578.
222 Tate, S.S., Thompson, G.A. and Meister, A. (1976) in Glutathione: Metabolism and Function (Arias, I.M. and Jakoby, W.B., eds.) pp. 45–61, Raven Press, New York.
223 Örning, L. and Hammarström, S. (1980) J. Biol. Chem. 255, 8023–8026.
224 Piper, P.J., Samhoun, M.N., Tippins, J.R., Williams, T.J., Palmer, M.A. and Peck, M.J. (1981) in SRS-A and Leukotrienes (Piper, P.J., ed.) pp. 81–99, John Wiley and Sons Ltd., Chichester, England.
225 Appelgren, L.-E. and Hammarström, S. (1982) J. Biol. Chem. 257, 531–535.
226 Hammarström, S., Bernström, K., Örning, L., Dahlén, S.-E., Hedqvist, P., Smedegård, G. and Revenäs, B. (1981) Biochem. Biophys. Res. Commun. 101, 1109–1115.
227 Jubiz, W., Rådmark, O., Malmsten, C., Hansson, G., Lindgren, J.Å., Palmblad, J., Udén, A.-M. and Samuelsson, B. (1982) J. Biol. Chem. 257, 6106–6110.
228 Borgeat, P., Picard, S., Vallerand, P. and Sirois, P. (1981) Prostaglandins Med. 6, 557–570.
229 Robinson, D.R., Dayer, J.M. and Krane, S.M. (1979) Ann. N.Y. Acad. Sci. 332, 279–294.
230 Lewis, G.P. (1979) Agents and Actions Suppl. (6), 7–15.
231 Trang, L. (1980) Sem. Arthr. Rheumat. 9, 153–190.
232 Flower, R.J. (1974) Pharmacol. Rev. 26, 33–67.
233 Zurier, R.B. and Sayadoff, D.M. (1975) Inflammation 1, 93–98.
234 Goldstein, I.M., Malmsten, C., Kindahl, H., Kaplan, H., Rådmark, O., Samuelsson, B. and Weissmann, G. (1978) J. Exp. Med. 148, 787–792.
235 O'Flaherty, J.T. (1980) Inflammation 4, 181–194.
236 Bokoch, G.M. and Reed, P.W. (1980) J. Biol. Chem. 255, 10223–10226.
237 Hutchroft, B.J. and Orange, R.P. (1980) Clin. Allergy 10, 565–574.
238 Stenson, W.F., Parker, C.W. (1979) J. Clin. Invest. 64, 1457–1465.
239 Rubin, R.P., Sink, L.E. and Freer, R.J. (1981) Biochem. J. 194, 497–505.
240 Walsh, C.E., De Chatelet, L.R., Thomas, M.J., O'Flaherty, J.T. and Waite, M. (1981) Lipids 16, 120–124.
241 Kitchen, E.A., Boot, J.R. and Dawson, W. (1978) Prostaglandins 16, 239–244.
242 Diaz-Perez, J.L., Goldyne, M.E. and Winkelman, R.K. (1976) J. Invest. Dermatol. 66, 149–152.
243 Goetzl, E.J., Hill, H.R. and Gorman, R.R. (1980) Prostaglandins 19, 71–85.
244 Hirata, F., Corcoran, B.A., Venkatasubramanian, K., Schiffman, E. and Axelrod, J. (1979) Proc. Natl. Acad. Sci. USA 76, 2640–2643.
245 Bray, M.A., Ford-Hutchinson, A.W., Shipley, M.E. and Smith, M.J.H. (1980) Br. J. Pharmacol. 71, 507–512.
246 Warne, P.J. and West, G.B. (1978) J. Pharm. Pharmacol. 30, 783–785.
247 Malmsten, C.L., Palmblad, J., Udén, A.-M., Rådmark, O., Engstedt, L. and Samuelsson, B. (1980) Acta Physiol. Scand. 110, 449–451.

248 Sato, M., Furuta, K. and Yamaguchi, A. (1980) Jpn. J. Pharmacol. 30, 919–921.
249 Palmblad, J., Malmsten, C.L., Udén, A.-M., Rådmark, O. and Samuelsson, B. (1981) Blood 58, 658–661.
250 Randall, R.W., Eakins, K.E., Higgs, G.A., Salmon, J.A. and Tateson, J.E. (1980) Agents and Actions 10, 553–555.
251 Bureau, J.P., Senelar, R. and Cupissol, D. (1980) Br. J. Exp. Pathol. 61, 479–485.
252 Goetzl, E.J., Brash, A.R., Tauber, A.I., Oates, J.A. and Hubbard, W.C. (1980) Immunology 39, 491–501.
253 Palmer, R.M., Stepney, R.J., Higgs, G.A. and Eakins, K.E. (1980) Prostaglandins 20, 411–418.
254 Goetzl, E.J. and Pickett, W.C. (1980) J. Immunol. 125, 1789–1791.
255 Smith, M.J., Ford-Hutchinson, A.W. and Bray, M.A. (1980) J. Pharm. Pharmacol. 32, 517–518.
256 Goetzl, E.J. and Pickett, W.C. (1981) J. Exp. Med. 153, 482–487.
257 Bray, M.A., Ford-Hutchinson, A.W. and Smith, M.J.H. (1981) Br. J. Pharmacol. 73, 259P.
258 Carr, S.C., Higgs, G.A., Salmon, J.A. and Spayne, J.A. (1981) Br. J. Pharmacol. 73, 253P.
259 Bhattacherjee, P., Eakins, K.E. and Hammond, B. (1981) Br. J. Pharmacol. 73, 254P.
260 Ford-Hutchinson, A.W., Bray, M.A., Cunningham, F.M., Davidson, E.M. and Smith, M.J.H. (1981) Prostaglandins 21, 143–152.
261 Sirois, P., Roy, S., Borgeat, P., Picard, S. and Corey, E.J. (1981) Biochem. Biophys. Res. Commun. 99, 385–390.
262 Pattison, J.D., Filer, D., Anderson, W.G., Gettingby, G. and Andersson, J.M. (1981) J. Clin. Lab. Immunol. 5, 191–194.
263 Takenchi, A. and Perseilin, R.H. (1981) Int. Arch. Allergy Appl. Immunol. 64, 171–180.
264 Van Oss, C.J., Absolom, D.R., Moore, L.L., Park, B.H. and Humbert, J.R. (1980) J. Reticuloendothel. Soc. 27, 561–567.
265 Goetzl, E.J., Valone, F.H., Reinhold, V.N. and Gorman, R.R. (1979) J. Clin. Invest. 63, 1181–1186.
266 Stenson, W.F. and Parker, C.W. (1979) Prostaglandins 18, 285–292.
267 Sha'afi, R.I., Naccache, P.H., Alubaidi, T., Molski, T.F.P. and Volpi, M. (1981) J. Cell Physiol. 106, 215–224.
268 Volpi, M., Naccache, P.H. and Sha'afi, R.I. (1980) Biochem. Biophys. Res. Commun. 92, 1231–1237.
269 Mottala, C., Dolzani, L. and Romeo, D. (1981) Cell Calcium 1, 371–380.
270 Keller, H.U., Wissler, J.H. and Dameran, B. (1981) Immunology 42, 379–384.
271 Zigmond, S.H. (1981) J. Cell Biol. 88, 644–648.
272 Goldstein, I.M. (1981) J. Lab. Clin. Med. 97, 599–601.
273 Dahinden, C. and Fehr, J. (1980) J. Clin. Invest. 66, 884–891.
274 Keller, H.U., Wilkinson, P.C., Abercrombie, M., Becker, E.L., Hirsch, J.G., Miller, M.E., Ramsey, W.S. and Zigmond, S.H. (1977) Cell Biol. Int. Rep. 1, 391–397.
275 Bradshaw, D., Giroud, J.P. and Roch-Arveiller, M. (1980) Br. J. Pharmacol. 68, 663–666.
276 Issekutz, A.C. and Biggar, W.D. (1977) Infect. Immun. 15, 212–220.
277 Nelson, R.D., Fiegel, V.D., Herron, M.J., Gracyk, J.M., Bauman, M.P., McCormack, R.T. and Simmons, R.L. (1981) Acta Physiol. Scand. suppl. 492, 31–42.
278 Perez, H.D., Weksler, B.B. and Goldstein, I.M. (1980) Inflammation 4, 313–328.
279 Petrone, W.F., English, D.K., Wong, K. and McCord, J.M. (1980) Proc. Natl. Acad. Sci. USA 77, 1159–1163.
280 Bragt, P.C. and Bonta, I.L. (1980) Agents and Actions 10, 563–569.
281 Boxer, L.A., Yoder, M., Bonsib, S., Schmidt, M., Ho, P., Jersild, R. and Baehner, R.L. (1979) J. Lab. Clin. Med. 93, 506–514.
282 Goldstein, I.M. (1979) J. Lab. Clin. Med. 93, 13–16.
283 Naccache, P.H., Showell, H.J., Becker, E.L. and Sha'afi, R.I. (1977) J. Cell Biol. 75, 635–649.
284 Showell, H.J., Freer, R.J., Zigmond, S.H., Schiffman, E., Aswanikumar, S., Corcoran, B. and Becker, E.L. (1976) J. Exp. Med. 143, 1154–1169.
285 Rubin, R.P., Sink, L.E., Schrey, M.P., Day, A.R., Liao, C.S. and Freer, R.J. (1979) Biochem. Biophys. Res. Commun. 90, 1364–1370.
286 Waite, M., De Chatelet, L.R., King, L. and Shirley, P.S. (1979) Biochem. Biophys. Res. Commun. 90, 984–992.

287 Rubin, R.P., Lynn, E.S. and Freer, R.J. (1981) Mol. Pharmacol. 19, 31–37.

288 Naccache, P.H., Showell, H.J., Becker, E.L. and Sha'afi, R.I. (1979) Biochem. Biophys. Res. Commun. 87, 292–299.

289 O'Flaherty, J.T., Showell, H.J., Ward, P.A. and Becker, E.L. (1979) Am. J. Pathol. 96, 799–810.

290 O'Flaherty, J.T., Showell, H.J., Becker, E.L. and Ward, P.A. (1979) Am. J. Pathol. 95, 433–444.

291 Walenga, R.W., Showell, H.J., Feinstein, M.B. and Becker, E.L. (1980) Life Sci. 27, 1047–1053.

292 Showell, H.J., Naccache, P.H., Sha'afi, R.I. and Becker, E.L. (1980) Life Sci. 27, 421–426.

293 Hafström, I., Palmblad, J., Malmsten, C., Rådmark, O. and Samuelsson, B. (1981) FEBS Lett. 130, 146–148.

294 Palmer, R.M.J. and Yeates, D.A. (1981) Br. J. Pharmacol. 73, 260P.

295 Weissman, G., Smolen, J.E. and Korchak, H.M. (1980) N. Engl. J. Med. 303, 27–34.

296 Smolen, J.E. and Weissmann, G. (1980) Biochim. Biophys. Acta 672, 197–206.

297 Grant, L. (1973) in: The Inflammatory Process, Vol. 2 (Zweifach, B.W., Grant, L. and McCluskey, R.T., eds.) pp. 205–249, Academic Press, New York.

298 Craddock, P.R., Hammerschmidt, D., White, J.G., Dalmasso, A.P. and Jacob, H.S. (1977) J. Clin. Invest. 60, 260–264.

299 O'Flaherty, J.T., Kreutzer, D.L. and Ward, P.A. (1977) J. Immunol. 119, 232–239.

300 O'Flaherty, J.T., Showell, H.J., Becker, E.L. and Ward, P.A. (1978) Am. J. Pathol. 92, 155–166.

301 O'Flaherty, J.T., Showell, H.J., Becker, E.L. and Ward, P.A. (1979) Prostaglandins 17, 915–927.

302 O'Flaherty, J.T., Showell, H.J., Becker, E.L. and Ward, P.A. (1979) Inflammation 3, 431–436.

303 Ford-Hutchinson, A.W., Bray, M.A. and Smith, M.J.H. (1979) J. Pharm. Pharmacol. 31, 868–869.

304 O'Flaherty, J.T. (1980) Inflammation 4, 45–53.

305 O'Flaherty, J.T., De Chatelet, L.R., McCall, C.E. and Bass, D.H. (1980) Proc. Soc. Exp. Biol. Med. 165, 225–232.

306 Nakamura, M., Baxter, C.R. and Masters, B.S.S. (1981) Biochem. Biophys. Res. Commun. 98, 743–751.

307 Light, D.R., Walsh, C., O'Collagnan, A.M., Goetzl, E.J. and Tauber, A.I. (1981) Biochemistry 20, 1468–1475.

308 Cross, A.R., Jones, O.T.G., Harper, A.M. and Segal, A.W. (1981) Biochem. J. 194, 599–606.

309 Bokoch, G.M. and Reed, P.W. (1979) Biochem. Biophys. Res. Commun. 90, 481–487.

310 Beswick, P.H. and Kay, A.B. (1981) Clin. Exp. Immunol. 43, 399–407.

311 Zabucchi, G., Berton, G. and Soranzo, M.R. (1981) FEBS Lett. 125, 165–169.

312 Nelson, R.D., Herron, M.J., Gracyk, J.M. and Simmons, R.L. (1981) J. Infect. Dis. 143, 94–100.

313 Smith, R.J. and Iden, S.S. (1981) J. Reticuloendoth. Soc. 29, 215–226.

314 Flower, R. (1978) in Advances in Prostaglandin and Thromboxane Research, Vol. 3 (Galli, C., Galli, G. and Porcellati, G., eds.), pp. 105–112, Raven Press, New York.

315 Levine, P.H., Hardin, J.C., Scoon, K.L. and Krinski, N.I. (1981) Inflammation 5, 19–28.

316 Nelson, D.H., Wennhold, A.R. and Murray, D.K. (1981) J. Steroid Biochem. 14, 321–326.

317 Min-Fu Tsan (1980) J. Cell Physiol. 105, 327–334.

318 Kensler, K.W. and Trusn, M.A. (1980) Cancer Res. 41, 216–222.

319 English, D., Roloff, J.S. and Lukens, J.N. (1981) J. Immunol. 126, 165–173.

320 McPhail, L.C., Henson, P.M. and Johnston, R.B. (1981) J. Clin. Invest. 67, 710–716.

321 Humes, J.L., Bonney, R.J. and Peleus, L. (1977) Nature 269, 149–151.

322 Stenson, W.F. and Parker, C.W. (1980) J. Immunol. 125, 1–5.

323 Scott, W.A., Zrike, J.M., Hamill, A.L., Kempe, J. and Cohn, Z.A. (1980) J. Exp. Med. 152, 324–333.

324 Bonney, R.J., Davies, P., Kuehl, F.A. and Humes, J.L. (1980) J. Reticuloendothel. Soc. 28 suppl., 1135.

325 Goetzl, E.J., Derian, C. and Valone, F.H. (1980) J. Biol. Chem. 255, 11828–11831.

326 Hunninghake, G.W., Gadek, J.E., Fales, H.M. and Crystal, R.G. (1980) J. Clin. Invest. 66, 473–483.

327 Merrill, W.W., Naegel, G.P., Matthay, R.A. and Reynolds, H.Y. (1980) J. Clin. Invest. 65, 268–276.

328 Davies, P., Bonney, R.J., Humes, J.L. and Kuehl, F.A. (1980) J. Invest. Dermatol. 74, 292–296.

329 Smith, R.L. and Weidemann, M.J. (1980) Biochem. Biophys. Res. Commun. 97, 973–980.

330 Parker, C.W., Kelly, J.P., Falkenhein, S.F. and Huber, M.G. (1979) J. Exp. Med. 149, 1487–1503.

331 Kelly, J.P. and Parker, C.W. (1979) J. Immunol. 122, 1556–1562.
332 Kelly, J.P., Johnson, M.C. and Parker, C.W. (1979) J. Immunol. 122, 1563–1571.
333 Goodman, M.G. and Weigle, W.O. (1980) J. Supramol. Structure 13, 373–384.
334 Goodman, M.G., Brunton, L.L. and Weigle, W.O. (1981) Cell Immunol. 58, 85–96.
335 Bray, M.A. and Smith, M.J.H. (1980) Int. J. Immunopharmacol. 2, 256.
336 Panush, R.S. (1981) J. Clin. Lab. Immunol. 5, 113–120.
337 McCarty, J. and Goetzl, E.J. (1979) Cell Immunol. 43, 103–112.
338 Newball, H.H., Meier, H.L. and Lichtenstein, L.M. (1980) J. Invest. Dermatol. 74, 344–348.
339 Yecies, L.D., Wedner, H.J. and Parker, C.W. (1979) J. Immunol. 123, 2814–2816.
340 Marone, G., Sobotka, A.K. and Lichtenstein, L.M. (1979) J. Immunol. 123, 1669–1677.
341 Sobotka, A.K., Marone, G. and Lichtenstein, L.M. (1979) Monogr. Allergy 14, 285–287.
342 Marone, G., Hammarström, S. and Lichtenstein, L.M. (1980) Clin. Immunol. Immunopathol. 17, 117–122.
343 Schleimer, R.P., Gillespie, E. and Lichtenstein, L.M. (1981) J. Immunol. 126, 570–574.
344 Crews, F.T., Morita, Y., Hirata, F., Axelrod, J. and Siraganian, R.P. (1980) Biochem. Biophys. Res. Commun. 93, 42–49.
345 Kay, A.B., Stechschulte, D.J. and Austen, K.F. (1971) J. Exp. Med. 133, 602–619.
346 Kimura, I., Yamamoto, S. and Yamura, T. (1979) Int. Arch. Allergy Appl. Immunol. 60, 465–468.
347 König, W., Frickhofen, N. and Tesch, H. (1979) Immunology 36, 733–742.
348 Tesch, H., König, W. and Frickhofen, N. (1979) Int. Arch. Allergy Appl. Immunol. 58, 436–446.
349 Tesch, H. and König, W. (1980) Scand. J. Immunol. 11, 409–418.
350 Czarnetzki, B.M. and Zimmerman, R.E. (1981) Int. Arch. Allergy Appl. Immunol. 65, 23–26.
351 Wasserman, S.I. (1980) Environ. Health Perspect. 35, 153–164.
352 Augstein, J., Farmer, J.B., Lee, T.B., Sheard, P. and Tattersall, M.L. (1973) Nat. New Biol. 245, 215–217.
353 Sheard, P., Lee, T.B. and Tattersall, M.L. (1977) Monogr. Allergy 12, 245–249.
354 Hanna, C.J., Bach, M.K., Pare, P.D. and Schellenberg, R.R. (1981) Nature 290, 343–344.
355 Dahlén, S.-E., Hedqvist, P., Hammarström, S. and Samuelsson, B. (1980) Nature 288, 484–486.
356 Schneider, M.W. and Drazen, J.M. (1980) Am. Rev. Respir. Dis. 121, 835–842.
357 Sirois, P., Borgeat, P., Jeansson, A., Roy, S. and Girard, G. (1980) Prostaglandins Med. 5, 429–444.
358 Sirois, P., Roy, S. and Borgeat, P. (1981) Prostaglandins Med. 6, 153–160.
359 Folco, C.G., Omini, C., Vigano, T., Brunelli, G., Rossini, G. and Berti, F. (1982) in Advances in Prostaglandin, Thromboxane and Leukotriene Research, Vol. 9 (Samuelsson, B. and Paoletti, R., eds.) pp. 153–167, Raven Press, New York.
360 Hansson, G., Dahlén, S.-E. and Granström, E. (1983) in Leukotrienes and Prostacyclin (Berti, F., ed.) NATO-ASI series, Plenum Press, New York, Vol. 54, pp. 65–80.
361 Schiantarelli, P., Borgrani, S. and Folco, G. (1981) Eur. J. Pharmacol. 73, 363–366.
362 Feuerstein, N., Foegh, M. and Ramwell, P. (1981) Br. J. Pharmacol. 72, 389–392.
363 Folco, G.C., Hansson, G. and Granström, E. (1981) Biochem. Pharmacol. 30, 2491–2493.
364 Omini, C., Sautebin, L., Galli, G., Folco, G.C. and Berti, F. (1980) in Advances in Prostaglandin and Thromboxane Research, Vol. 7 (Samuelsson, B., Ramwell, P. and Paoletti, R., eds.) pp. 927–933, Raven Press, New York.
365 Turk, J., Wyche, A. and Needleman, P. (1980) Biochem. Biophys. Res. Commun. 95, 1628–1634.
366 Brigham, K.L., Bowers, R.E. and Haynes, J. (1979) Circ. Res. 45, 292–297.
367 Brigham, K.L., Woolverton, W., Blake, L. and Staub, N. (1974) J. Clin. Invest. 54, 792–804.
368 Ogletree, M.L. and Brigham, K.L. (1980) J. Appl. Physiol. 48, 581–586.
369 Williams, T.J. and Piper, P.J. (1980) Prostaglandins 19, 779–789.
370 DelMaestro, F.F., Thaw, H.H., Björk, J., Planker, M. and Arfors, K.E. (1980) Acta Physiol. Scand. suppl. 492, 43–57.
371 Bray, M.A., Cunningham, F.M., Ford-Hutchinson, A.W. and Smith, M.J.H. (1981) Br. J. Pharmacol. 72, 483–486.
372 Bray, M.A., Cunningham, F.M., Ford-Hutchinson, A.W. and Smith, M.J.H. (1981) Br. J. Pharmacol. 73, 258P.

373 Wedmore, C.V. and Williams, T.J. (1981) Nature 289, 646–649.
374 Flick, M.R., Perel, A. and Staub, N.C. (1981) Circ. Res. 48, 344–351.
375 Wedmore, C.V. and Williams, T.J. (1981) Br. J. Pharmacol. 73, 209P.
376 Holme, G., Brunet, G., Piechuta, H., Masson, P., Girard, Y. and Rokach, J. (1980) Prostaglandins 20, 717–728.
377 Findlay, S.R., Lichtenstein, L.M., Siegel, H. and Triggle, D.J. (1981) J. Immunol. 126, 1728–1730.
378 Drazen, J.M., Lewis, R.A., Austen, K.F., Toda, M., Brion, F., Marfat, A. and Corey, E.J. (1981) Proc. Natl. Acad. Sci. USA 78, 3195–3198.
379 Sirois, P., Borgeat, P. and Jeansson, A. (1981) J. Pharm. Pharmacol. 33, 468–469.
380 Ueno, A., Tanaka, K., Katori, M., Hayashi, M. and Arai, Y. (1981) Prostaglandins 21, 637–648.
381 Eling, T., Warnock, R., Dick, D. and Tainer, B. (1980) Prostaglandins Med. 5, 345–355.
382 Osborne, D.J. (1981) Abstract book: International Symposium on Leukotrienes and other Lipoxygenase Products, Florence, Italy, June 1981, p. 77.
383 Bild, G.S., Ramadoss, C.S., Lim, S. and Axelrod, B. (1977) Biochem. Biophys. Res. Commun. 74, 949–954.
384 Bergström, S., Ryhage, R., Samuelsson, B. and Sjövall, J. (1963) J. Biol. Chem. 238, 3555–3564.
385 Hamberg, M., Svensson, J. and Samuelsson, B. (1974) Proc. Natl. Acad. Sci. USA 71, 3824–3828.
386 Levine, L., Alam, I., Gjika, H., Carty, T.J. and Goetzl, E.J. (1980) Prostaglandins 20, 923–934.
387 Eskra, J.D., Levine, L. and Carty, T.J. (1980) Prostaglandins Med. 5, 201–207.
388 Hwang, D.H. and Bryant, R.W. (1981) Abstract book: International Symposium on Leukotrienes and other Lipoxygenase Products, Florence, Italy, June 1981, p. 59.
389 Levine, L., Morgan, R.A., Lewis, R.A., Austen, K.F., Clark, D.A., Marfat, A. and Corey, E.J. (1981) Proc. Natl. Acad. Sci. USA 78, 7692–7696.
390 Tappel, A.L. (1961) in Autooxidation and Antioxidants, Vol. 1 (Lundberg, W.O., ed.), p. 325, Wiley (Interscience), New York.
391 Downing, D.T., Aheen, D.G. and Bachta, M. (1970) Biochem. Biophys. Res. Commun. 40, 218–223.
392 Blain, J.A. and Shearer, G. (1965) J. Sci. Food Agric. 16, 373–378.
393 Tobias, L.D. and Hamilton, J.G. (1978) Lipids 14, 181–193.
394 Baumann, J., v. Bruchhausen, F. and Wurm, G. (1980) Prostaglandins 20, 627–639.
395 Robak, J. and Dunice, Z. (1980) Biochim. Biophys. Acta 620, 59–62.
396 Vanderhoek, J.Y., Makheja, A.N. and Bailey, J.M. (1980) Biochem. Pharmacol. 29, 3169–3173.
397 Makheja, A.N., Vanderhoek, J.Y., Bryant, R.W. and Bailey, J.M. (1980) in Advances in Prostaglandins and Thromboxane Research, Vol. 6, (Samuelsson, B., Ramwell, P. and Paoletti, R., eds.) pp. 309–312, Raven Press, New York.
398 Hammarström, S. (1977) Biochim. Biophys. Acta 487, 517–519.
399 Sun, F.F., McGuire, J.C., Morton, D.R., Pike, J.E., Sprecher, H. and Kunan, W.H. (1981) Prostaglandins 21, 333–343.
400 Wilhelm, T.E., Sankarappa, S.K., Van Rollins, M. and Sprecher, H. (1981) Prostaglandins 21, 323–332.
401 Walker, J.R. and Dawson, W. (1979) J. Pharm. Pharmacol. 31, 778–780.
402 Walker, J.R., Boot, J.R., Beverley, C. and Dawson, W. (1980) J. Pharm. Pharmacol. 32, 866–867.
403 Sun, F.F., McGuire, J.C., Wallach, D.P. and Brown, V.R. (1980) in Advances in Prostaglandin and Thromboxane Research, Vol. 6 (Samuelsson, B., Ramwell, P. and Paoletti, R., eds.) pp. 111–113, Raven Press, New York.
404 Vanderhoek, J.Y., Bryant, R.W. and Bailey, J.M. (1980) J. Biol. Chem. 255, 5996–5998.
405 Blackwell, G.J. and Flower, R.J. (1978) Prostaglandins 16, 417–427.
406 Higgs, G.A., Flower, R.J. and Vane, J.R. (1979) Biochem. Pharmacol. 28, 1959–1961.
407 Rådmark, O., Malmsten, C. and Samuelsson, B. (1980) FEBS Lett 110, 213–215.
408 Ford-Hutchinson, A.W., Bray, M.A., Shipley, M.E., Doig, M.V. and Smith, M.J.H. (1980) in Inflammation: Mechanisms and Treatment, Vol. 4 (Willoughby, D.A. and Giraud, J.P., eds.) pp. 241—248, MTP Press Limited, Lancaster, England.
409 Chand, N. (1979) Agents and Actions 9, 133–140.
410 Lee, T.H., Walport, M.J., Wilkinson, A.H., Turner-Warwick, M. and Kay, A.B. (1981) Lancet, 304–305.

411 Welton, A.F., Hope, W.C., Tobias, L.D. and Hamilton, J.G. (1981) Biochem. Pharmacol. 30, 1378–1382.
412 Sheard, P., Holroyde, M.C., Ghelani, A.M., Bantick, J.R. and Lee, T.B. (1982) in Advances in Prostaglandin, Thromboxane and Leukotriene Research, Vol. 9 (Samuelsson, B. and Paoletti, R., eds.) pp. 229–235, Raven Press, New York.
413 Holroyde, M.C., Altounyan, R.E.C., Cole, M., Dixon, M. and Elliott, E.V. (1982) in Advances in Prostaglandin, Thromboxane and Leukotriene Research, Vol. 9 (Samuelsson, B. and Paoletti, R., eds.) pp. 237–242, Raven Press, New York.
414 Ashack, R.J., McCarty, L.P., Malek, R.S., Goodman, F.R. and Peet, N.P. (1980) J. Med. Chem. 23, 1022–1026.
415 Pace-Asciak, C.R., Mizuno, K. and Yamamoto, S. (1981) Biochim. Biophys. Acta 665, 352–354.
416 Pace-Asciak, C.R., Mizuno, K. and Yamamoto, S. (1982) Biochim. Biophys. Acta 712, 142–145.
417 Pace-Asciak, C.R., Granström, E. and Samuelsson, B. (1983) J. Biol. Chem., in press.

CHAPTER 5

Enzymes in the arachidonic acid cascade

SHOZO YAMAMOTO

Department of Biochemistry,
Tokushima University School of Medicine, Kuramoto-cho, Tokushima 770, Japan

1. Introduction

In this chapter the arachidonate cascade will be reviewed from an enzymological point of view. Most steps of the cascade are enzyme-catalyzed reactions although some steps have only been implicated to involve enzymes. Several but not all enzymes have been purified and their properties extensively investigated; the reaction mechanisms have been discussed in detail. A number of review articles dealing with PG biosynthesis and metabolism have been published [1–12] although only a few of these describe and discuss the current status of studies on the enzymes responsible for each of the individual steps of the arachidonate cascade.

2. Prostaglandin endoperoxide-synthesizing enzymes

Starting with arachidonic acid, the initial step of PG and TX biosynthesis is an oxygenative cyclization to produce PGG_2 which contains both an endoperoxide and a hydroperoxide moiety (Fig. 1). The enzyme responsible for this reaction is generally referred to as fatty acid cyclooxygenase [13], a term which describes the specific reaction catalyzed. However, care should be taken in the general use of this term. As will be described later, the same enzyme also catalyzes the second step of PG biosynthesis, i.e. the conversion of the 15-hydroperoxide of PGG_2 to a 15-hydroxyl group to form another endoperoxide intermediate, PGH_2 (Fig. 1). These two successive reactions are often referred to as the fatty acid cyclooxygenase reaction although this term is often confusing and misleading. Consequently, for clarity, the enzyme preparation which contains these two enzyme activities has been termed PG endoperoxide synthetase [14] or PGH synthase [15].

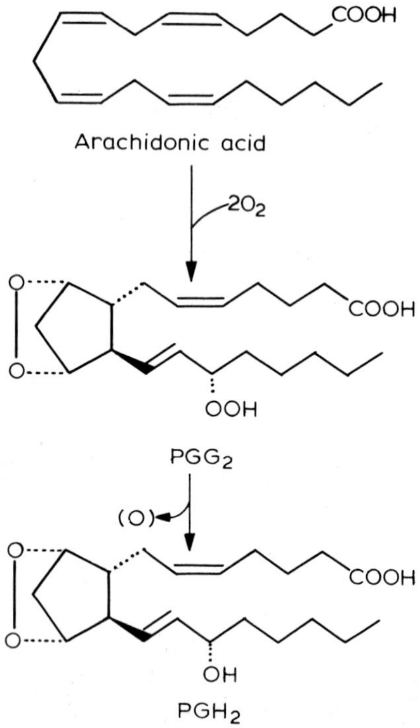

Fig. 1. Fatty acid cyclooxygenase and prostaglandin hydroperoxidase reactions.

(a) Fatty acid cyclooxygenase

i. Distribution and subcellular localization

The enzyme system responsible for the conversion of eicosapolyenoic acid into PGE is located in a particulate fraction of ovine [16,17] and bovine [18,19] vesicular gland, and can be obtained by centrifugation at 100 000 × *g*. The fatty acid cyclooxygenase is thus located in the microsomal fraction of a cell homogenate. Although particulate bound this enzyme can be solubilized from microsomes with detergent [20]. Through use of monoclonal antibodies, the enzyme was localized in the endoplasmic reticulum and nuclear membrane of Swiss mouse 3T3 fibroblast, but not in the mitochondrial or plasma membrane [21]. The biosynthetic activity of PGE was extensively screened in various tissues of various animals, and the result suggests a ubiquitous distribution of fatty acid cyclooxygenase [22]. In addition to ovine and bovine vesicular gland the enzyme can be solubilized from the microsomes of bovine [23] and human [24] platelets, rabbit kidney medulla [25] and rat brain [26].

ii. Molecular properties

The enzyme can be purified from the microsomes of bovine vesicular gland through DEAE-cellulose column chromatography, isoelectrofocusing and Sepharose column chromatography. The purified enzyme shows an apparent homogeneity upon polyacrylamide disc gel electrophoresis [14]. Molecular weight of the enzyme is 300 000–350 000 as estimated by gel filtration although a value of 71 000 is obtained by polyacrylamide disc gel electrophoresis in 0.1% SDS [27]. The specific activity of the purified enzyme is about 2.4 μmol of fatty acid consumed/min/mg [14]. The purified enzyme shows no significant absorption in the visible region indicating no content of either heme or flavin [27]. Atomic absorption spectrophotometry shows the content of less than 0.1 mol of iron or copper per mol of enzyme based on a molecular weight of 71 000 [27]. The enzyme is reasonably stable when handled below room temperature, and there is no appreciable loss of enzyme activity during storage at $-70°C$ for many months [14].

The purification of the enzyme from ovine vesicular gland has been reported by two groups using essentially similar procedures [28,29]. Molecular weight is 70 000 [28] or 72 000 [29], the latter including the value of carbohydrate contained in an amount of 3.4%. The specific enzyme activity is 46 μmol of oxygen consumed/min/mg protein [28] or 7.70 μmol of fatty acid converted/min/mg protein [29]. Amino acid composition of the enzyme is known, and the *N*-terminal amino acid is alanine [29]. Conflicting results have been reported for heme content in the purified enzyme preparation. Van der Ouderaa et al. reported negligible absorbance in the visible region [29] while Hemler et al. reported a minor absorption peak at 412 nm with varying intensities from preparation to preparation [28]. A significant amount of nonheme iron is present in the preparation of Hemler et al. [28] whereas only 0.15 [29] or 0.04–0.12 [30] mol of iron per mol of enzyme was observed by Van der Ouderaa et al.

The enzyme can be purified also from human platelet microsomes to a specific enzyme activity of 1.39 μmol/min/mg of protein [24].

iii. Catalytic properties

The fatty acid cyclooxygenase reaction is a bis-dioxygenation of the polyunsaturated fatty acid. As shown in Fig. 1, using arachidonic acid as substrate, the enzyme produces PGG_2 by incorporation of two molecules of oxygen. One molecule is retained as a peroxide linking C_9 and C_{11} while the second molecule of oxygen appears as a hydroperoxide at C_{15}. ^{18}O experiments have indicated that both oxygen atoms at 9- and 11- positions originated from the same molecule of oxygen, demonstrating that the incorporation of oxygen involves a dioxygenase reaction [31]. A hypothetical reaction mechanism has been proposed (Fig. 2), in which two dioxygenase reactions incorporated oxygen at the 11- and 15-positions [16,31,32]. Although the intermediacy of the 11-hydroperoxide has not been proven directly, experiments using a pseudo-substrate support this mechanism. Thus, when the enzyme reacts with 11,14-eicosadienoic acid, a dioxygenation at the 11-position occurs with the consumption of an equimolar amount of oxygen [33].

The stoichiometry of the cyclooxygenase reaction has been investigated with an ovine microsomal preparation. A 1 : 2 ratio of fatty acid conversion and oxygen consumption was demonstrated [34,35]. The enzyme is saturated with 30 μM oxygen, the K_m for which is about 5 μM [36]. Either arachidonic acid or 8,11,14-eico-

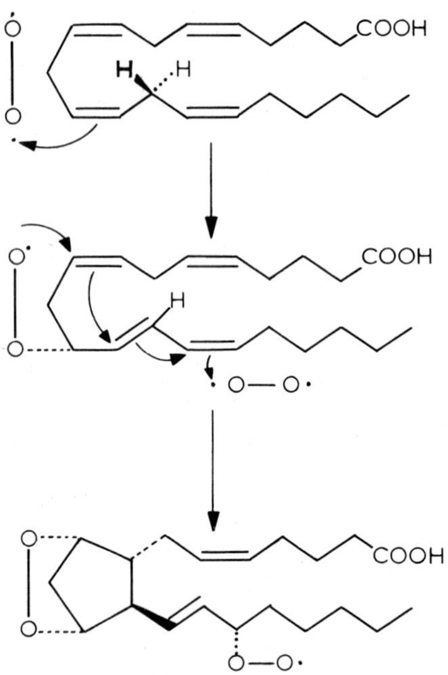

Fig. 2. Hypothetical mechanism of fatty acid cyclooxygenase reactions.

satrienoic acid are normally used as substrate for routine enzyme assays. The relative reaction velocity of the enzyme with these two substrates is essentially the same, i.e. $C_{20:3}/C_{20:4} = 223/251$ as determined with an electronic differentiator connected to an oxygen electrode [37]. The enzyme activity with 5,8,11,14,17-eicosapentaenoic acid, a fatty acid of nutritional interest, is 21 : 38 over arachidonic acid when a sufficient amount of hydroperoxide is present in the reaction mixture to activate the enzyme; in the absence of hydroperoxide activator eicosapentaenoic acid is not a substrate [37]. The role of the hydroperoxide activator is described in Chapter 6 of this volume.

In an effort to identify an activator which had earlier been found in the high-speed supernatant of a homogenate of sheep vesicular gland [17], hemoglobin was found to be the active principle in the overall PGE_2 synthesizing system of bovine vesicular gland although hematin was equally active [18]. The activity of hematin and hemoglobin was also confirmed with the purified enzyme [20], and it is now well established that heme is required as a cofactor for both cyclooxygenase and hydroperoxidase reactions with enzymes of bovine [14,27,38] and ovine [29,39] vesicular gland, bovine [23] and human [24] platelet, rabbit kidney [25] and rat brain [26].

A heme-free form of the bovine or the ovine enzyme purified by van der Ouderaa et al. [29] is essentially inactive unless heme is added to the reaction mixture, and the addition of about 1 μM hematin gives a maximum enzyme activity [14,29]. On the other hand, with the ovine preparation of Hemler et al. [28] as an acetone powder of microsomes or as the solubilized enzyme, the enzyme activity is not affected by the addition of heme, although the purified enzyme is stimulated 3–5 fold [40]. The results suggest that heme, which may be a native cofactor, may be lost during the purification procedures [28].

It should be noted that in addition to hematin the cofactor function is also observed with various protein-bound hemes including hemoglobin [14,18,27,40] and myoglobin [14,18,27]. However, it remains unclear how the heme moiety of hemoglobin or myoglobin can stimulate the enzyme. Hematoheme, the prosthetic group of cytochrome *c* is inactive [14,27]. Manganese protoporphyrin, in which the iron moiety of heme is replaced by manganese, is also active although its activity is specific for cyclooxygenase and inactive for the hydroperoxidase reaction [27,41].

Another effect of the heme cofactor is in the inactivation of the enzyme. When the bovine enzyme is mixed with hematin or hemoglobin, enzyme activity is lost rather rapidly. The rate of enzyme inactivation depends on the heme/enzyme ratio. As the amount of heme is raised beyond the equimolar quantity, the inactivation occurs faster. The half life of the enzyme is approximately 30 min when incubated with 5-fold excess of hematin or of hemoglobin at 24°C, pH 7.4. All the active heme compounds including the mangano analogue inactivate the enzyme. Both the cyclooxygenase and hydroperoxidase activities are lost in parallel [27]. A similar effect is observed with the ovine enzyme, and peroxide is presumed to participate in the heme-induced inactivation [39]. Such an enzyme-destroying action of heme hampers the purification and kinetic studies of the enzyme. Fortunately, however, the enzyme is protected from the heme-induced inactivation by the simultaneous presence of tryptophan, epinephrine, hydroquinone [27], phenol [27,39] and other compounds, all of which are cofactors for the hydroperoxidase reaction (see below).

These observations are suggestive of a hemoprotein nature for this enzyme despite the purified enzyme being almost heme-free and requiring the presence of exogenous heme for its activity. When the enzyme and heme are mixed and an aliquot of the mixture is removed and diluted before the enzyme is inactivated by its interaction with heme, the enzyme retains almost full activity even if the final concentration of heme is far below its saturation level in the assay mixture. This finding suggests that heme is bound to the enzyme protein before activation of the enzyme [27]. Furthermore, when hematin is added to a solution of the ovine enzyme and a difference spectrum is recorded between enzyme plus heme versus heme alone, an absorption at 408 nm is observed which increases as more hematin is added. A parallel increase in cyclooxygenase and hydroperoxidase activities are seen. At maximal enzyme activity, the saturation value of heme is 1.8 mol per mol of enzyme on the basis of a molecular weight of 70 000. An enzyme-heme complex can be prepared by equilibrium ultrafiltration. The trivalent state of the enzyme shows an absorption peak at 408 nm, while the divalent form gives α-band at 558 nm, β-band at 530 nm and γ-band at 424 nm [30]. Another study on the same ovine enzyme reported a conflicting result regarding heme binding. The enzyme can be purified in the presence of flufenamic acid as a stabilizer, and an active apo-enzyme can be prepared by the use of a heme-binding peptide of cytochrome b_5. Titration of this enzyme preparation with heme supports a 1 : 1 stoichiometry of the heme-binding [41a]. Another technique to prepare an active apo-enzyme is the anaerobic treatment of holo-enzyme with dithionite followed by the addition of oxygen [15].

Since the dissociation of the enzyme-heme complex occurs in the presence of non-ionic detergent, it is believed that the enzyme releases its heme prosthetic group during solubilization with a non-ionic detergent resulting in a heme-depleted enzyme preparation [30]. The bovine enzyme is presumed to have a looser binding of heme [42]. The function of the heme cofactor in the cyclooxygenase reaction will be discussed later together with that in the hydroperoxidase reaction.

Another peculiar characteristic of the cyclooxygenase is the time course of enzyme reaction. In most other enzymes the reaction proceeds at a constant rate exhibiting a linear time course when the enzyme is saturated with substrate,and then slows down as the substrate decreases below the saturating concentration. In sharp contrast, the cyclooxygenase reaction slows down gradually as soon as the reaction is started and ceases after 1–2 min. Therefore, it is difficult to determine a precise initial velocity of the cyclooxygenase reaction. This is possible, however, with a specially designed electronic differentiator [43]. Kinetic studies on the cyclooxygenase reaction are very much hampered by this unusual property of the enzyme. The cessation of the reaction is neither due to the exhaustion of substrate nor the accumulation of an inhibitor since the reaction can be resumed by the addition of fresh enzyme, but not by the further supply of substrate. Such a phenomenon has been observed by many investigators [14,27,34,35], and is referred to as "self-catalyzed destruction" [34] or "self-deactivation" [35]. Both the cyclooxygenase and hydroperoxidase reactions show a similar time course [27]. The reaction rate increases in proportion to the amount of enzyme only over a limited range [27]. The extent of reaction, i.e. the amount of product accumulating over the lifetime of the enzyme, is in proportion to the amount of enzyme [27,34].

The mechanism of destruction of the enzyme has been discussed and several attempts to elucidate this mechanism have been made. First, although interaction of cyclooxygenase and heme causes inactivation of the enzyme, the rate of the self-inactivation of enzyme is higher and the enzyme destruction occurs even in the presence of tryptophan which protects the enzyme from the inactivation by heme [27]. Second, the heme cofactor, either enzyme-bound or dissociated, may be destroyed by the peroxide product. When the absorption of heme is followed during the reaction, a loss of heme is observed, but heme destruction proceeds at a slower rate than the rate of enzyme inactivation [39]. Third, the enzyme may be inactivated by an active oxygen species which is presumably released during the hydroperoxidase reaction. Reduction of the 15-hydroperoxide group of PGG_2 to a hydroxyl group may produce an active oxygen species if the hydroperoxide is not fully reduced to water. This oxygen species is presumed to be a radical which would destroy the enzyme protein or the surrounding tissue as an inflammatory agent [35]. The mechanism will be mentioned later in more detail, although this hypothesis for the self-destruction of enzyme is believed to be insufficient for the manganese protoporphyrin-assisted reaction of cyclooxygenase which also shows enzyme in-

TABLE 1
Effect of various compounds on fatty acid cyclooxygenase and prostaglandin hydroperoxidase

Numbers in parentheses indicate most informative references.

	Fatty acid cyclooxygenase (Arachidonic acid → PGG_2)	Prostaglandin hydroperoxidase (PGG_2 → PGH_2)
Heme	1) prosthetic group-like activity (14, 27, 30, 42) 2) enzyme inactivation (27, 41)	1) prosthetic group-like activity (38) 2) enzyme inactivation (27)
Manganese protoporphyrin	1) prosthetic group-like activity (27) 2) enzyme inactivation (27, 41)	1) no prosthetic group-like activity (27) 2) enzyme inactivation (27, 41)
Peroxide	1) initiator of reaction (41, 45)	1) substitute for PGG as substrate (29, 38) 2) generator of active oxygen species to inactivate enzyme (35)
Aromatic compounds Tryptophan Phenol Hydroquinone, etc.	1) protection of enzyme from heme-induced inactivation (27, 41) 2) acceleration (39)	1) hydrogen donor in peroxidase reaction (29, 38) 2) protection of enzyme from heme-induced inactivation (27, 41)
Anti-inflammatory drugs Aspirin Indomethacin, etc.	inhibition (46)	no inhibition (46)

activation despite the absence of the hydroperoxidase activity [39]. The fourth hypothesis attributes the enzyme inactivation to an intermediate species which may arise during enzyme catalysis [39].

There are other factors which affect the activity of the enzyme. As reported with the ovine enzyme, the cyclooxygenase reaction is inhibited by glutathione peroxidase [34,44], indicating that the cyclooxygenase reaction requires some form of peroxide. When the oxygen consumption is followed continuously, a lag phase appears before the enzyme shows its full activity. The lag phase is more obvious if the reaction mixture is preincubated with sodium diethyldithiocarbamate (to remove any contaminating peroxide) or if the heme cofactor is replaced by manganese protoporphyrin [41,45]. The addition of 1 μM PGG_2 diminishes the lag period and accelerates the early state of oxygen consumption while PGH_2 has little effect [41]. Hydroperoxides of eicosatrienoic acid and arachidonic acid (soybean lipoxygenase products) are also active [45]. Based on these findings the cyclooxygenase reaction is presumed to be triggered and accelerated by the accumulating PGG, the reaction product of the enzyme [41,45].

The inhibition of cyclooxygenase by non-steroidal anti-inflammatory drugs is well-known and will be treated in the following chapter. It should be noted that indomethacin [14,46], aspirin [46,47] and other non-steroidal anti-inflammatory drugs [46] inhibit cyclooxygenase specifically, but not the hydroperoxidase component.

The diverse effects of various compounds which either activate or inhibit cyclooxygenase are summarized in Table 1.

(b) Prostaglandin hydroperoxidase

i. Glutathione peroxidase

The conversion of PGG to PGH had formerly been thought to be catalyzed by glutathione peroxidase. This enzyme catalyzes the dehydrogenation of glutathione (GSH) with various hydroperoxides (ROOH) as hydrogen acceptors, although it is non-specific in terms of hydrogen-accepting peroxide (Fig. 3). Because of the ubiquitous distribution of the enzyme and the stimulation of the overall synthesis of PGE_2 from arachidonic acid by glutathione, this enzyme activity was assigned to the PGG to PGH step [48–50].

The purified enzyme from bovine vesicular gland catalyzes the conversion of PGG to PGH in the presence of tryptophan. If tryptophan is replaced by glutathione, there is essentially no conversion of PGG to PGH. The purified enzyme is free of glutathione peroxidase activity as tested with glutathione and cumene hydroperoxide [38]. Thus, glutathione peroxidase is not involved in the conversion of PGG to PGH so far as it is catalyzed by the PG hydroperoxidase activity of PG endoperoxide synthetase.

ii. Association with cyclooxygenase

The conversion of PGG to PGH is carried out by an enzyme which is associated with the cyclooxygenase activity [38]. The two enzymes appear at the same pH region upon isoelectrofocusing. Both enzymic reactions show indistinguishable pH and temperature inactivation profiles. Both activities show an identical specificity

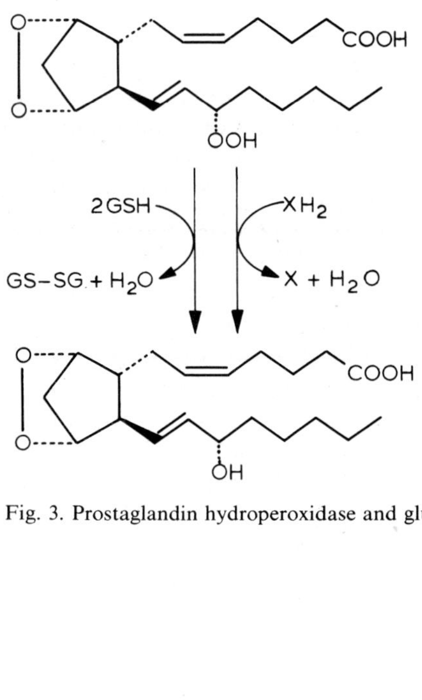

Fig. 3. Prostaglandin hydroperoxidase and glutathione peroxidase.

towards heme requirement except for manganese protoporphyrin, which is active only with cyclooxygenase. Both reactions proceed in the unusual time-course described above. Various attempts to resolve the two enzymes as two separate proteins have so far been unsuccessful. The close association of the two enzyme activities is also observed with the enzyme from ovine vesicular glands [29]. The current concept is that the two different enzyme activities are due to the same enzyme protein [29,39] although the possibility that the two separate enzyme proteins are tightly bound cannot be ruled out.

iii. Hydrogen donors

Various aromatic compounds stimulate the overall synthesis of PGE from arachidonic acid. The following activators have been reported (Fig. 4); hydroquinone [16,29], tetrahydrofolic acid [17], phenol [39,51], *p*-aminophenol [19], epinephrine [19], serotonin [19], tryptophan [14,20,38], uric acid [52], tetramethylphenylenediamine [29], benzidine [38] and guaiacol [38]. Most of these compounds behave as hydrogen donors in the peroxidatic reaction. Therefore, it is likely that these compounds are dehydrogenated during conversion of PGG to PGH. Actually, with epinephrine and guaiacol the dehydrogenation occurs in a stoichiometric amount when PGG_1 is converted to PGH_1 [38]. However, such a stoichiometric transformation is not observed with tryptophan as hydrogen donor [38].

iv. Hydrogen acceptors

Various hydroperoxides (in addition to PGG) can serve as hydrogen acceptors during the dehydrogenation of guaiacol or epinephrine by the bovine enzyme, e.g.

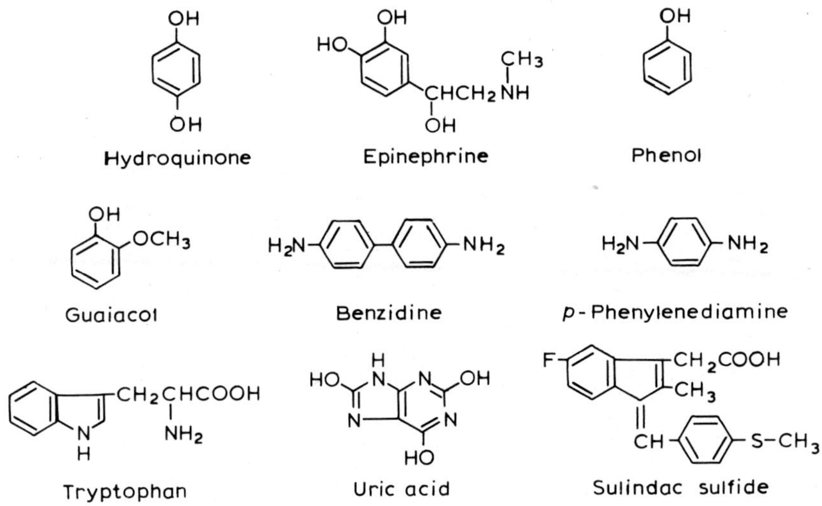

Fig. 4. Aromatic cofactors for PG hydroperoxidase.

15-hydroperoxy-PGE_1, 15-hydroperoxy-8,11,13-eicosatrienoic acid, hydrogen peroxide, *t*-butyl hydroperoxide, *p*-methane hydroperoxide and cumene hydroperoxide. Among these hydroperoxides PGG is the most active in terms of V_{max} and K_m. This is followed by 15-hydroperoxy-PGE_1 and 15-hydroperoxy-8,11,13-eicosatrienoic acid. Thus, the enzyme has a broad specificity for hydroperoxide requirement, but higher activity and affinity are observed with hydroperoxides of PG-like structure [38]. The ovine enzyme also has a peroxidase activity as tested with tetramethylphenylenediamine and hydrogen peroxide [29]. An "unusual" peroxidase activity with a wide peroxide specificity which is capable of oxidizing cofactors of PG biosynthesis has been demonstrated with the ovine vesicular gland microsomes [53].

v. Co-oxygenation

In the conversion of PGG to PGH the bond between two oxygen atoms of the 15-hydroperoxide moiety is cleaved. Electrons must be supplied for hydroperoxide reduction. As shown in Fig. 5, the two-electron reduction (XH_2) produces a hydroxyl group which is attached to the PG molecule and a molecule of water. This is a typical peroxidatic reaction occurring in the epinephrine- or guaiacol-assisted conversion of PGG to PGH by PG hydroperoxidase and also in the glutathione peroxidase reaction with PGG as hydrogen acceptor (see above). Another possible way for hydroperoxide cleavage is to trap one oxygen atom by a trapping agent (Y in Fig. 5) rather than its two-electron reduction to water. For example, oxygenation of 1,3-diphenylisobenzofuran, luminol, benzo(a)pyrene and cholesterol takes place during the reaction of arachidonic acid with ovine vesicular gland microsomes. This co-oxygenation can be stimulated by PGG_2 and 15-hydroperoxy-5,8,11,13-eicosatetraenoic acid [54]. The co-oxygenation of benzo(a)pyrene produces the 1,6-, 3,6-

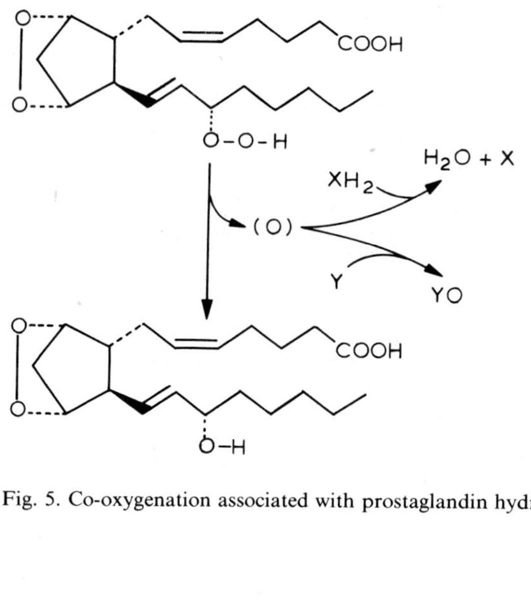

Fig. 5. Co-oxygenation associated with prostaglandin hydroperoxidase reaction.

and 6,12-quinones [55]. When diphenylisobenzofuran is incubated with ^{18}O-labeled 15-hydroperoxy-5,8,11,13-eicosatetraenoic acid, the oxygen incorporated into *o*-dibenzylbenzene does not derive from the hydroperoxy oxygen but rather from atmospheric oxygen [56]. *N*-[4-(5-Nitro-2-furyl)-2-thiazolyl]formamide (FANFT) a urinary bladder carcinogen, is also co-oxygenated in the hydroperoxidase reaction, and the co-oxygenation is reduced in the absence of atmospheric oxygen [57]. In contrast to benzo(a)pyrene and FANFT, ^{18}O atom is transferred from 15-hydroperoxy-PGE_2 to sulindac sulfide (*cis*-5-fluoro-2-methyl-1-[*p*-(methylthio)-benzilidine] indene-3-acetic acid) [58]. This compound is known to be co-oxygenated at its disulfide to produce a sulfoxide in a stoichiometric amount concomitant with the reduction of the hydroperoxy group of 15-hydroperoxy-PGE_1 [59]. An identical oxygen transfer from hydroperoxide occurs in the cooxygenation of methyl phenyl sulfide to its sulfoxide [59a].

vi. Chemiluminescence

Light emission is known to accompany some enzymatic reactions involving singlet oxygen or certain activated species of reactant or product. When eicosapolyenoic acids are incubated with a microsomal preparation of sheep vesicular gland capable of PGE synthesis, light is emitted [60]. The light emission is associated with the co-oxygenation of luminol coincident with the microsomal transformation of arachidonate. Addition of PGG_2 in place of arachidonic acid also produces the luminescence [54]. The luminol-induced luminescence is inhibited by superoxide dismutase, catalase and hydroxyl radical scavengers. This observation is interpreted as an interaction of luminol and hydroxyl radicals formed in a Haber-Weiss reaction during the catalysis of heme [61]. Light emission is also observed in the reaction of purified bovine enzyme with PGG_2 or other hydroperoxides [62]. It should be noted that the luminescence produced by the bovine enzyme is specific for tryptophan or other indole compounds. The emission spectrum has peaks around 500, 550, and 610 nm, which is distinguishable from the reported spectrum of singlet oxygen yet similar to the emission spectrum of tryptophan presumably due to its triplet state formed under ultraviolet irradiation [63].

(c) Summary

As described above, a number of compounds participate in the reactions of cyclooxygenase and hydroperoxidase. Some of them stimulate these reactions while others are inhibitory. The complex effects of these activators and inhibitors on the cyclooxygenase and hydroperoxidase reactions are summarized in Table 1. Many things remain to be investigated before the precise reaction mechanism of the enzyme can be understood. Particularly the role of heme must be studied at the level now available for cytochrome oxidase, horseradish peroxidase and cytochrome *P*-450. Although available evidence strongly suggests that the enzyme is a hemoprotein like other oxygenases, the enzyme has not been isolated and purified as a hemoprotein as has been done with fungal lipoxygenase [64].

A hypothetical reaction mechanism was proposed by Hemler and Lands to harmonize various observations so far reported with ovine and bovine enzymes [39]. In this mechanism interaction of a hydroperoxide (PGG_2 in a normal catalysis) and the enzyme-bound ferriheme produces a hydroperoxy radical. This radical abstracts the 13-S-hydrogen from arachidonic acid. The resulting alkyl radical acts as an activated form of arachidonic acid and reacts with an oxygen molecule (a biradical) at C-11. This is followed by cyclization of the hydrocarbon chain and incorporation of another molecule of oxygen at C-15. The resulting 15-hydroperoxy radical ends the sequence by abstracting a hydrogen atom from the enzyme-bound hydroperoxide to form the end product, PGG_2. The inhibition by antioxidant at a higher concentration and the self-destruction of the enzyme during catalysis are related by these authors to an intermediate radical formed on the enzyme surface. The hydroperoxidase activity is attributed to the catalysis of the enzyme in which the iron moiety of the enzyme-bound heme undergoes a valency change reducing the hydroperoxide of PGG_2 to water with hydrogens abstracted from hydrogen-donating cofactor. A hypothesis was proposed for the interaction of heme and arachidonic acid [65]. The carboxyl group of arachidonic acid attaches to one ligand of heme, and the hydrocarbon chain curls around the outside of the heme ring. The oxygen molecule associated with the ligand of heme on the other side reacts with C-11, followed by the ring closure and the addition of another molecule of oxygen at C-15.

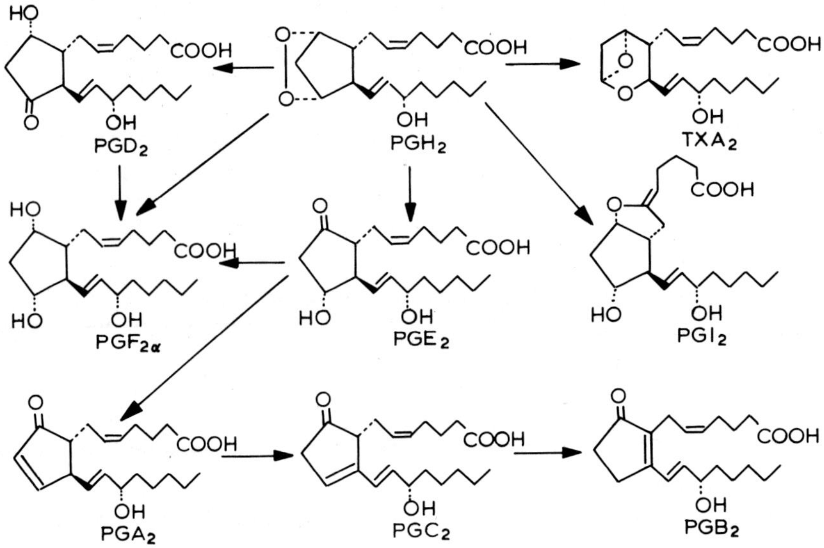

Fig. 6. Divergent biosynthetic pathways of PG and TX from PGH_2.

3. Prostaglandin endoperoxide-metabolizing enzymes

PGH_2 is at a pivotal stage in the divergent pathways leading to the synthesis of various types of PGs and TX (Fig. 6). Most of the enzymes utilizing PGH_2 as substrate, are isomerases which attack the 9,11-endoperoxide bridge of PGH_2. Their distribution in various tissues determines the tissue specificity for PG and TX biosynthesis. The particular isomerase present in any tissue determines which PG is to be formed presumably as an important factor in the regulation of some particular function in that tissue.

(a) TXA synthase

The biosynthesis of TXA_2 can be detected in a variety of tissues [11,66,67], including arterial tissues [67a,67b]. The enzyme which produces TXA_2 from PGH_2 is localized in a microsomal fraction of platelets [67–70], lung [67,71], spleen [67] and macrophage [67]. The enzyme can be solubilized with the aid of a non-ionic detergent from a microsomal fraction of bovine [23] and human [72] platelets and bovine [73] and porcine [73a] lung, and purified partially by the use of DEAE-cellulose. TXA_2 is extremely unstable and is readily transformed to a stable degradation product (TXB_2) when it is extracted with organic solvent from the reaction mixture. If the reaction of PGH_2 with the microsomes [68,74] or the solubilized enzyme [23] is performed for 30–60 s at 0°C, the formation of TXA_2 can be detected by its

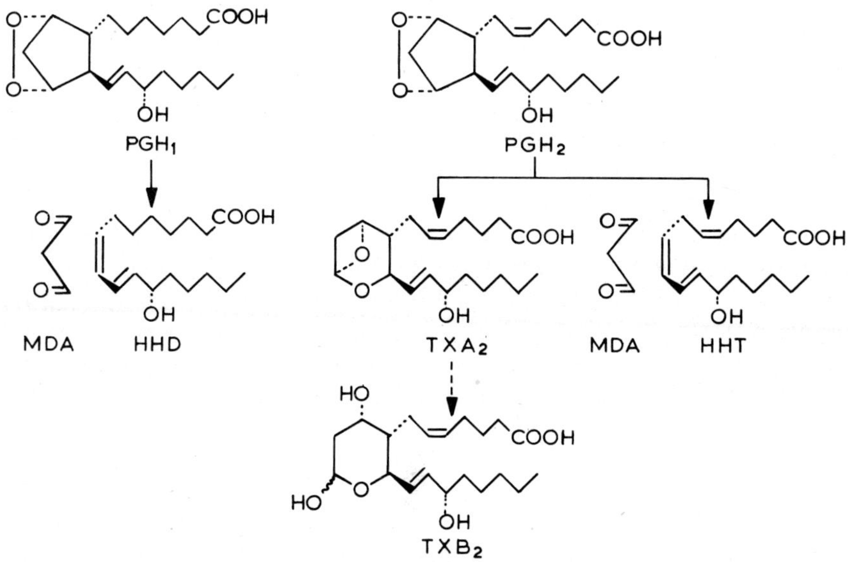

Fig. 7. Reactions of TXA synthase with PGH_1 and PGH_2.

pro-aggregatory or rabbit aorta contractile activity. Concomitant with TXA_2 formation the solubilized enzyme produces 12L-hydroxy-5,8,10-heptadecatrienoic acid (HHT) in a ratio of 1–2 : 1 over TXB_2 [23,72,73]. Malondialdehyde (MDA) is also presumably released. Since several compounds inhibit the formation of both TXB_2 and HHT in parallel, it is presumed that both are formed by the same enzyme [75,76]. HHT is considered to be produced directly from PGH_2 rather than via TXA_2 [75,77] (Fig. 7). A hypothesis was proposed that TXA synthase is not an isomerase but catalyzes a dismutase-type reaction [77]. An interesting observation is the reaction of the enzyme with PGH_1 [73,78]. As shown in Fig. 7, PGH_1 is converted predominantly to 12L-hydroxy-8,10-heptadecadienoic acid (HHD) with only a small amount of TXB_1 produced. Similar dose-inhibition curves are obtained in the inhibition of HHT and HHD formation by TXA synthase inhibitors, L-8027 and imidazole. The formation of HHD from PGH_1 is suppressed by PGH_2. These observations suggest that the same enzyme catalyzes the production of both HHT and HHD. On the basis of the previously known function of cytochrome *P*-450 as an oxene transferase, spectrophotometric study of platelet microsomes suggests the participation of cytochrome *P*-450 in the isomerization of 9,11-endoperoxide to produce TXA_2 from PGH_2 [78a]. In view of the pathological role of TXA_2 in the cardiovascular system, a variety of compounds have been tested as inhibitors of TXA synthase including imidazole [79] and its derivatives [80,81] and PG endoperoxide analogues [82].

(b) PGD synthase

The conversion of PGH_2 to PGD_2 is an isomerization of the 9,11-endoperoxide moiety to 9α-hydroxyl and 11-keto groups (Fig. 6). The activity of the enzyme which produces PGD_2 from either arachidonic acid or PGH_2 is detected in various tissues of rat; lung [48], stomach [48], small intestine [48], skin [48], brain [26,67,83], spleen [84] and mast cells [85]. As examined with rat brain, the enzyme is found predominantly in the cytosol, and can be purified to an apparent homogeneity [26]. The regional distribution of the enzyme was studied with rat brain, and the predominant occurrence of PGD synthase in neuroblastoma cells (an insignificant activity in glioma cells) suggested a neuromodulator function of PGD_2 [86]. However, there is a paper reporting the localization of PGD synthase in the microvasculature of rat cerebral cortex rather than neuronal and glial cells [86a]. A similar enzyme can be purified from the cytosol of rat spleen [84], and is also found in the cytosol of rat mast cells [85]. The brain enzyme does not require glutathione [26] whereas the enzyme from spleen [84] and mast cells [85] is stimulated by the addition of glutathione.

(c) PGE synthase

The conversion of PGH_2 to PGE_2 is an isomerization of the 9,11-endoperoxide to 9-keto and 11α-hydroxyl groups (Fig. 6). The enzyme system catalyzing the overall synthesis of PGE_2 from arachidonic acid was earlier referred to as prostaglandin synthase (EC 1.14.99.1). However, when the enzyme system was solubilized from microsomes of bovine vesicular gland, PGE synthase was separated from PG endoperoxide synthetase [20]. PGE synthase, which produces PGE_2 from PGH_2 in the presence of glutathione, is found in the microsomes of bovine vesicular gland [48] and rabbit kidney medulla [25]. The enzyme can be solubilized from microsomes of bovine vesicular gland and partially purified [87]. Although the enzyme is very unstable when it is solubilized from the microsomes, it can be protected from inactivation by various thiol compounds. Glutathione is required as a specific coenzyme for the reaction, but it is not oxidized in a stoichiometric amount. A hypothetical role of glutathione as a nucleophile in a 1,2-hydride shift during the isomerization of endoperoxide has been proposed [44].

(d) PGF synthase

As shown in Fig. 6, there are three possibilities for the synthesis of $PGF_{2\alpha}$. First, the endoperoxide of PGH_2 can be directly reduced as was proposed previously [32]. This proposal is primarily based on the finding that the 9-H of arachidonic acid is retained in $PGF_{2\alpha}$. Thus the overall reaction is a reductive cleavage of the 9,11-endoperoxide of PGH_2. The activity to synthesize $PGF_{2\alpha}$ from PGH_2 is found in the microsomes of cow and guinea pig uterus [88]. However, the nature of the enzyme and the reducing agent remains unclear. The second pathway is the conversion of PGE_2 into $PGF_{2\alpha}$. The 9-keto group of the former can be reduced to a hydroxyl group. This conversion occurs in various tissues [89–91]. The third mechanism of $PGF_{2\alpha}$ synthesis is the reduction of 11-keto group of PGD_2 [92–94].

(e) PGI synthase

The formation of PGI_2 is an isomerization of the 9,11-endoperoxide of PGH_2 into a 6,9-epoxide and an 11α-hydroxyl group (Fig. 8). PGI_2 is unstable especially at acidic pH and is readily transformed into 6-keto-$PGF_{1\alpha}$, a stable but biologically inactive product (see Chapter 3). The PGI synthase activity is detected in a variety of tissues; artery, vein, heart, lung, kidney, spleen, stomach and macrophage (ref. 66 and Table 2 in ref. 11). One paper reports the lack of PGI_2 synthesis in aortic tissue of chicken [94a]. The enzyme is localized in the microsomes of artery [95–97], lung [71], vesicular gland [98,99] and corpora lutea [100]. The enzyme can be solubilized from the microsomes of rabbit aorta [101] and pig aorta [102,103] with non-ionic detergents and partially purified. The primary production of PGI_2 rather than 6-keto-$PGF_{1\alpha}$ by the enzymatic reaction with PGH_2 has been shown by the isolation of the methyl ester of PGI_2 [101] which is more stable. The enzyme is inhibited by hydroperoxide of various unsaturated fatty acids [96,97,103]. HHT is produced in a small amount during PGI_2 synthesis, but unlike TXA synthase HHT formation is not attributed to PGI synthase [102]. On the other hand, the solubilized enzyme produces HHD from PGH_1 at a rate of about 70% of that of 6-keto-$PGF_{1\alpha}$

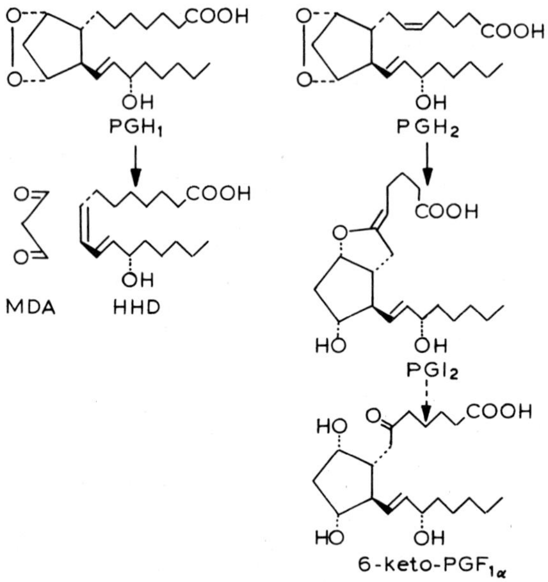

Fig. 8. Reactions of PGI synthase with PGH_1 and PGH_2.

production from PGH_2 [101] (Fig. 8). Like TXA synthase the participation of the oxene transferase activity of cytochrome *P*-450 was proposed for the endoperoxide isomerization from PGH_2 to PGI_2 [78a,103a].

(f) PGA synthase

As shown in Fig. 6, PGA_2 is a dehydration product of PGE_2. The enzyme responsible for this reaction has been reported in human serum [104].

(g) PGC synthase

PGC_2 is formed through an isomerization of the Δ^{10} of PGA_2 to Δ^{11} (Fig. 6). An enzyme previously referred to as PGA isomerase is present in the serum or plasma of human [104], rabbit [105], cat [105] pig [105], dog [105] and rat [105]. The cat enzyme has been partially purified [105].

(h) PGB synthase

The conversion of PGC_2 to PGB_2 occurs by an isomerization of Δ^{11} into $\Delta^{8(12)}$ (Fig. 6). This reaction is considered to be an enzymatic reaction and the enzyme is found in human and rabbit serum [104].

4. Prostaglandin and thromboxane-catabolizing enzymes

Studies on the catabolism of PG were initiated by the isolation and identification of catabolites in urine and plasma which established catabolic pathways especially of PGE and PGF [1,4]. Each step of the catabolic pathway is catalyzed by an enzyme. In this chapter only papers describing the properties of individual enzymes will be reviewed.

(a)15-Hydroxy-PG dehydrogenase

Since this enzyme was first isolated and purified from swine lung [106], a number of papers have been published reporting its occurrence in animal tissues, substrate specificity, enzyme inhibitors, reaction mechanism and physiological function. These papers have been anteceded by two comprehensive review articles [107,108].

i. NAD-linked dehydrogenase (Type I)

This enzyme is specific for the 15-hydroxyl group of the PG molecule, which is transformed into a 15-keto derivative as shown in Fig. 9. NAD serves as a specific hydrogen acceptor. No oxidation occurs with steroid alcohols, hydroxy acids or aliphatic alcohols [106]. The enzyme has been purified from pig lung [106,109], beef lung [110], monkey lung [111], human placenta [112], rat kidney [113] and porcine kidney [114]. Distribution of the enzyme in other tissues is described in refs. 107 and 108. Enzyme activity [106,109–114] is found either in the high-speed supernatant of a tissue homogenate or it is considered to be a cytosolic enzyme as judged from its behavior during purification.

Substrate specificity of different enzyme preparations is listed in Table V in ref.

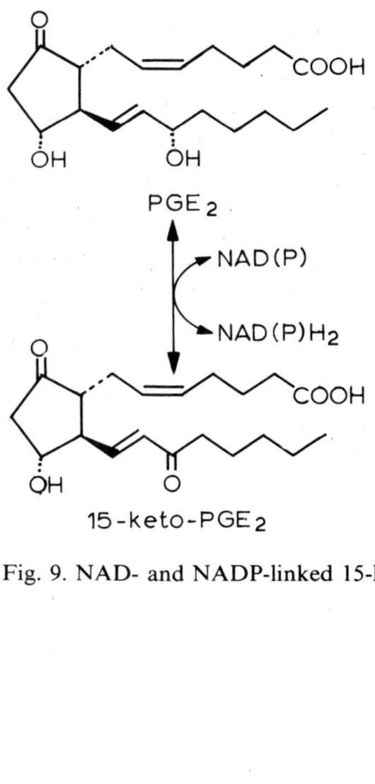

Fig. 9. NAD- and NADP-linked 15-hydroxy-PG dehydrogenase.

TABLE 2
Substrate specificity of 15-hydroxy-PG dehydrogenases for naturally occurring PGs

Enzyme source H-acceptor Parameter	Pig lung NAD Relative activity	Pig lung NAD Relative activity	Pig lung NAD Relative activity	Pig lung NAD Relative activity	Monkey lung NAD Relative activity	Monkey lung NAD K_m μM	Pig kidney NAD K_m μM	Human placenta NAD Relative activity	Human placenta NADP Relative activity	Human placenta NADP Relative activity	Rabbit kidney NADP Relative activity
PGE_1	100	100	100	100		14.5	1.2				
PGE_2	97	100	67	100	210	11.9	1.2	100	0.5	0.1	4.1
PGE_3	60	90	34								
$PGF_{1\alpha}$	75	69		58		95	19.2	34			
$PGF_{2\alpha}$	62	66		76	100	56	12.5	97		0.4	2.2
$PGF_{3\alpha}$	62										
PGA_1	45	86	52				1.7	65	8.4	29	
PGA_2	33	48	50	82	135		4.6				
PGB_1	0	0						0	100	100	
PGB_2	0	0			0		inactive				
PGD_1								4	1.6		
PGD_2				8	0						
PGG_2					0						
PGH_2					189						
PGI_2				91		7.4	5.0	73	0.9		100
6-keto-$PGF_{1\alpha}$				88			5.1	48	0.9		1.7
TXB_2							400	0	1.7		0
Reference	106	115	116	117	111	119	114	118	118	129	134

107 and Table III in ref. 108. As listed in Table 2 in this chapter, which includes recent findings, PGE, PGF and PGA are active substrates for all the NAD-linked dehydrogenases, while PGB and PGD are either poor or inactive substrates. As examined with some enzyme preparations, PGI_2 and 6-keto-$PGF_{1\alpha}$ are also active substrates whereas TXB_2 is a poor substrate. The structure-activity relationship of various PGs and their derivatives was reviewed in ref. 107. The reaction of 15-hydroxy-PG dehydrogenase is known to be reversible; i.e. 15-keto-PGE_1 is reduced back to PGE_1 using NADH as a hydrogen donor [112,120,121]. The optimum pH for the forward reaction is 8.8 or higher, and that for the backward reaction is 5.5 [121]. Since the metabolic deactivation of biologically active PGs is catalyzed by 15-hydroxy-PG dehydrogenases [122], a number of studies on the inhibitors of the enzyme have been reported and reviewed in references 107, 108 and 123. The Type I dehydrogenase has been shown to change markedly in its activity as a function of the state of the animal and during development. It has been studied in vitro in the kidney [160] and lung [161] of the developing rat, the kidney [162], lung [163], brain [164] and liver [165] of the fetal sheep, and in lungs from pregnant rabbit [166,167,168] and rat [169]. This has been reviewed in ref. 165. In some organs, activity is several fold greater during the fetal or postnatal period than in the adult, in others it is lower, reaching adult levels of activity at a well defined period in fetal or postnatal life.

ii. NADP-linked dehydrogenase (Type II)

This enzyme catalyzes the oxidation of the 15-hydroxyl group of PG with NADP as a more effective hydrogen acceptor than NAD (Fig. 9). The enzyme was first found in monkey and human brain, erythrocytes and in swine kidney [124]. It has been purified from swine kidney [125,126], chicken kidney [127], human erythrocyte [128] and human placenta [129]. As shown in Table 2, PGB is a better substrate of this enzyme than PGE and PGF in contrast to the NAD-linked enzyme [118,129]. It should be noted that this enzyme also exhibits PG 9-keto reductase activity [126,128,130]. The two enzymes cannot be separated from each other during purification from human erythrocyte [128] and human placenta [130]. Both activities of the latter enzyme are inhibited by ethacrynic acid, furosemide and indomethacin [130]. The enzyme purified to homogeneity from swine kidney shows essentially the same sensitivities of the two enzyme activities to heat treatment and indomethacin inhibition [126]. Thus, the enzyme catalyzes four types of reactions; 9-keto reduction ($PGE_2 \rightarrow PGF_{2\alpha}$), 9-hydroxy dehydrogenation ($PGF_{2\alpha} \rightarrow PGE_2$), 15-keto reduction (15-keto-$PGF_{2\alpha} \rightarrow PGF_{2\alpha}$) and 15-hydroxy dehydrogenation ($PGE_2 \rightarrow$ 15-keto-PGE_2) using NADPH or NADP [126].

iii. PGA-specific dehydrogenase

An NAD-linked 15-hydroxy-PG dehydrogenase specific for A-type PGs is found in a soluble fraction of rabbit kidney papilla. The enzyme is active with PGA_1 ($K_m = 15\ \mu M$) and PGA_2 ($K_m = 6\ \mu M$) but neither PGE_1, PGE_2, $PGF_{1\alpha}$, $PGF_{2\alpha}$ or PGB_1 is an active substrate [131].

iv. PGD-specific dehydrogenase

An NADP-linked 15-hydroxy-PG dehydrogenase specific for D-type PG can be partially purified from the cytosol of swine brain [132]. PGA_2, PGB_2, PGD_2, PGE_2 and $PGF_{2\alpha}$ are poor substrates. As shown in Fig. 10, the reaction product is 15-keto-PGD_2 which is unstable and is readily converted into an enolate anion under alkaline condition. 15-keto-PGD_2 is enzymatically converted into 13,14-dihydro-15-keto-PGD_2 by an NADPH-linked reductase which is present in the partially purified preparation.

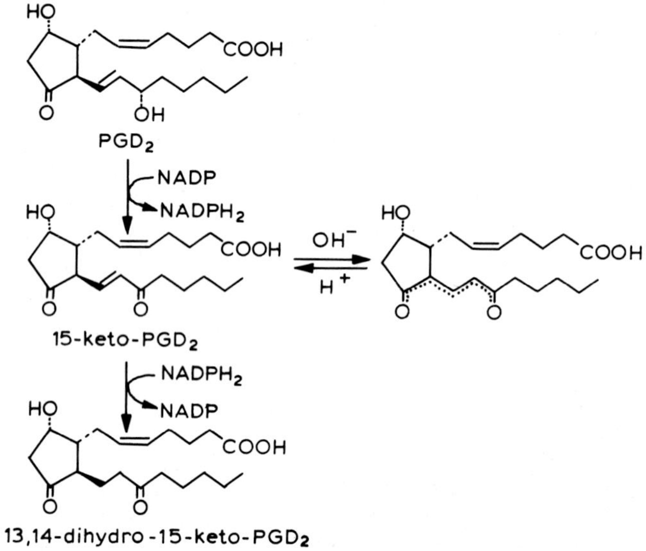

Fig. 10. 15-Hydroxy dehydrogenation and Δ^{13}-reduction of PGD_2.

v. PGI-specific dehydrogenase

An NADP-linked 15-hydroxy-PG dehydrogenase specific for PGI_2 can be purified from an ultracentrifuged homogenate of rabbit kidney [133,134]. PGE_2, $PGF_{2\alpha}$, 6-keto-$PGF_{1\alpha}$ and TXB_2 are oxidized with reaction rates less than 4% that of PGI_2. The enzyme catalyzes oxido-reduction more rapidly at C-15 than at C-9. NAD is inactive as hydrogen acceptor [134]. The enzyme is purified to homogeneity and has a molecular weight of 56000–62000 containing no flavin [170].

(b) 9-Hydroxy-PG dehydrogenase

The enzyme which attacks specifically the 9-hydroxyl group of the PG molecule with NAD as a hydrogen acceptor was first found in the cytosol of adult rat kidney [135,136]. As shown in fig. 11, the rat kidney enzyme purified to homogeneity oxidizes the 9-hydroxyl group of 15-keto-13,14-dihydro-$PGF_{2\alpha}$ and 15-keto-$PGF_{2\alpha}$

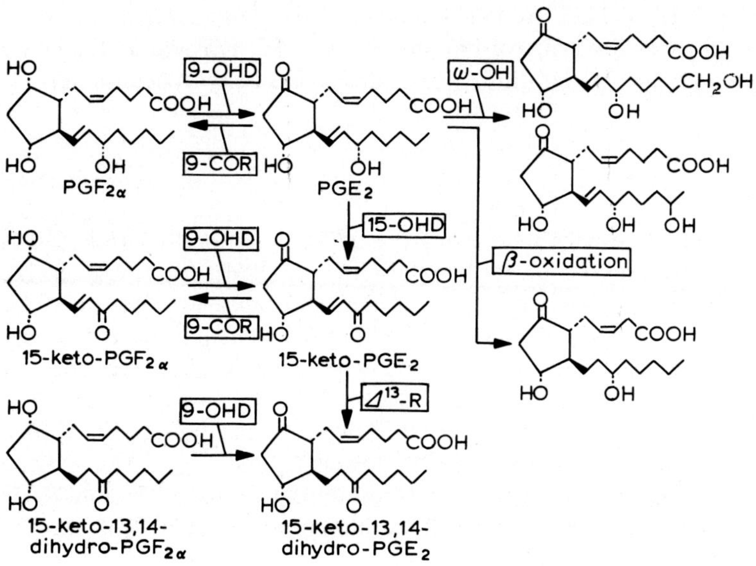

Fig. 11. Enzymes involved in PG metabolism. 15-OHD, 15-hydroxy-PG dehydrogenase; Δ^{13}R, PG Δ^{13} reductase; 9-OHD, 9-hydroxy-PG dehydrogenase; 9-COR, PG 9-keto reductase; ω-OH, ω-hydroxylase.

and $PGF_{2\alpha}$ with relative V_{max} of 100 : 64.7 : 15.0 [137]. A similar enzyme which oxidizes $PGF_{2\alpha}$ and $PGF_{1\alpha}$ was also found in rabbit kidney [138,139], stomach [139] and ileum [139]. Since the enzyme is much more active with NAD than NADP as cofactor and specific for the A-side of NAD, the enzyme reaction is distinguishable from the reversal of the PG-9-keto reductase reaction [137].

(c) PG 9-keto reductase

The enzyme which transforms PGE_2 to $PGF_{2\alpha}$ by the reduction of the 9-keto group of the former, was first found in heart, kidney, brain and liver of rat [140]. This enzyme uses NADPH more effectively and is located in the cytosol of pigeon heart, brain, lung, liver and other mammalian tissues while the enzyme utilizing NADH more effectively is found in the microsomes of monkey liver [141]. The NADPH-linked enzyme can be partially purified from chicken heart and resolved into two enzyme fractions [142]. Many other papers reported the occurrence of PG 9-keto reductase in various mammalian tissues: liver of guinea-pig, rabbit and horse and heart of horse [91], rabbit kidney [143,144], human [145] and rat [146] testis, rat and human skin [147], pig kidney [125,126], chicken kidney [127], human placenta [130] and human erythrocyte [128]. As shown in Fig. 11, the purified enzyme from chicken heart catalyzes the reduction from PGE_2 to $PGF_{2\alpha}$ and from 15-keto-PGE_2 to 15-keto-$PGF_{2\alpha}$ [142]. A finding of pharmacological importance is the bradykinin-enhanced conversion of PGE to PGF by PG 9-keto reductase [148]. Furthermore, as described in the section of 15-hydroxy-PG dehydrogenase, PG-9-keto reductase activity is associated with the NADP-linked 15-hydroxy-PG dehydrogenase activity [126,128,130].

(d) PG Δ^{13}-reductase

The occurrence of a reductase which saturates the Δ^{13} double bond of 15-keto-PG was presumed from structures of urinary metabolites of PGE and PGF. Swine tissues including kidney, lung, liver, intestine, adrenal and brain were screened for Δ^{13} reductase activity [149]. The enzyme purified from chicken heart [150] uses NADPH as a hydrogen donor while NADH is almost ineffective. The reduction of Δ^{13} occurs specifically with 15-keto-PGE_2 and 15-keto-$PGF_{2\alpha}$, but not PGE_2 and $PGF_{2\alpha}$ (Fig. 11). In contrast, the purified enzyme from bovine lung [151] utilizes both NADH (higher K_m and V_{max}) and NADPH (lower K_m and V_{max}). The enzyme reaction is irreversible when examined with 13,14-dihydro-15-keto-PGE_1 and NAD or NADP [151]. The highly purified enzyme from human placenta [152] is specific for NADH while NADPH is inactive, and relative V_{max} of various 15-keto-PGs is as follows: 15-keto-PGE_2, 100%; 15-keto-PGE_1, 55%; 15-keto-$PGF_{2\alpha}$, 56%; 15-keto-PGA_1, 108%; 15-keto-PGB_1, 79%. The enzyme reaction is irreversible.

(e) β-Oxidation

The β-oxidation system of rat liver mitochondria [153] is capable of shortening the α-side chain of various PGs, PGE_1, PGB_1, $PGF_{1\alpha}$ and $PGF_{2\alpha}$, into the corresponding C_{18} homologues (Fig. 11). PGA_1, 11α,15-dihydroxy-9-ketoprostanoic acid and 11α-hydroxy-9,15-diketoprostanoic acid are transformed into both C_{16} and C_{18} homologues. In the neonatal rat in vivo, the β-oxidation system is already active at 7 days after birth as determined by intravenous infusion of tritiated $PGF_{2\alpha}$ and monitoring of the urinary metabolites [172].

(f) ω-Oxidation

The occurrence of 19-hydroxylated PGA_1, A_2, B_1 and B_2 in human seminal plasma [154] suggested the involvement of an ω-hydroxylase system in the synthesis of these compounds. Later 19-hydroxylated PGE_1 and PGE_2 were isolated from fresh human seminal plasma [155] or from seminal plasma that had been subjected to *O*-methyloxime hydrochloride treatment [156]. These results suggested that the previously identified 19-hydroxy-PGA and 19-hydroxy-PGB were artifacts [155]. 19-Hydroxy-$PGF_{1\alpha}$ and 19-hydroxy-$PGF_{2\alpha}$ were also isolated [157]. Earlier 19- and 20-hydroxylation of PGA_1 was demonstrated with microsomes of guinea pig liver in the presence of NADPH, while hydroxylation of PGE_1 occurred only in small amount [158]. On the other hand, analysis of urinary metabolites of PGs revealed the formation of ω-oxidized PGs [1,4]. In the presence of NADPH a particulate fraction from lung of pregnant rabbit hydroxylates the C-20 of PGE_1, PGE_2, $PGF_{2\alpha}$, 13,14-dihydro-15-keto-PGE_2 and 13,14-dihydro-15-keto-$PGF_{2\alpha}$ [159]. The participation of the hepatic microsomal *P*-450 system in the ω-hydroxylation of PG is suggested from studies with guinea pig liver microsomes [173]. PGA_1 and PGE_1 are hydroxylated primarily ($>95\%$) at the (ω-1)-carbon and to a minor extent ($<5\%$) at the ω position (Fig. 11). Inhibitors of *P*-450 (SKF 525A, metyrapone, nicotinamide and carbon monoxide) and antibody against NADPH-cytochrome *c* reductase inhibit the hydroxylation. Microsomes of guinea pig kidney cortex hydroxylate PGE_1 in a similar manner [174]. Microsomes of both liver and kidney of pig catalyze the (ω-1)- and ω-hydroxylation of PGA_1 and PGE_1, but only PGA_1 is ω-hydroxylated by a reconstituted system of pig kidney [175]. Incubation of arachidonic acid with the microsomes of rabbit renal cortex produces 19- and 20-hydroxy-arachidonic acid in the presence of NADPH. Since carbon monoxide inhibits formation of these compounds, they are likely formed by the microsomal cytochrome *P*-450 system of rabbit renal cortex [171]. The activity of the ω-oxidation system has been studied in the developing rat through analysis of tritiated metabolites appearing in the urine after tritiated $PGF_{2\alpha}$ infusion. While little or no ω-oxidized products were detected before 24 days of age, adult-like activity was observed by 34 days postnatally [172].

5. *Lipoxygenases*

In addition to fatty acid cyclooxygenase (11,15-bis-lipoxygenase) there are several other lipoxygenases in mammalian tissues (Fig. 12). Leukocytes and mast cells contain a 5-lipoxygenase which leads to the biosynthesis of leukotrienes from arachidonic acid [176,177]. 12-Lipoxygenase, rich in platelets, initiates a biosynthetic

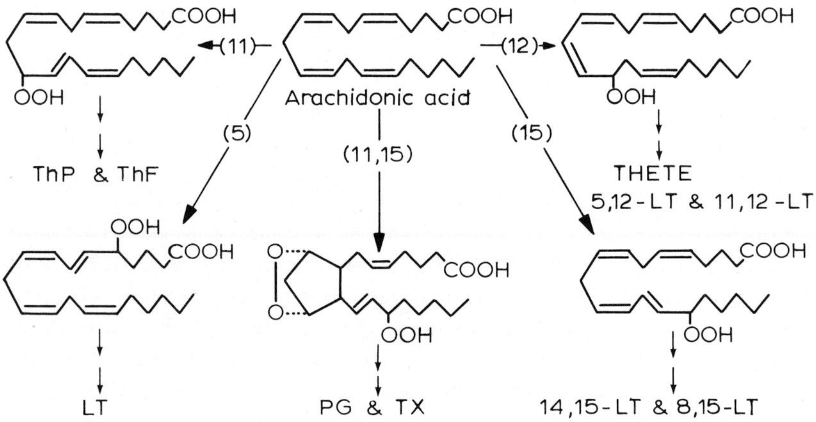

Fig. 12. Mammalian lipoxygenases. PG, prostaglandin; TX, thromboxane, LT, leukotriene; THETE, trihydroxyeicosatetraenoic acid; ThP, tetrahydropyranyl compound; ThF, tetrahydrofuranyl compound.

TABLE 3
Occurrence of lipoxygenases in mammalian cells

Enzyme	Animal	Tissue	References
5-Lipoxygenase	Human	Lymphocyte	208
		Polymorphonuclear leukocyte	196
	Horse	Eosinophil	207
	Rabbit	Polymorphonuclear leukocyte	194, 195
		Alveolar macrophage	210
	Murine	Mastocytoma cell	201
	Rat	Mononuclear cell	203
		Basophilic leukemia cell	205, 206
	Guinea pig	Peritoneal leukocyte	199
8-Lipoxygenase	Human	Neutrophil	196
9-Lipoxygenase	Human	Neutrophil	196
11-Lipoxygenase	Human	Neutrophil	196
	Sheep	Vesicular gland	193
	Guinea pig	Lung	209
	Rabbit	Alveolar macrophage	210
12-Lipoxygenase	Human	Platelets	185–187, 198
	Horse, cow pig and sheep }	Platelets	187
	Rabbit	Aorta	189
	Guinea pig	Lung	188
		Spleen	188
	Human	Neutrophil	196
		Lymphocyte	208
	Mouse	Peritoneal macrophage	190
	Rat	Mast cell	191
		Lung	180
	Pig	Polymorphonuclear leukocyte	200
15-Lipoxygenase	Human	Polymorphonuclear leukocyte	182, 195
		Lung	192
	Guinea pig	Lung	209
	Sheep	Vesicular gland	193
	Rabbit	Polymorphonuclear leukocyte	211
		Reticulocyte	213

pathway from arachidonic acid towards formation of several trihydroxy fatty acids [178,179,180] and leukotrienes [181]. 15-Lipoxygenase produces another group of leukotrienes [182] while an 11-lipoxygenase may open the way to the synthesis of tetrahydrofuranyl and tetrahydropyranyl compounds [183,184]. Most of these lipoxygenases have still to be purified, and little is known about their properties. Table 3 lists various mammalian lipoxygenases whose occurrence has been proved by the isolation of the enzyme or implicated by the isolation of arachidonic acid derivatives hydroxylated at the appropriate position.

(a) 12-Lipoxygenase

The occurrence of 12-lipoxygenase was shown during the synthesis of TXA_2 [185]. The enzyme activity is found in the high speed supernatant of broken platelets of various animals (horse, cow, sheep, pig and man), and a partially purified enzyme produces a hydroperoxy acid [187]. Stereochemically labeled arachidonic acid has been used to show that elimination of the "L" hydrogen from C-10 may be the initial reaction in the formation of 12-hydroperoxy eicosatetraenoic acid [197]. A similar enzyme is found in the particulate fraction of human platelets [186]. The enzyme of human platelet cytosol can be partially purified. Two separate lipoxygenase activities are detected upon gel filtration and ion-exchange chromatography. One of the two fractions (molecular weight 100 000) has little or no peroxidase activity producing predominantly 12-hydroperoxy-eicosatetraenoic acid. The other fraction (molecular weight 160 000) contains both 12-lipoxygenase and peroxidase activities and may be a functional complex of the two enzymes thereby producing 12-hydroxy acid [198]. Another 12-lipoxygenase is found in the cytosol of porcine polymorphonuclear leukocytes and can be partially purified to a peroxidase-free preparation. In addition to arachidonic acid the enzyme is active with 5-hydroxy-6,8,11,14-eicosatetraenoic acid (a 5-lipoxygenase product from arachidonic acid) producing 5S,12S-dihydroxy-(E, Z, E, Z)-6,8,10,14-eicosatetraenoic acid [199,200].

(b) 5-Lipoxygenase

The occurrence of 5-lipoxygenase was implicated from the isolation of 5-hydroxy-6,8,11,14-eicosatetraenoic acid produced from arachidonic acid by rabbit polymorphonuclear leukocytes [194]. The enzyme is now known to initiate the biosynthetic pathway of some leukotrienes, and is considered to occur in various leukotriene-synthesizing tissues: rabbit peritoneal polymorphonuclear leukocytes [194], murine mastocytoma cells [201], human polymorphonuclear leukocytes [202], rat peritoneal mononuclear cells [203,204], rat basophilic leukemia cells [205,206], and horse eosinophils [207]. The $10\,000 \times g$ supernatant of rat basophilic leukemia cells produces 5-hydroxy arachidonic acid, and the reaction requires the presence of calcium ion and glutathione [206]. The $100\,000 \times g$ supernatant of guinea pig peritoneal polymorphonuclear leukocytes contains a 5-lipoxygenase, which also requires calcium ion and produces 5-hydroperoxy acid in the absence of glutathione [199].

(c) 15-Lipoxygenase

This enzyme is found in the cytosol of rabbit peritoneal polymorphonuclear leukocytes and can be purified about 250-fold. The reaction product from arachidonic acid is 15-hydroperoxy-5,8,11,13-eicosatetraenoic acid which undergoes non-enzymatic degradation to 15-hydroxy-, 15-keto-, 13-hydroxy-14,15-epoxy- and 11,14,15-trihydroxy derivatives [211].

(d) Reticulocyte lipoxygenase

A unique lipoxygenase was isolated and purified from rabbit reticulocytes [212]. The purified enzyme with a molecular weight of 78 000 contains two moles of iron per enzyme molecule. The enzyme is identical with the previously known protein factors which inhibit the respiratory chain. The purified lipoxygenase causes a loss of acid-labile sulfur from mitochondrial electron transfer particles and acts preferably on the mitochondrial membrane. The enzyme is considered to work in the lysis of mitochondria during the maturation of erythrocytes. The major product from arachidonic acid is 15S-hydroperoxy-5,8,11,13-eicosatetraenoic acid, although the 12S-hydroperoxy derivative is produced as a minor product [213].

(e) PG production by soybean lipoxygenase

Lipoxygenase-2, an isozyme distinct from the well-known soybean 15-lipoxygenase (lipoxygenase-1), transforms arachidonic acid into a product which is reduced to $PGF_{2\alpha}$ by dithionite reduction and is presumed to be PGG_2 [214].

6. Cytochrome P-450

Arachidonic acid is oxygenated by either of two types of cytochrome *P*-450, and the reaction is dependent on the presence of NADPH, oxygen and NADPH-cytochrome *P*-450 reductase. The product profile is unique for the type of cytochrome *P*-450, the result suggesting an enzyme-directed oxygenation of a specific site of arachidonic acid [215]. Among the products by rat liver microsomes are 9-, 11-, 12- and 15-monohydroxy derivatives of arachidonic acid [216]. Compounds known to inhibit cytochrome *P*-450 reduce the amount of the oxygenated products. The stoichiometric utilization of NADPH and oxygen conforms to a monooxygenase reaction [217]. In addition to the monohydroxy acids, four types of epoxy acids are produced; 5,6-epoxy-8,11,14-, 8,9-epoxy-5,11,14-, 11,12-epoxy-5,8,14- and 14,15-epoxy-5,8,11-eicosatrienoic acids [218]. Rabbit liver microsomes also catalyze oxygenation of arachidonic acid. The reaction requires NADPH and oxygen, and is inhibited by carbon monoxide. The products identified are 14,15- and 11,12-dihydroxy-eicosatrienoic acids [219]. Furthermore, four epoxide derivatives are found; 5(6)oxido-8,11,14-, 8(9)oxido-5,11,14-, 11(12)oxido-5,8,14- and 14(15)oxido-5,8,11-eicosatrienoic acids. These compounds are converted to the corresponding *vic*-diols by the action of epoxide hydrolase. In contrast to the lipoxygenase pathway described above in which the hydroperoxide product is transformed to an epoxide and further to a diol, the hepatic microsomal system may monooxygenate arachidonic acid directly to epoxy derivatives. These epoxides may be rapidly hydrolyzed by epoxide hydrolase to *vic*-diols [220].

Acknowledgments

This review was supported in part by grants-in-aid for scientific research from the Ministry of Education, Science and Culture of Japan and the Intractable Disease Division, Public Health Bureau, Ministry of Health and Welfare of Japan.

References

1 Samuelsson, B. (1972) Fed. Proc. 31, 1442–1450.
2 Hinman, J.W. (1972) Annu. Rev. Biochem. 41, 161–178.
3 Sih, C.J. and Takeguchi, C.A. (1973) in The Prostaglandins (Ramwell, P.W., ed.) Vol. 1, pp. 83–100, Plenum Press, New York.
4 Samuelsson, B., Granström, E., Gréen, K., Hamberg, M. and Hammarström, S. (1975) Annu. Rev. Biochem. 44, 669–695.
5 Yamamoto, S., Ogino, N., Ohki, S., Yoshimoto, T., Bhat, S.G., Oka, J. and Hayaishi, O. (1977) in Biochemical Aspects of Prostaglandins and Thromboxanes (Kharasch, N. and Fried, J., eds.) pp. 1–13, Academic Press, New York.
6 Gibson, K.H. (1977) Chem. Soc. Rev. 6, 489–510.
7 Maclouf, J., Sors, H. and Rigaud, M. (1977) Biomedicine 26, 362–375.
8 Pace-Asciak, C.R. (1977) Prostaglandins 13, 811–817.
9 Samuelsson, B., Goldyne, M., Granström, E., Hamberg, M., Hammarström, S. and Malmsten, C. (1978) Annu. Rev. Biochem. 47, 997–1029.
10 Lands, W.E.M. (1979) Annu. Rev. Physiol. 41, 633–652.
11 Moncada, S. and Vane, J.R. (1979) Pharmacol. Rev. 30, 293–331.
12 Kindahl, H. (1980) J. Am. Vet. Med. Assoc. 176, 1173–1177.
13 Hamberg, M., Svensson, J., Wakabayashi, T. and Samuelsson, B. (1974) Proc. Natl. Acad. Sci. USA 71, 345–349.
14 Miyamoto, T., Ogino, N., Yamamoto, S. and Hayaishi, O. (1976) J. Biol. Chem. 251, 2629–2636.
15 Titus, B.G., Kulmacz, R.J. and Lands, W.E.M. (1982) Arch. Biochem. Biophys. 214, 824–828.
16 Nugteren, D.H., Beerthuis, R.K. and van Dorp, D.A. (1966) Rec. Trav. Chim. 85, 405–419.
17 Samuelsson, B. (1967) Progr. Biochem. Pharmacol. 3, 59–70.
18 Yoshimoto, A., Ito, H. and Tomita, K. (1970) J. Biochem. 68, 487–499.
19 Takeguchi, C., Kohno, E. and Sih, C.J. (1971) Biochemistry 10, 2372–2376.
20 Miyamoto, T., Yamamoto, S. and Hayaishi, O. (1974) Proc. Natl. Acad. Sci. USA 71, 3645–3648.
21 Rollins, T.E. and Smith, W.L. (1980) J. Biol. Chem. 255, 4872–4875.
22 Christ, E.J. and van Dorp, D.A. (1972) Biochim. Biophys. Acta 270, 537–545.
23 Yoshimoto, T., Yamamoto, S., Okuma, M. and Hayaishi, O. (1977) J. Biol. Chem. 252, 5871–5874.
24 Ho, P.P.K., Towner, R.D. and Esterman, M.A. (1980) Prep. Biochem. 10, 597–613.
25 Bhat, S.G., Yoshimoto, T., Yamamoto, S. and Hayaishi, O. (1978) Biochim. Biophys. Acta 529, 398–408.
26 Shimizu, T., Yamamoto, S. and Hayaishi, O. (1979) J. Biol. Chem. 254, 5222–5228.
27 Ogino, N., Ohki, S., Yamamoto, S. and Hayaishi, O. (1978) J. Biol. Chem. 253, 5061–5068.
28 Hemler, M., Lands, W.E.M. and Smith, W.L. (1976) J. Biol. Chem. 251, 5575–5579.
29 van der Ouderaa, F.J., Buytenhek, M., Nugteren, D.H. and van Dorp, D.A. (1977) Biochim. Biophys. Acta 487, 315–331.
30 van der Ouderaa, F.J., Buytenhek, M., Slikkerveer, F.J. and van Dorp, D.A. (1979) Biochim. Biophys. Acta 572, 29–42.
31 Samuelsson, B. (1965) J. Am. Chem. Soc. 87, 3011–3013.
32 Hamberg, M. and Samuelsson, B. (1967) J. Biol. Chem. 242, 5336–5343.
33 Hemler, M.E., Crawford, C.G. and Lands, W.E.M. (1978) Biochemistry 17, 1772–1779.

34 Smith, W.L. and Lands, W.E.M. (1972) Biochemistry 121, 3276–3285.
35 Egan, R.W., Paxton, J. and Kuehl, F.A. (1976) J. Biol. Chem. 251, 7329–7335.
36 Lands, W.E.M., Sauter, J. and Stone, G.W. (1978) Prostaglandins and Medicine 1, 117–120.
37 Culp, B.R., Titus, B.G. and Lands, W.E.M. (1979) Prostaglandins and Medicine 3, 269–278.
38 Ohki, S., Ogino, N., Yamamoto, S. and Hayaishi, O. (1979) J. Biol. Chem. 254, 829–836.
39 Hemler, M.E. and Lands, W.E.M. (1980) J. Biol. Chem. 255, 6253–6261.
40 Rome, L.H. and Lands, W.E.M. (1975) Prostaglandins 10, 813–824.
41 Hemler, M.E., Graff, G. and Lands, W.E.M. (1978) Biochem. Biophys. Res. Commun. 85, 1325–1331.
41 a. Roth, G.J., Machuga, E.T. and Strittmatter, P. (1981) J. Biol. Chem. 256, 10018–10022.
42 Hemler, M.E. and Lands, W.E.M. (1980) Arch. Biochem. Biophys. 201, 586–593.
43 Cook, H.W., Ford, G. and Lands, W.E.M. (1979) Anal. Biochem. 96, 341–351.
44 Lands, W., Lee, R. and Smith, W. (1971) Ann. N.Y. Acad. Sci. 180, 107–122.
45 Hemler, M.E., Cook, H.W. and Lands, W.E.M. (1979) Arch. Biochem. Biophys. 193, 340–345.
46 Mizuno, K., Yamamoto, S. and Lands, W.E.M. (1982) Prostaglandins 23, 743–757.
47 van der Ouderaa, F.J., Buytenhek, M., Nugteren, D.H. and van Dorp, D.A. (1980) Eur. J. Biochem. 109, 1–8.
48 Nugteren, D.H and Hazelhof, E. (1973) Biochim. Biophys. Acta 326, 448–461.
49 Samuelsson, B. and Hamberg, M. (1974) in Prostaglandin Synthetase Inhibitors (Robinson, H.J. and Vane, J.R., eds.) pp. 107–119, Raven Press, New York.
50 Chan, J.A., Nagasawa, M., Takeguchi, C. and Sih, C.J. (1975) Biochemistry 14, 2987–2991.
51 Smith, W.L. and Lands, W.E.M. (1971) J. Biol. Chem. 246, 6700–6702.
52 Ogino, N., Yamamoto, S., Hayaishi, O. and Tokuyama, T. (1979) Biochem. Biophys. Res. Commun. 87, 184–191.
53 O'Brien, P.J. and Rahimtula, A. (1976) Biochem. Biophys. Res. Commun. 70, 832–838.
54 Marnett, L.J., Wlodawer, P. and Samuelsson, B. (1975) J. Biol. Chem. 250, 8510–8517.
55 Marnett, L.J., Reed, G.A. and Johnson, J.T. (1977) Biochem. Biophys. Res. Commun. 79, 569–576.
56 Marnett, L.J., Bienkowski, M.J. and Pagels, W.R. (1979) J. Biol. Chem. 254, 5077–5082.
57 Zenser, T.V., Mattammal, M.B. and Davis, B.B. (1980) J. Pharmacol. Exp. Ther. 214, 312–317.
58 Egan, R.W., Gale, P.H., VandenHeuvel, W.J.A., Baptista, E.M. and Kuehl, F.A. (1980) J. Biol. Chem. 255, 323–326.
59 Egan, R.W., Gale, P.H. and Kuehl, F.A. (1979) J. Biol. Chem. 254, 3295–3302.
59 a. Egan, R.W., Gale, P.H., Baptista, E.M., Kennicott, K.L., VandenHeuvel, W.J.A., Walker, R.W., Fagerness, P.E. and Kuehl, F.A. (1981) J. Biol. Chem. 256, 7352–7361.
60 Marnett, L.J., Wlodawer, P. and Samuelsson, B. (1974) Biochem. Biophys. Res. Commun. 60, 1286–1294.
61 O'Brien, P.J. and Hulett, L.G. (1980) Prostaglandins 19, 683–691.
62 Yoshimoto, T., Yamamoto, S., Sugioka, K., Nakano, M., Takyu, C., Yamagishi, A. and Inaba, H. (1980) J. Biol. Chem. 255, 10199–10204.
63 Vladimirov, Y.A., Roshchupkin, D.I. and Fesenko, E.E. (1970) Photochem. Photobiol. 11, 227–246.
64 Matsuda, Y., Satoh, T., Beppu, T. and Arima, K. (1976) Agr. Biol. Chem. 40, 963–976.
65 Peterson, D.A. and Gerrard, J.M. (1979) Medical Hypotheses 5, 683–694.
66 Pace-Asciak, C.R. and Rangaraj, G. (1977) Biochim. Biophys. Acta 486, 579–582.
67 Sun, F.F., Chapman, J.P. and McGuire, J.C. (1977) Prostaglandins 14, 1055–1074.
67 a. Ingerman-Wojenski, C., Silver, M.J., Smith, J.B. and Macarak, E. (1981) J. Clin. Invest. 67, 1292–1996.
67 b. Salzman, P.M., Salmon, J.A. and Moncada, S. (1980) J. Pharmacol. Exp. Ther. 215, 240–247.
68 Needleman, P., Moncada, S., Bunting, S., Vane, J.R., Hamberg, M. and Samuelsson, B. (1976) Nature 261, 558–560.
69 Ho, P.P.K., Walters, C.P. and Sullivan, H.R. (1976) Prostaglandins 12, 951–970.
70 Tai, H.-H. and Yuan, B. (1978) Biochim. Biophys. Acta 531, 286–294.
71 Tai, H.-H., Yuan, B. and Wu, A.T. (1978) Biochem. J. 170, 441–444.
72 Hammarström, S. and Falardeau, P. (1977) Proc. Natl. Acad. Sci. USA 74, 3691–3695.
73 Wlodawer, P. and Hammarström, S. (1978) Biochem. Biophys. Res. Commun. 80, 525–532.

73 a. Hall, E.R. and Tai, H.-H. (1981) Biochim. Biophys. Acta 665, 498–503.
74 Svensson, J., Hamberg, M. and Samuelsson, B. (1976) Acta Physiol. Scand. 98, 285–294.
75 Diczfalusy, U., Falardeau, P. and Hammarström, S. (1977) FEBS Lett. 84, 271–274.
76 Raz, A., Aharony, D. and Kenig-Wakshal, R. (1978) Eur. J. Biochem. 86, 447–454.
77 Anderson, M.W., Crutchley, D.J., Tainer, B.E. and Eling, T.E. (1978) Prostaglandins 16, 563–570.
78 Diczfalusy, U. and Hammarström, S. (1979) FEBS Lett. 105, 291–295.
78 a. Ullrich, V., Castle, L. and Haurand, M. (1982) in Oxygenases and Oxygen Metabolism (Nozaki, M., Yamamoto, S., Ishimura, Y., Coon, M.J., Estabrook, R.W. and Ernster, L., eds.), Academic Press, New York, in press.
79 Moncada, S., Bunting, S., Mullane, K., Thorogood, P., Vane, J.R., Raz, A. and Needleman, P. (1977) Prostaglandins 13, 611–618.
80 Tai, H.-H. and Yuan, B. (1978) Biochem. Biophys. Res. Commun. 80, 236–242.
81 Yoshimoto, T., Yamamoto, S. and Hayaishi, O. (1978) Prostaglandins 16, 529–540.
82 Gorman, R.R., Bundy, G.L., Peterson, D.C., Sun, F.F., Miller, O.V. and Fitzpatrick, F.A. (1977) Proc. Natl. Acad. Sci. USA 74, 4007–4011.
83 Abdel-Halim, M.S., Hamberg, M., Sjöquist, B. and Änggård, E. (1977) Prostaglandins 14, 633–643.
84 Christ-Hazelhof, E. and Nugteren, D.H. (1979) Biochim. Biophys. Acta 572, 43–51.
85 Steinhoff, M.M., Lee, L.H. and Jakschik, B.A. (1980) Biochim. Biophys. Acta 618, 28–34.
86 Shimizu, T., Mizuno, N., Amano, T. and Hayaishi, O. (1979) Proc. Natl. Acad. Sci. USA 76, 6231–6234.
86 a. Gerritsen, M.E. and Printz, M.P. (1981) Prostaglandins 22, 553–566.
87 Ogino, N., Miyamoto, T., Yamamoto, S. and Hayaishi, O. (1977) J. Biol. Chem. 252, 890–895.
88 Wlodawer, P., Kindahl, H. and Hamberg, M. (1976) Biochim. Biophys. Acta 431, 603–614.
89 Hamberg, M. and Israelsson, U. (1970) J. Biol. Chem. 245, 5107–5114.
90 Leslie, C.A. and Levine, L. (1973) Biochem. Biophys. Res. Commun. 52, 717–724.
91 Hensby, C.N. (1975) Biochim. Biophys. Acta 409, 225–234.
92 Wong, P.Y.-K. (1981) Biochim. Biophys. Acta 659, 169–178.
93 Reingold, D.F., Kawasaki, A. and Needleman, P. (1981) Biochim. Biophys. Acta 659, 179–188.
94 Watanabe, K., Shimizu, T. and Hayaishi, O. (1981) Biochem. Intern. 2, 603–610.
94 a. Claeys, M., Wechsung, E., Herman, A.G. and Nugteren, D.H. (1981) Prostaglandins 21, 739–749.
95 Moncada, S., Gryglewski, R., Bunting, S. and Vane, J.R. (1976) Nature 263, 663–665.
96 Gryglewski, R.J., Bunting, S., Moncada, S., Flower, R.J. and Vane, J.R. (1976) Prostaglandins 12, 685–713.
97 Salmon, J.A., Smith, D.R., Flower, R.J., Moncada, S. and Vane, J.R. (1978) Biochim. Biophys. Acta 523, 250–262.
98 Chang, W.-C. and Murota, S. (1977) Biochim. Biophys. Acta 486, 136–144.
99 Cottee, F., Flower, R.J., Moncada, S., Salmon, J.A. and Vane, J.R. (1977) Prostaglandins 14, 413–423.
100 Wallach, D.P. (1978) Prostaglandins 15, 671–684.
101 Watanabe, K., Yamamoto, S. and Hayaishi, O. (1979) Biochem. Biophys. Res. Commun. 87, 192–199.
102 Wlodawer, P. and Hammarström, S. (1979) FEBS Lett. 97, 32–36.
103 Wlodawer, P. and Hammarström, S. (1980) Prostaglandins 19, 969–976.
103 a. Ullrich, V., Castle, L. and Weber, P. (1981) Biochem. Pharmacol. 30, 2033–2036.
104 Polet, H. and Levine, L. (1975) J. Biol. Chem. 250, 351–357.
105 Jones, R.L., Cammock, S. and Horton, E.W. (1972) Biochim. Biophys. Acta 280, 588–601.
106 Änggård, E. and Samuelsson, B. (1966) Arkiv Kemi 25, 293–300.
107 Marrazi, M.A. and Andersen, N.H. (1974) in The Prostaglandins (Ramwell, P.W., ed.), Vol. 2, pp. 99–155, Plenum Press, New York.
108 Hansen, H.S. (1976) Prostaglandins 12, 647–679.
109 Marrazi, M.A. and Matschinsky, F.M. (1972) Prostaglandins 1, 373–388.
110 Saeed, S.A. and Roy, A.C. (1972) Biochem. Biophys. Res. Commun. 47, 96–102.
111 Sun, F.F., Armour, S.B., Bockstanz, V.R. and McGuire, J.C. (1976) Adv. Prostaglandin Thromboxane Res. 1, 163–169.

112 Braithwaite, S.S. and Jarabak, J. (1975) J. Biol. Chem. 250, 2315–2318.
113 Wright, J.T., Corder, C.N. and Taylor, R. (1976) Biochem. Pharmacol. 25, 1669–1673.
114 Kung-Chao, D.T.Y. and Tai, H.H. (1980) Biochim. Biophys. Acta 614, 1–13.
115 Nakano, J., Änggård, E. and Samuelsson, B. (1969) Eur. J. Biochem. 11, 386–389.
116 Vonkeman, H., Nugteren, D.H. and van Dorp, D.A. (1969) Biochim. Biophys. Acta 187, 581–583.
117 Ohno, H., Morikawa, Y. and Hirata, F. (1978) J. Biochem. 84, 1485–1494.
118 Jarabak, J. and Fried, J. (1979) Prostaglandins, 18, 241–246.
119 McGuire, J.C. and Sun, F.F. (1978) Arch. Biochem. Biophys. 189, 92–96.
120 Marrazi, M.A., Shaw, J.E., Tao, F.T. and Matschinsky, F.M. (1972) Prostaglandins 1, 389–395.
121 Yamazaki, M. and Sasaki, M. (1975) Biochem. Biophys. Res. Commun. 66, 255–261.
122 Änggård, E. (1966) Acta Physiol. Scand. 66, 509–510.
123 Flower, R.J. 91974) Pharmacol. Rev. 26, 33–67.
124 Lee, S.-C. and Levine, L. (1975) J. Biol. Chem. 250, 548–552.
125 Lee, S.-C., Pong, S.-S., Katzen, D., Wu, K.-Y. and Levine, L. (1975) Biochemistry 14, 142–145.
126 Chang, D.G.-B., Sun, M. and Tai, H.-H. (1981) Biochem. Biophys. Res. Commun. 99, 745–751.
127 Hassid, A. and Levine, L. (1977) Prostaglandins 13, 503–516.
128 Kaplan, L., Lee, S.-C. and Levine, L. (1975) Arch. Biochem. Biophys. 167, 287–293.
129 Westbrook, C., Lin, Y.-M. and Jarabak, J. (1977) Biochem. Biophys. Res. Commun. 76, 943–949.
130 Lin, Y.-M. and Jarabak, J. (1978) Biochem. Biophys. Res. Commun. 81, 1227–1234.
131 Oien, H.G., Ham, E.A., Zanetti, M.E., Ulm, E.H. and Kuehl, F.A. (1976) Proc. Natl. Acad. Sci. USA 73, 1107–1111.
132 Watanabe, K., Shimizu, T., Iguchi, S., Wakatsuka, H., Hayashi, M. and Hayaishi, O. (1980) J. Biol. Chem. 255, 1779–1782.
133 Korff, J. and Jarabak, J. (1980) Prostaglandins 20, 111–125.
134 Korff, J.M. and Jarabak, J. (1981) Prostaglandins 21, 719–725.
135 Pace-Asciak, C. (1975) J. Biol. Chem. 250, 2789–2794.
136 Pace-Asciak, C. and Domazet, Z. (1975) Biochim. Biophys. Acta 380, 338–343.
137 Yuan, B., Tai, C.L. and Tai, H.-H. (1980) J. Biol. Chem. 255, 7439–7443.
138 Hoult, J.R.S. and Moore, P.K. (1977) Br. J. Pharmacol. 61, 615–626.
139 Moore, P.K. and Hoult, J.R.S. (1978) Biochim. Biophys. Acta 528, 276–287.
140 Leslie, C.A. and Levine, L. (1973) Biochem. Biophys. Res. Commun. 52, 717–724.
141 Lee, S.-C. and Levine, L. (1974) J. Biol. Chem. 249, 1369–1375.
142 Lee, S.-C. and Levine, L. (1975) J. Biol. Chem. 250, 4549–4555.
143 Stone, K.J. and Hart, M. (1975) Prostaglandins 10, 273–288.
144 Toft, B.S. and Hansen, H.S. (1979) Biochim. Biophys. Acta 574, 33–38.
145 Carpenter, M.P., Robinson, R.D. and Thuy, L.P. (1978) Lipids 13, 308–311.
146 Thuy, L.P. and Carpenter, M.P. (1978) Biochem. Biophys. Res. Commun. 81, 322–328.
147 Ziboh, V.A., Lord, J.T. and Penneys, N.S. (1977) J. Lipid Res. 18, 37–43.
148 Wong, P.Y.-K., Terragno, D.A., Terragno, N.A. and McGiff, J.C. (1977) Prostaglandins 13, 1113–1125.
149 Änggård, E., Larsson, C. and Samuelsson, B. (1971) Acta Physiol. Scand. 81, 396–404.
150 Lee, S.-C. and Levine, L. (1974) Biochem. Biophys. Res. Commun. 61, 14–21.
151 Hansen, H.S. (1979) Biochim. Biophys. Acta 574, 136–145.
152 Westbrook, C. and Jarabak, J. (1978) Arch. Biochem. Biophys. 185, 429–442.
153 Hamberg, M. (1968) Eur. J. Biochem. 6, 135–146.
154 Hamberg, M. and Samuelsson, B., (1967) in Prostaglandins (Bergström, S. and Samuelsson, B., eds.) p. 63–70, Almqvist and Wiksell, Stockholm.
155 Jonsson, H.T., Middleditch, B.S. and Desiderio, D.M. (1975) Science 187, 1093–1094.
156 Taylor, P.L. and Kelly, R.W. (1974) Nature 250, 665–667.
157 Taylor, P.L. and Kelly, R.W. (1975) FEBS Lett. 57, 22–25.
158 Israelsson, U., Hamberg, M. and Samuelsson, B. (1969) Eur. J. Biochem. 11, 390–394.
159 Powell, W.S. and Solomon, S. (1978) J. Biol. Chem. 253, 4609–4616.
160 Pace-Asciak, C. (1975) J. Biol. Chem. 250, 2795–2800.

161 Pace-Asciak, C. and Miller, D. (1973) Prostaglandins 4, 351–362.
162 Pace-Asciak, C. (1977) Prostaglandins 13, 649–660.
163 Pace-Asciak, C. (1977) Prostaglandins 13, 661–668.
164 Pace-Asciak, C. and Rangaraj, G. (1976) J. Biol. Chem. 251, 3381–3385.
165 Pace-Asciak, C.R. (1980) Seminars perinatol. 4, 15–21.
166 Sun, F.F. and Armour, S.B. (1974) Prostaglandins 7, 327–338.
167 Egerton-Vernon, J.M. and Bedwani, J.R. (1975) Eur. J. Pharmacol. 33, 405–408.
168 Bedwani, J.R. and Marley, P.B. (1975) Br. J. Pharmacol. 53, 547–554.
169 Carminati, P., Luzzani, F. and Lerner, L.J. (1974) Prostaglandins 8, 205–211.
170 Korff, J.M. and Jarabak, J. (1982) J. Biol. Chem. 257, 2177–2181.
171 Oliw, E.H., Lawson, J.A., Brash, A.R. and Oates, J.A. (1981) J. Biol. Chem. 256, 9924–9931.
172 Pace-Asciak, C.R. and Edwards, N.S. (1980) J. Biol. Chem. 255, 6106–6110.
173 Kupfer, D., Navarro, J. and Piccolo, D.E. (1978) J. Biol. Chem. 253, 2804–2811.
174 Navarro, J., Piccolo, D.E. and Kupfer, D. (1978) Arch. Biochem. Biophys. 191, 125–133.
175 Masters, B.S.S., Parkhill, L.K., Yasukochi, Y., Okita, R.T., Theoharides, A.D. and Kupfer, D. (1980) in Biochemistry, Biophysics and Regulation of Cytochrome *P*-450 (Gustafsson, J.Å., et al., eds) p. 101–104, Elsevier/North-Holland Biomedical Press, Amsterdam.
176 Samuelsson, B., Hammarström, S., Murphy, R.C. and Borgeat, P. (1980) Allergy 35, 375–381.
177 Borgeat, P. and Sirois, P. (1981) J. Med. Chem. 24, 121–126.
178 Jones, R.L. Kerry, P.J., Poyser, N.L., Walker, I.C. and Wilson, N.H. (1978) Prostaglandins 16, 583–589.
179 Bryant, R.W. and Bailey, J.M. (1979) Prostaglandins 17, 9–18.
180 Pace-Asciak, C.R., Mizuno, K. and Yamamoto, S. (1981) Biochim. Biophys. Acta 665, 352–354.
181 Samuelsson, B. (1983) in Advances in Prostaglandins and Thromboxane Research (Samuelsson, B., Paoletti, R. and Ramwell, P., eds.) Raven Press, New York, Vol. 11, pp. 1–13.
182 Lundberg, U., Rådmark, O., Malmsten, C. and Samuelsson, B. (1981) FEBS Lett. 126, 127–132.
183 Pace-Asciak, C. and Wolfe, L.S. (1970) Chem. Commun. 1235–1236.
184 Pace-Asciak, C. (1971) Biochemistry 10, 3664–3669.
185 Hamberg, M. and Samuelsson, B. (1974) Proc. Natl. Acad. Sci. USA 71, 3400–3404.
186 Ho, P.P.K., Walters, P. and Sullivan, H.R. (1977) Biochem. Biophys. Res. Commun. 76, 398–405.
187 Nugteren, D.H. (1975) Biochim. Biophys. Acta 380, 299–307.
188 Hamberg, M. (1976) Biochim. Biophys. Acta 431, 651–654.
189 Greenwald, J.E., Bianchine, J.R.a and Wong, L.K. (1979) Nature 281, 588–589.
190 Rigaud, M., Durand, J. and Breton, J.C. (1979) Biochim. Biophys. Acta 573, 408–412.
191 Roberts, L.J., Lewis, R.A., Oates, J.A. and Austen, K.F. (1979) Biochim. Biophys. Acta 575, 185–192.
192 Hamberg, M., Hedqvist, P. and Rådegran, K. (1980) Acta Physiol. Scand. 110, 219–221.
193 Hamberg, M. and Samuelsson, B. (1967) J. Biol. Chem. 242, 5344–5354.
194 Borgeat, P., Hamberg, M. and Samuelsson, B. (1976) J. Biol. Chem. 251, 7816–7820.
195 Borgeat, P. and Samuelsson, B. (1979) Proc. Natl. Acad. Sci. USA 76, 2148–2152.
196 Goetzl, E.J. and Sun, F.F. (1979) J. Exp. Med. 150, 406–411.
197 Hamberg, M. and Hamberg, G. (1980) Biochem. Biophys. Res. Commun. 95, 1090–1097.
198 Siegel, M.I., McConnell, R.T., Porter, N.A. and Cuatrecasas, P. (1980) Proc. Natl. Acad. Sci. USA 77, 308–312.
199 Yamamoto, S., Yoshimoto, T., Ochi, K., Miyamoto, Y., Miyamoto, T. and Taniguchi, K. (1982) in Oxygenases and Oxygen Metabolism (Nozaki, M., Yamamoto, S., Ishimura, Y., Coon, M.J., Ernster, L. and Estabrook, R.W., eds.) pp. 619–629, Academic Press, New York.
200 Yoshimoto, T., Miyamoto, Y., Ochi, K. and Yamamoto, S. (1982) Biochim. Biophys. Acta 713, 638–646.
201 Murphy, R.C., Hammarström, S. and Samuelsson, B. (1979) Proc. Natl. Acad. Sci. USA 76, 4275–4279.
202 Hansson, G. and Rådmark, O. (1980) FEBS Lett. 122, 87–90.
203 Bach, M.K., Brashler, J.R., Hammarström, S. and Samuelsson, B. (1980) J. Immunol. 125, 115–117.

204 Doig, M.V. and Ford-Hutchinson, A.W. (1980) Prostaglandins 20, 1007–1019.
205 Morris, H.R., Taylor, G.W., Piper, P.J., Samhoun, M.N. and Tippins, J.R. (1980) Prostaglandins 19, 185–201.
206 Jakschik, B.A. and Lee, L.H. (1980) Nature 287, 51–52.
207 Jörg, A., Henderson, W.R., Murphy, R.C. and Klebanoff, S.J. (1982) J. Exp. Med. 155, 390–402.
208 Parker, C.W., Stenson, W.F., Huber, M.G. and Kelly, J.P. (1979) J. Immunol. 122, 1572–1577.
209 Hamberg, M. and Samuelsson, B. (1974) Biochem. Biophys. Res. Commun. 61, 942–949.
210 Valone, F.H., Franklin, M., Sun, F.F. and Goetzl, E.J. (1980) Cell Immunol. 54, 390–401.
211 Narumiya, S., Salmon, J.A., Cottee, F.H., Weatherly, B.C. and Flower, R.J. (1981) J. Biol. Chem. 256, 9582–9592.
212 Rapoport, S.M., Schewe, T., Wiesner, R., Halangk, W., Ludwig, P., Janicke-Höhne, M., Tannert, C., Hiebsch, C. and Klatt, D. (1979) Eur. J. Biochem. 96, 545–561.
213 Bryant, R.W., Bailey, J.M., Schewe, T. and Rapoport, S.M. (1982) J. Biol. Chem. 257, 6050–6055.
214 Bild, G.S., Bhat, S.G., Ramadoss, C.S. and Axelrod, B. (1978) J. Biol. Chem. 253, 21–23.
215 Capdevila, J., Parkhill, L., Chacos, N., Okita, R., Masters, B.S.S. and Estabrook, R.W. (1981) Biochem. Biophys. Res. Commun. 101, 1357–1363.
216 Capdevila, J., Marnett, L.J., Chacos, N., Prough, R.A. and Estabrook, R.W. (1982) Proc. Natl. Acad. Sci. USA 79, 767–770.
217 Capdevila, J., Chacos, N., Werringloer, J., Prough, R.A. and Estabrook, R.W. (1981) Proc. Natl. Acad. Sci. USA 78, 5362–5366.
218 Chacos, N., Falck, J.R., Wixtrom, C. and Capdevila, J. (1982) Biochem. Biophys. Res. Commun. 104, 916–922.
219 Oliw, E.H. and Oates, J.A. (1981) Biochim. Biophys. Acta 666, 327–340.
220 Oliw, E.H., Guengerich, F.P. and Oates, J.A. (1982) Proc. Natl. Acad. Sci USA 257, 3771–3779.

CHAPTER 6

Inhibitors and activators of prostaglandin biosynthesis

WILLIAM E.M. LANDS and ARTHUR M. HANEL

Department of Biological Chemistry, University of Illinois at Chicago, Chicago, IL 60612, U.S.A.

1. Introduction

The enzyme reaction which converts polyunsaturated fatty acids to prostaglandins is a complex polyatomic reaction. It inserts two moles of oxygen into the polyunsaturated fatty acid to give five new chiral centers with no definite recognized reaction intermediate. The insertion of the 4 oxygen atoms by the cyclooxygenase activity requires no additional cosubstrates, and is achieved by a *bis*-dioxygenation process in which both oxygen-oxygen bonds are kept intact [1]. The resultant endoperoxide hydroperoxy derivative, PGG, is readily reduced by peroxidase activity to the endoperoxide hydroxy derivative, PGH. Both the cyclooxygenase and the peroxidase activities appear to be catalyzed by the same purified protein which is named prostaglandin H synthase. The enzyme has been purified to homogeneity [2,3,4] and it appears to be similar in many tissues of many different species. Cyclooxygenase activity has attracted much interest since the time that it was recognized to be the site of action for non-steroidal antiinflammatory agents such as aspirin and other aspirin-like drugs [5]. It is the cyclooxygenase activity which appears to be responsible for the wide range of pathophysiologic events that are now recognized to be due to excessive prostaglandin generation. Exposure of the enzyme to some antiinflammatory agents can completely inactivate the cyclooxygenase activity while leaving peroxidase activity relatively unaffected [3,4]. Developing a rationale for how the wide variety of different pharmaceutical agents exert their effect requires some detailed understanding of the mechanism whereby cyclooxygenase action occurs. The following sections are intended to examine several aspects of activation of cyclooxygenase action for use in the subsequent interpretations of the action of the inhibitors.

The formation of prostaglandins from polyunsaturated fatty acids appears to be a lipid hydroperoxide-initiated free radical chain reaction in which positive feedback

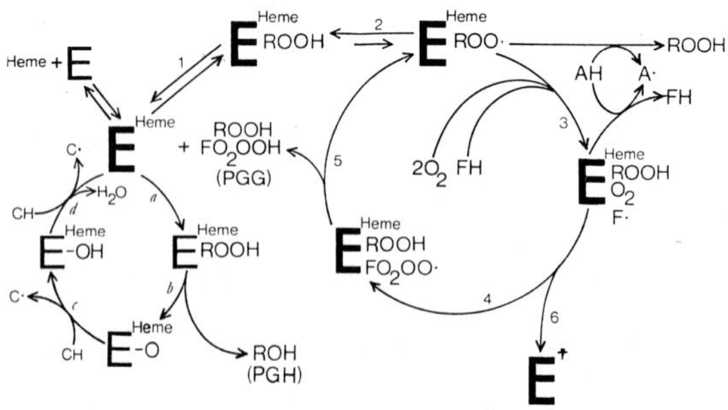

Fig. 1. Proposed mechanisms for prostaglandin H synthase. The holoenzyme catalyzes both the cyclooxygenase reaction (at the right) and the peroxidase reaction (at the left).

aspects of product activation are countered with negative feedback features of self-catalyzed inactivation [6]. These complex features make traditional kinetic analyses somewhat oversimplified and inadequate. As a result, attempts to interpret the mechanism of a given inhibition or activation of cyclooxygenase activity have sometimes produced disconcerting paradoxes. Fig. 1 helps interpret the site of action of the activators and inhibitors to be discussed. Reaction steps 1–6 represent steps related to the cyclooxygenase activity and steps a–d represent those catalyzed by the peroxidase activity. The likelihood of paradoxical situations being generated is evident in the relationship whereby the product of reaction 5 can be the activator for reaction 1 and yet it is destroyed in the process of reaction b. Thus, we recognize that the PGH synthase has the ability to generate and to destroy lipid peroxides that are necessary for its own activity.

The design and conduct of experimental protocols which can elaborate on these mechanistic features represent a difficult challenge encountered by laboratories around the world. When the cyclooxygenase reaction is initiated in the presence of small amounts of lipid hydroperoxide, the overall consumption of oxygen proceeds at a rapidly accelerating rate as reaction 5 generates more activating lipid hydroperoxide. The oxygenation reaction reaches an optimum velocity value and then deccelerates as a result of the self-catalyzed inactivation (indicated as step 6) until finally no further oxygenation occurs. Many kinetic details are not apparent when investigators only isolate the products that have accumulated within 60 or 120 seconds. As a result, some mechanistic features of activation and inhibition are not adequately treated in many reports although general overall phenomena are reproducibly observed by most investigators. The following discussion of activators involves three different types of factors that enhance prostaglandin production; heme, peroxidase cosubstrates and lipid hydroperoxide. These three activators act in concert with the enzymic protein and the two substrates, oxygen and fatty acid, to form prostaglandins. All are essential except the peroxidase cosubstrates, which are probably abundant in vivo and which appear to be stimulatory only in certain conditions in vitro. It seems likely that the major physiologic aspects of controlling prostaglandin biosynthesis in tissues are the regulation of the availability of both the substrate fatty acid and the activator hydroperoxide.

2. *Activators of prostaglandin biosynthesis*

(a) Heme

Heme is an essential component of fully active cyclooxygenase [2,3,4]. It binds tightly to the apoenzyme [2,6,7] but can be removed during purification procedures, especially in the presence of detergents [7]. Binding of heme to PGH synthase has no definite stoichiometry, and catalytically inactive heme was bound in amounts up to 4 moles per 70 000 daltons [2,8] when excess heme was present. This was 5 to 10 times that which was actually needed for full catalytic action [6,8]. Crude acetone powder preparations of sheep seminal vesicles contain both apo (heme-free) and holo (heme-containing) forms of the enzyme, and they exhibit a time-dependent increase in total activity while standing in buffered systems that contain a stabilizing agent such as phenol [9,10]. This progressive increase in enzyme activity has been attributed to a slow transfer of heme from other microsomal proteins to the apocyclooxygenase [11]. The purified apoenzyme that is free from other competing proteins is activated immediately by added hematin. The slow activation noted with acetone powders [9] raises the question of whether heme supply could be limiting prostaglandin formation in vivo. The answer will require knowing the intracellular location of the cyclooxygenase in various tissues and the amount of heme available at those loci. The primary site for the enzyme in the endoplasmic reticulum [12] has an abundance of heme that makes it less likely that heme availability is generally limiting the biosynthesis of prostaglandins in most tissues. Nevertheless, specialized cells that synthesize only limited amounts of heme may be limited in a full expression of their apoenzyme potential because of competition for heme among the various hemeproteins.

An interesting feature of the mangano-protoporphyrin analog of PGH synthase is its ability to perform cyclooxygenase reactions while providing no measurable peroxidase activity [13]. This finding has allowed study of the cyclooxygenase activity separate from that of the peroxidase [14] whereas both activities occur simultaneously when the enzyme is assisted by Fe protoporphyrin.

(b) Peroxidase cosubstrates

Peroxidase cosubstrates, particularly phenolic agents, have been reported to increase the synthesis of prostaglandins in vitro [9,15,16]. This activation of cyclooxygenase action generally increases the optimal rate of biosynthesis in vitro several fold, thereby providing larger yields of prostaglandins in the same period of time. The customary explanation of the stimulation of horseradish peroxidase by reducing agents [17] seems appropriate also for the prostaglandin peroxidase activity, and it helps interpret the manner in which stimulating prostaglandin peroxidase action can aid cyclooxygenase action. Peroxidase action cleaves peroxide bonds while forming metastable oxidized forms of the enzyme noted as "compound I" and "compound II". The hypothesis is that the reducing agents serve as peroxidase cosubstrates to speed the return of intermediate oxidized heme forms of the enzyme back to the initial state (reactions C and D, Fig. 1). These steps restore the enzyme to forms that can then participate in the cyclooxygenase process. Support for this concept derives from the finding that the oxygenation catalyzed by the mangano-protoporphyrin form of the enzyme (which has no peroxidase activity) was not stimulated by the peroxidase cosubstrate [6]. Also, when peroxidase activity of the ferriprotoporphyrin enzyme is blocked by cyanide, added phenol no longer stimulates cyclooxygenase activity [6].

Phenolic agents which activate cyclooxygenase activity often manifest a stimulation at low concentrations and an inhibition at high concentrations [6]. This biphasic response creates a paradoxical situation since the same agent may cause either stimulation or inhibition depending upon its concentration or upon the environment of the cyclooxygenase. Phenolic agents vary in their relative tendencies to activate and inhibit [16,18], and some have proved useful in modifying pathophysiologic conditions associated with the overproduction of prostaglandins. This section is directed to activators of prostaglandin synthesis, and the inhibitory action of phenolic agents such as Tylenol and MK-447 will be reviewed after examining the role of hydroperoxide activators. The inhibitory action of phenolic agents is particularly dependent upon the availability of hydroperoxide activator which is discussed in the following section.

(c) Lipid hydroperoxides

Lipid hydroperoxides serve as essential activators of both of the known purified fatty acid oxygenases: soybean lipoxygenase [19] and cyclooxygenase [20,21]. A wide variety of hydroperoxides can facilitate prostaglandin biosynthesis [22], and the demonstrated effectiveness of the generated intermediate hydroperoxide, PGG, provides an explanation for the rapid initial acceleration noted in some experimental conditions [23]. The observed cessation of the fatty acid oxygenation reaction by removal of hydroperoxide indicates a need for the continued presence of this activator even after the reaction has been initiated. When PGG was added to slowly accelerating systems it eliminated the lags whereas the hydroxyl analog, PGH, had no effect [24]. The fact that acceleration was observed during fatty acid oxygenation was important kinetic evidence for the enzymatic generation of an essential activator of the overall oxygenation reaction with both lipoxygenase and cyclooxygenase. Removal of hydroperoxides by added glutathione peroxidase can slow their accumulation rate and increase the time required for the enzyme system to reach an optimum velocity of oxygenation. Such lag times can become more pronounced for the cyclooxygenase in the presence of phenolic agents (see Fig. 5 in ref. 6) which appear to terminate radical intermediates of the cyclooxygenase-catalyzed reaction and thereby greatly decrease the rate of hydroperoxide generation relative to hydroperoxide destruction.

The ability of PGH synthase to effectively catalyze oxygenation while simultaneously removing much of the hydroperoxide activator by peroxidatic action indicates that the oxygenation reaction has a greater affinity than the peroxidase for hydroperoxide. This is further supported by the fact that glutathione peroxidase alone does not appreciably inhibit the PGH synthase but is inhibitory only when an additional inhibitor (such as phenol or cyanide) is present to synergistically slow the rate of accumulation of activator. Overall, the results indicate that about 10^{-8} M hydroperoxide can trigger the oxygenation catalyzed by PGH synthase [25]. Since this amount represents 0.01% of the polyunsaturated fatty acid in a 10^{-4} M solution, it is easy to understand how most experiments contain enough hydroperoxide so that the requirement is not observed with in vitro protocols. Nevertheless, cells of most tissues normally contain appreciable amounts of peroxidase activity and essentially undetectable amounts of hydroperoxides. Thus, in vivo, the supply of these activators tends to be low so that very small increases in their content could have a major activating action on cellular cyclooxygenase activity in the presence of substrate fatty acid.

3. Inhibitors of prostaglandin biosynthesis

(a) General aspects

There are four important components involved in the PGH synthase reaction: enzyme, two substrates and activator. An agent which interferes with the availability or functioning of any of these components would necessarily inhibit the oxygenation reaction to some degree. Thus, for this discussion, we have divided the inhibitors into four types depending on whether they interfere with: enzyme availability; fatty acid availability; oxygen availability; or hydroperoxide availability.

i. Enzyme availability

The question of the availability of active enzyme includes the availability of the protein portion, or apoenzyme, as well as the availability of the heme cofactor that binds to the protein. At the present time, there are no major recognized selective therapeutic inhibitors of protein synthesis, nor are there recognized selective therapeutic tactics which interfere with the binding of the iron protoporphyrin to the apoenzyme. Both the process of protein synthesis and of heme-protein interaction are so general as to make it unlikely that effective therapeutic agents would be available to selectively inhibit only the cyclooxygenase-related processes. A report of the presence in plasma of an endogenous inhibitor of the prostaglandin H synthase noted that it was located in the haptoglobin fraction [26]. Its mode of action and physiologic importance is not clear, but it may be altering enzyme or heme availability. Recent reports indicate that cyclooxygenase activity can be induced in mastocytoma cells by sodium butyrate [27,28]. This inducible nature of the enzyme opens the possibility that selective inhibition of the induction could be examined in these cells, but no clear evidence for a selective inhibitor or inducer is available at the present time.

One technique in altering the availability of the active enzyme at a tissue site is the irreversible inactivation [9] by certain antiinflammatory agents which bind at the substrate site and irreversibly inactivate the enzyme. Restoration of activity presumably requires synthesis of new catalytically active protein within the cell. This type of enzyme loss when applied selectively to platelets relative to vascular endothelial cells may have benefits in antithrombotic preventive therapy [29].

One important mechanism of limiting the availability of active holoenzyme in a tissue is prevention of the appearance of cells that contain large amounts of active cyclooxygenase. Thus, a number of antiinflammatory agents which limit the total amount of hydroperoxide synthesized in a tissue prevent the migration to the inflammatory site of cells which contain appreciable amounts of cyclooxygenase activity [30]. This inhibition of migration could be achieved by several methods, including blocking the cellular chemotactic receptors or blocking synthesis of the chemotactic agents. Such indirect modes of limiting prostaglandin biosynthesis need to be evaluated when comparing observed in vivo inhibitions of hydroperoxide biosynthesis with results obtained in vitro.

ii. Fatty acid availability

Evaluation of fatty acid availability can be divided into two aspects: the availability of the non-esterified fatty acid in the immediate microenvironment of the cyclooxygenase, and the effective binding of that fatty acid at the active site of the cyclooxygenase. The local availability is regulated predominantly by the nutritional supply of the acid to the cell and by the activity of acylhydrolases and acyltransferases. Some cellular acylhydrolase activity appears to be suppressed by a polypeptide which is formed in greater amounts when induced by antiinflammatory steroids [31]. This seems to be a major mechanism by which steroids lower the amount of substrate available to the cyclooxygenase. The effectiveness of substrate acid binding to the cyclooxygenase active site can be diminished by a variety of physiologic and pharmacologic competitive agents discussed below.

Prostaglandins are synthesized from an essential polyunsaturated fatty acid which cannot be synthesized de novo in mammalian tissues. As a result, the dietary supply of polyunsaturated acid is an important modulating factor in making the appropriate substrate available to the enzyme. The two major types of polyunsaturated fatty acids in mammals are derived from linoleic acid (the (n-6) type) and linolenic acid (the (n-3) type). Arachidonic acid (20 : 4n-6), derived from linoleic acid (18 : 2n-6), is the most common twenty-carbon polyunsaturated fatty acid in human tissues. It is an essential fatty acid in mammals, and it is a major mediator of pathophysiologic events as it is converted to the dienoic prostaglandins and thromboxanes and the tetraenoic leukotrienes [32,33]. Our daily diet usually contains appreciable amounts of grain and cereal products rich in the n-6 fatty acids, and human deficiencies of the n-6 acids are not common.

Eicosapentaenoic acid (20 : 5n-3) which is of the linolenic (n-3) family has attracted much attention recently. This fatty acid is particularly abundant in marine organisms and constitutes a major polyunsaturated fatty acid in the diet of individuals in coastal fishing villages [34]. It is incorporated into tissue lipids in a manner like arachidonate, competing for esterification at the 2-position of the phosphoglycerides. The incidence of myocardial infarction in Greenland Eskimos [35] appears to be a manifestation of the inhibition of prostaglandin synthesis [36] by the long-chain polyunsaturated acids of the linolenic series (20 : 5n-3, 22 : 5n-3 and 22 : 6n-3). Although cyclooxygenase activity can convert eicosapentaenoic acid to triene prostaglandins in vitro [37,38,39], considerable evidence shows that abnormally high peroxide levels are necessary to activate reaction with this acid [25,40]. Thus, under conditions of low peroxide concentrations more closely resembling the physiologic levels in tissues, we find that polyunsaturated acids of the linolenic type (n-3) are unable to be oxygenated by cyclooxygenase activity, and therefore, they serve principally as competitive substrate analogues which block the synthesis of prostaglandins from arachidonate. The fatty acids with longer chain length and greater number of double bonds are most effective in competing for binding [36]. Presumably the reduced incidence of thrombosis in Eskimos is due to competition by the n-3 fatty acids at the active site of cyclooxygenase within blood platelets. Competitive inhibition by the linolenic type of polyunsaturated acid [36] appears to be a more significant mechanism of inhibition of prostaglandin formation than the proposed role of the linolenic type in serving as precursor for trienoic prostaglandins [39].

iii. Oxygen availability

Although two moles of oxygen combine with arachidonate in forming PGG_2 at the catalytic site, there is no clear evidence for oxygen binding to the enzyme or for it being blocked by analogs such as carbon monoxide [6,41]. Cyanide can inhibit cyclooxygenase activity when present at high concentrations, but such levels are much higher than that needed to inhibit other heme proteins. Estimation of the affinity for oxygen indicated that the cyclooxygenase activity was essentially saturated with oxygen above 10 μM O_2 [42]. This value is similar to that reported for cytochrome oxidase [43]. Thus, at all levels of oxygen availability that permit cell respiration, prostaglandin biosynthesis can be expected to function. Oxygen availability in tissue may become limiting in regions 50 μ from the capillary or among vigorously respiring cells. In those conditions, the oxygen availability may also limit prostaglandin biosynthesis.

iv. Hydroperoxide availability

The essential role of hydroperoxides in promoting prostaglandin biosynthesis has been generally overlooked, and few reports explicitly describe the ways by which peroxides may become more or less available to the cyclooxygenases. In the same manner that more cyclooxygenase activity is made available, the recruitment of peroxide forming cells to a site can elevate lipid hydroperoxides. These cells are stimulated to produce peroxides by a variety of conditions [44,45]. Factors that limit either the recruitment or the stimulation of these cells could limit prostaglandin formation.

A second method for maintaining low levels of lipid hydroperoxide activator is prevention of its synthesis. Lipid hydroperoxides are formed in phagocytic cells as a result of the attack of reactive oxygen products on saturated fatty acids [46], and they are also formed by lipoxygenases [47]. In an inflamed lesion, phagocytosing leukocytes have an accelerated generation of superoxide anions as a consequence of their increased NAD(P)H oxidase activity [48]. The hydrogen peroxide and superoxide anion formed by various oxidases [49] can lead to the formation of more reactive oxygen species which, in turn, initiate lipid peroxidation, thus making these cells a potential source for the activator lipid hydroperoxide. Superoxide dismutase, catalase and radical scavengers may act to limit the formation of lipid hydroperoxides [49], and antioxidants such as vitamin E (tocopherol) [50] may also be important in this regard. Hydroxyl radical scavengers such as mannitol and benzoate [51] have also been reported to limit lipid hydroperoxide formation in vitro. Likewise, β-carotene [52] and furan derivatives [53] can limit the formation of lipid hydroperoxides.

Lipid hydroperoxides are also produced enzymatically by lipoxygenase activity. Preparations of purified [54] or semi-purified lipoxygenase [47] allowed isolation of the hydroperoxy acid. However, most reports of tissue lipoxygenase action describe only the production of hydroxy acids by intact cell or crude homogenates [55–59] that rapidly reduce the hydroperoxy acid to the hydroxy acid [47]. Cook and Lands [21] have suggested that there is continuous physiological control by cytosolic factors, glutathione and glutathione peroxidase, which rapidly destroy the lipid hydroperoxide activator.

Glutathione peroxidase is the primary mechanism in cells for lipid hydroperoxide removal [60]. Glutathione peroxidase activity is a function of the level of enzyme, which may be induced by prolonged exposure to increased lipid hydroperoxide levels [61], and a function of the level of reduced glutathione, which is a cosubstrate in the reduction of the lipid hydroperoxide. Glutathione peroxidase activity requires selenium, and a dietary deficiency in this metal can increase the tendency of tissues to form peroxides. Though manipulation to enhance glutathione peroxidase activity seems unlikely in the near future, therapeutic advances in limiting lipid hydroperoxide abundance by using radical scavengers and antioxidants may prove fruitful.

(b) Mechanisms of inhibitor action

i. Competitive substrate analogs

All long chain fatty acids have some ability to mimic arachidonate and bind at the substrate site of prostaglandin H synthase. Thus, competitive inhibition has been described by several laboratories [62,63,64] with stronger binding and inhibition occurring for the more highly unsaturated acids [36,65]. The conjugated analogs (5,8,12,14- and 8,12,14-) are stronger inhibitors than the natural non-conjugated forms [63]. As noted in the general comments above on fatty acid availability, the esterification and release of various dietary acids can affect the binding of arachidonate to the catalytic site. This may give physiologic suppression of prostaglandin formation as suggested by model studies with animals [66,67] and the low incidence of heart attacks in Eskimos [68].

Some aromatic acids are also capable of selective, competitive interaction at the substrate site. These arylacetic and 2-phenylpropionic analogs are members of a large set of non-steroidal anti-inflammatory agents now recognized as anti-cyclooxygenase agents. The two most widely used agents, aspirin and indomethacin, bind competitively at the substrate site [10,69] and additionally cause irreversible inactivation of cyclooxygenase activity (see Section ii below). Many other agents of the arylacetic acid type exhibit a reversible, competitive inhibition of the cyclooxygenase activity. In cases where there is an asymmetric center next to the carboxyl group, the more active stereoisomer tends to have the S-configuration [70]. The chiral influence is variable with a 6-fold preference for dextrorotatory pirprofen and a 130-fold one for dextrorotatory naproxen [71]. The reversible binding of these agents provided classical competitive Lineweaver-Burk plots [72–75] although some reports noted linearity only at substrate concentrations above 60–100 μM [72,73]. Non-linear features below 50 μM indicated a greater degree of inhibition than expected for a classical Michaelis kinetic formulation [72,73]. This effect at low substrate levels is predicted by the complex enzyme mechanism reflecting the need for the cyclooxygenase to generate its own activating hydroperoxide when it is not provided exogenously (see section 3c below). Reviews of the optimal structural characteristics (e.g. refs. 76, 77) emphasized a biplanar array for the substrate site following earlier suggestions of Shen [78]. Recent computer-assisted modelling studies [79] led Shen to reaffirm some of the prior concepts while emphasizing a probable carboxyl binding locus below the plane of the "ring binding region". Another computer study produced a different concept: that the inhibitors may relate closer to the geometry of the peroxyradical [80] that forms during the reaction. Such heuristic examinations of structure activity relationships may develop clearer alternatives for the dimensions of the hypothetical complementary active site.

Acetylenic fatty acids are substrate analogs which provide unusual insight into the interaction of fatty acids with the cyclooxygenase active site. They exhibit both competitive and non-competitive aspects. All of the 18- and 20-carbon acetylenic acids examined [81,10] exhibited a reversible interaction at the active site competitive with arachidonate ($K_I \simeq 2$ to 20 μM).

The tetrayne analog of arachidonate irreversibly inhibited prostaglandin formation [82] and a 9,12-diynoic analog of linoleate was effective against both cyclooxygenase and lipoxygenase activity [83]. In the latter study, no other positional isomers of the diynoic acids and none of the 15 isomers of octadecanoic acid were reported to be effective [83]. In a detailed reexamination of the inhibitory characteristics of the monoynoic substrate analogs, a time-dependent, irreversible inactivation of the cyclooxygenase activity was found for only two isomers: the 10- and 13-octadecynoic acids [81].

The first order rate constants for the irreversible inactivation by various acetylenic analogs ranged from 0.08 to 0.26 min^{-1} [81], and the affinity for the active site was comparable to that of arachidonate ($K_m \simeq 5$ μM). The acetylenic analogs could still inactivate the cyclooxygenase activity when glutathione peroxidase was added to remove peroxides [10]. However, when the enzyme-phenol complex was formed, the irreversible inactivation did not occur in the presence of glutathione peroxidase. This result is analogous to that for substrate-mediated inactivation in that the enzyme-phenol complex (Ea, ref. 20) does not sustain the self-inactivating cyclooxygenase reaction in the presence of glutathione peroxidase [20]. The ability of catalase to prevent the time-dependent inactivation by the acetylene acids suggests that H_2O_2 may serve in the generation of a transient intermediate radical that destroys the catalytic site [84]. Apparently, certain acetylenic isomers react in part as a substrate even though there is no measurable consumption of oxygen. Perhaps these positional isomers form a metastable intermediate of oxygen with the acetylenic bond that leads to destructive side reactions which inactivate the catalytic site rather than providing oxygen consumption and continued turnover at the catalytic site. The high selectivity of this event indicates a strict orientational arrangement with the radical generating part of the catalytic site and certain positions of the acyl chain.

ii. Irreversible time-dependent agents

Soon after the action of antiinflammatory agents upon cyclooxygenase activity was recognized [5], we observed that indomethacin [9,10] and aspirin [10] caused a progressive, irreversible inhibition when left in contact with the enzyme. These agents also compete with arachidonate for the cyclooxygenase substrate site, but their binding constants are not exceptionally strong [10,69]. Their inhibitory potency appeared more dependent upon their rate of inactivation (k') and the length of exposure (t) than upon their binding affinity (K_I) for the active site [69]. The effectiveness of these relatively weak binding agents creates a paradox in comparing the time-dependent, concentration-dependent, irreversible loss of activity to the inhibition by simpler competitive binding agents. Many reports of inhibitors of prostaglandin biosynthesis are based upon the amount of product accumulated over a period of time (often 2 to 20 min) rather than upon the rate of enzyme action. Since the enzyme is exposed to the agent throughout that period of time, and in many cases for a period of time prior to adding substrate, a lower amount of product accumulated may be due not only to competitive binding, but also to an irreversible loss of enzyme. The apparent K_I value obtained in such assays can be appreciably lower than that due to the actual affinity of the agent for the active site. Because of the inactivation phenomenon, agents of similar binding affinity can have very different effectiveness. As an example, 0.3 μM of the irreversible inactivator, flurbiprofen, can rapidly become more inhibitory than 50 μM ibuprofen which has a similar binding constant at the substrate site, but is fully reversible (ref. 69, Fig. 1). Inactivation thus creates a paradoxical behaviour that is very dependent upon the degree of exposure of the enzyme to drug prior to assaying the product formed.

Irreversible drugs like aspirin and indomethacin [9] are prevented from inactivating the cyclooxygenase in a competitive manner by *o*-phenanthroline [9,10], docosahexaenoic acid [10] and arachidonic acid [64]. All of these compounds appear to bind to the complementary active site for substrate described in 3b(i) above. Thus irreversible inactivation by indomethacin and aspirin can be prevented by any reversible competitive inhibitor which binds to that hydrophobic site. Furthermore, since the substrate, arachidonate, can bind more tightly than aspirin or indomethacin [64,69], little inhibition is observed when the drug is added to the enzyme at the same time as substrate. On the other hand, a very brief exposure of the enzyme to low levels of an irreversible agent prior to adding substrate will give extensive inhibition of prostaglandin formation. Thus, a very low level of the irreversible agent indomethacin (0.16 μM) with seminal vesicle microsomes for 2 minutes gave 53% inhibition which was reduced to 24% in the presence of 330 μM of salicyclic acid and prevented completely by 660 μM salicylate [85]. These results confirm the more detailed results with *o*-phenanthroline blocking the irreversible action of indomethacin that were described earlier [10].

Although the 660 μM salicylate could effectively compete against the 0.16 μM indomethacin (when the concentration of [I] was less than the K_I value), it could not appreciably inhibit at 110 μM arachidonate (when [S] was 10 to 20 times the K_s value). Similarly, the ability of 8 μM of the reversible inhibitor diflunesal to block the irreversible action of 0.16 μM indomethacin is predictable since IC_{50} considerations (see Table 1) indicate that diflunesal was present at 3 to 8 times its K_I value whereas indomethacin was present at much lower amounts relative to its binding constant. The assignment of an extremely low value (0.16 μM) for the apparent "K_I" of the irreversible agent, indomethacin, illustrates the paradoxical effect of inadequate kinetic treatments. Thus the recent attribution of the antagonized inhibition that is described above to a putative supplementary site on the enzyme [85] needs a careful reassessment.

Detailed structure-activity studies showed that small structural differences in the agents determined whether or not they caused irreversible inactivation. Particularly striking was the conversion of the free carboxylic acid to the methyl ester which gave an agent that had a similar binding affinity [86], but appeared to be completely devoid of ability to irreversibly inactivate the cyclooxygenase activity. The value of the apparent inactivation constants (K') for the acidic forms of the compounds ranged from zero for ibuprofen and mefenamic acid to 0.0003, 0.04, 0.4 and 1.1 M^{-1} min^{-1} for aspirin, indomethacin, meclofenamate and flurbiprofen, respectively [86].

iii. Non-competitive radical trapping agents

The phenolic inhibitors which can serve as radical trapping agents provide a major paradoxical effect; stimulating cyclooxygenase activity in conditions when relatively high amounts of peroxide occur, and inhibiting when the amount of peroxide is relatively low [6]. This biphasic character seems most likely due to the separate actions of these agents in stimulating peroxidase activity (via CH action, Fig. 1) and also inhibiting the cyclooxygenase activity (via AH action, Fig. 1). Thus, when testing for stimulatory (coenzyme) activity, several dihydroxynapthalenes were observed to be potent inhibitors [87]. The inhibition of cyclooxygenase exerted by phenolic antioxidants was not correlated with either their general antioxidant potency or with their ability to inhibit soybean lipoxygenase [88].

Phenolic inhibitors and their general inhibitory actions were reviewed recently by Dewhirst [18]. Their efficacy in numerous over-the-counter preparations may reflect their ability to inhibit cyclooxygenase activity, and some stringent structural requirements indicate a probable direct interaction with the catalytic protein [18]. Several irreversible phenolic inhibitors appeared to be equal to or more potent than indomethacin in preventing platelet aggregation [18]. Alternatively, this result could reflect a possible lack of irreversible action by indomethacin on cyclooxygenase activity in platelets. In such a case, the apparent "K_I" of indomethacin would resemble the higher value of the "true" K_I. The report [18] noted, however, that longer preincubation times could give lower IC_{50} (or K_I) values for the irreversible agent.

Xylenols and tricresol were effective in blocking prostaglandin formation by 3T3 fibroblasts in culture [89]. Inhibition of aggregation and prostaglandin formation from arachidonate was also described, although the substituted phenols did not block aggregation induced by PGG. Thus, the phenolic agents could inhibit arachidonate oxidation without preventing the conversion of PGG to thromboxane.

A recent provocative interpretation of the role of PGG in inflammation [90] suggested that PGG may act by forming a free radical (tentatively identified as a hydroxyl radical). Support for the concept was based on the effective suppression of inflammation by agents regarded to stimulate the peroxidase-catalyzed conversion of PGG_2 to PGH_2. Since studies showed that prostaglandin synthase activity in vitro could be stimulated by phenol and MK-447, a paradox evolved from the observation that both inhibitors and stimulators of the formation of prostaglandins can suppress inflammatory responses. Resolution of the paradox may come from the fact that phenolic agents do not stimulate when peroxide levels are low in vitro or when prostaglandin peroxidase activity is absent [6]. This reflects again the biphasic effect of agents that have both CH and AH activities (see Fig. 1). Emphasis on the CH activity of some agents [90,91] omits consideration of the inhibitory action (AH) on cyclooxygenase that can be expected with low hydroperoxide levels that do occur in vivo.

(c) IC_{50} concepts and concerns

Published evaluations of the effectiveness of inhibitors of prostaglandin biosynthesis have produced varied quantitative values for a given compound. The preceding sections on the mechanism of action of the enzyme with its activators and inhibitors indicate some of the complex and apparently contradictory aspects of prostaglandin biosynthesis that can occur. This section is designed to review some of the quantitative relationships among the enzyme, substrates, activators and inhibitors that are important in assessing fully the effectiveness of an inhibitor. In many cases, the level of peroxides in in vitro assay systems exceed that necessary for full enzyme activation ($P > K_p$) and no evidence for their requirement is observed. Thus, the general kinetic formulation (I) for the early phases of oxygenase action [92] can be represented in an abbreviated form (II), deleting terms dependent upon hydroperoxide, P. This indicates that the customary Michaelis kinetic formulation can represent the early phases of the oxygenase reaction when adequate hydroperoxide is present.

$$\nu_t = \frac{k_3[E_t]}{1 + \frac{K_S^S}{S_t}\left(1 + \frac{I}{K_I^S}\right) + \frac{K_P^P}{P_t - k_8(P_t)}\left[1 + \frac{I}{K_I^P} + \frac{K_S^S}{S_t}\left(1 + \frac{I}{K_I^S} + \frac{I}{K_I^P} + \frac{I^2}{K_I^P K_I^S}\right)\right]} \tag{I}$$

$$\nu_t = \frac{K_3[E]}{1 + \frac{K_S^S}{S_t}\left(1 + \frac{I}{K_I^S}\right)} \tag{II}$$

An earlier review of these relationships provides more details [86], and this section focuses upon the way that the commonly reported dimension of IC_{50} relates to the molecular events.

i. Substrate related inhibitors

A classical competitive inhibitor binds reversibly to the enzyme at the substrate binding site to form an EI complex with an inhibition constant, K_I, that is the dissociation constant for the enzyme-inhibitor complex:

$$E + I \rightleftharpoons EI \qquad K_I = \frac{[E][I]}{[EI]} \qquad \text{(Scheme 1)}$$

Equation II, which is the classical relationship for a simple competitive system, illustrates that at constant [S] and [I], the more potent inhibitor, producing a smaller ν, will have a smaller observed K_I. The K_I values (dissociation constants) are useful measures of affinity for competitive inhibitors, and they can be obtained easily in the laboratory by recording reaction velocities at a number of inhibitor concentrations at different levels of substrate. The fractional remaining uninhibited velocity (ν_i/ν) in a competitively inhibited system will be

$$\nu_i/\nu = \frac{[S] + K_S}{[S] + K_S(1 + [I]/K_I)} \tag{a}$$

In this case, the fractional uninhibited velocity depends upon the substrate concentration, ranging from (a) at very high [S] to $1/(1 + [I]/K_I)$ at very low [S] values. Thus, reported IC_{50} values for such an agent may vary appreciably although the K_I value is constant.

Non-competitive inhibitors presumably bind at a locus on the enzyme other than the substrate site to form the inactive EI and EIS.

$$\begin{array}{ccccc} E & + S \rightleftharpoons & ES & \xrightarrow{k_3} & E + \text{Product} \\ + & & + & & \\ I & & I & & \\ \downarrow\uparrow & & \uparrow\downarrow & & \\ EI & & EIS & & \end{array} \qquad \text{(Scheme 2)}$$

$$K_I = [E][I]/[EI] \qquad\qquad K_I' = [ES][I]/[ESI]$$

$$v = \frac{k_3[E]\ \text{total}}{(1 + K_S/[S])(1 + [I]/K_I)} \qquad \text{(b)}$$

When binding of either [I] or [S] does not affect the affinity for the other, $K_I' = K_I$, and equation (b) indicates that a lower velocity will be associated with a small K_I value. In this type of inhibition, the fractional uninhibited velocity will be $v_i/v = 1/(1 + [I]/K_I)$, and the IC_{50} values should be constant and independent of substrate concentration.

Table 1 lists the predicted IC_{50} values for an agent with a K_I of 1 μM acting either competitively or non-competitively on an enzyme system for which the substrate has a K_m value of 5 μM.

TABLE 1
The effect of assay conditions on IC_{50} values

Substrate concentration (μM)	Predicted IC_{50} value (μM)	
	Competitive	Non-Competitive
1	1.2	1
5	2.0	1
10	3.0	1
50	11.0	1
100	21.0	1
300	31.0	1

ii. Time-dependent (irreversible) inhibitors

Many of the inhibitors that react with cyclooxygenase in a time-dependent irreversible manner do so by reversibly forming an EI complex at the substrate site which then leads irreversibly by a first-order process to an inactive form of the enzyme, $E^{\dagger}$. The overall scheme of such a competitive, time-dependent inhibitor is then:

$$E + S \rightleftharpoons ES \xrightarrow{k_3} E + P$$

$$E + I \rightleftharpoons EI \xrightarrow{k_3} E^{\dagger}$$

In this example, there is a K_I value for the binding of inhibitor, and the rate of enzyme inactivation is $d[E^{\dagger}]/dt = k[EI]$, where k is the rate constant for the inactivating event (reviewed in ref. 86).

$$v_{obs} = \frac{k_3[E]\exp(-k[I]t/K_I([S]/K_s + [I]/K_I + 1))}{1 + K_s(1 + [I]/K_I)/[S]} \quad \text{(c)}$$

This equation is similar to the rate equation for a classical competitive inhibitor except for the exponential term that modifies the total amount of functional enzyme at any given time. Two constants in equation (c) define the time-dependent activity of the inhibitor: K_I and k. Like the classical competitive example above, the K_I represents the dissociation constant for the enzyme-inhibitor complex. Both ligands, S and I, compete for the catalytic site, and the smaller the value of the K_s and K_I, the greater is the affinity of the enzyme for the substrate and inhibitor, respectively. The rate constant for enzyme destruction, k, generally has dimensions of $\min^{-1}$ for the first order process. A larger numerical value for the k indicates a faster conversion of the EI complex to inert enzyme.

When experiments are performed to estimate either K_I or IC_{50} values, the results will depend on the time, t, at which the velocity is observed as well as upon the concentration of substrate. When t is relatively small, the expression simplifies to equation II, the classical formation. However, as it becomes larger, the velocity falls significantly in a manner dependent upon $k.I.t$. Many investigators have used an averaged velocity based on the amount of product accumulated in one or two minutes without regard for the widely varied velocities that occur during this time. Such an approach simplifies the effort needed and accommodates a pragmatic priority for the recognition of relatively effective drugs irrespective of mechanism. The comparative IC_{50} values obtained may show inconsistencies when applied to interpretations of in vivo effectiveness (see also variable IC_{50} values in Table 2). Failure to account for irreversible inactivation of the enzyme makes uncertain some interpretations (e.g. ref. 85).

Incubation of enzyme and inhibitor in the absence of substrate (often called preincubation) provides a simpler system in which the apparent rate constant for irreversible enzyme loss will be:

$$k_{app} = \frac{k[I]}{K_I + [I]} \quad \text{(d)}$$

This equation predicts higher values for the apparent destruction constant, k_{app}, at higher concentrations of inhibitor. At very low levels of inhibitor ($[I] < K_I$) the value for the k_{app} will vary directly with [I] in a manner similar to curves published for indomethacin and aspirin [10]. In this case, the term $k_{app}/[I]$ which is subsequently defined as k' in this discussion will be approximately equal to k/K_I in magnitude and constant for different [I] values (see Fig. 2a).

Thus, the k' values reported for several recognized antiinflammatory agents had dimensions of min^{-1} μM^{-1} [42]. These were obtained in studies that had small amounts of irreversible inhibitor relative to that needed for binding (K_I value). The inhibitory action followed the pattern illustrated in Fig. 2A. At levels of inhibitor that are in the same concentration range as the K_I, both the k_{app} and the k' values will vary with [I] (Fig. 2B). At very high levels of inhibitor ([I] > K_I) the values for k_{app} from the graph will be nearly independent of [I] and approximately equal to k (Fig. 2C) in a manner similar to curves reported for the acetylenic inhibitors [81]. In that report, the k_{app} values were conveniently expressed as min^{-1}.

iii. Peroxide antagonists

The phenolic radical trapping agents exhibit properties of both non-competitive and competitive inhibition, yielding curvilinear double reciprocal plots that make "simple Michaelis-Menten" analysis unreliable. Thus, Vanderhoek and Lands [88] noted that estimates of K_I were difficult at times for the antioxidants tested because of non-linear responses. A general kinetic formulation of fatty acid oxygenase action that included terms for peroxide activation gave very close agreement with the actual observed behavior of both soybean lipoxygenase [93] and sheep cyclooxygenase [23] activities. That algebraic formulation used equilibrium binding affinities to describe enzyme interactions with the substrate (K_s) and the hydroperoxide (K_p) in the system. When this equation was used to evaluate the inhibition of cyclooxygenase by acetamidophenol, it allowed assignment of K_I values for 1.2 mM and 0.4 mM at the substrate site and hydroperoxide activator site, respectively [23]. These K_I values provide pragmatic summaries of the interactions of enzyme with inhibitor, and in this case, they direct attention to an apparently stronger interference of acetamidophenol with the hydroperoxide activator site. The graphical display of the expected and observed relationship between substrate and inhibitor concentration and reaction velocity showed that interference with hydroperoxide activation gave curvilinear plots with a greater degree of inhibition than was expected for interference only with the substrate binding. Antagonists of the peroxide activation caused increased lag times in the initial phase of the reaction reflecting the need for greater amounts of peroxide to overcome the antagonism [23]. The IC_{50} values are

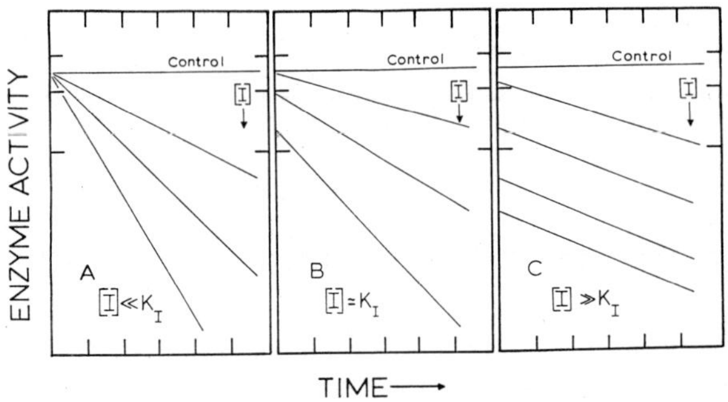

Fig. 2. Kinetic patterns of cyclooxygenase activity loss by irreversible inactivators.

thus very dependent upon the prevailing steady state level of hydroperoxide activator [92]. Thiol analogs of prostaglandins, resembling in part the activating hydroperoxide PGG, were reported to be reversible, noncompetitive (rather than competitive) inhibitors [94]. These seem likely to be capable of serving as hydroperoxide antagonists, and they could be expected to be increasingly effective at lower surrounding concentrations of hydroperoxide activator.

(d) General data available

The preceding section illustrated how the three different types of inhibitory process can produce IC_{50} values that have different relationships to substrate and activator levels. Thus, it is not surprising that the reported values of IC_{50} for a given agent can vary widely (see Table 2) in a way that partially reflects the different substrate concentrations and assay conditions used. For example, IC_{50} values of 0.7, 2, 6.3 and 15 μM were reported from different laboratories for mefenamic acid using substrate concentrations of 1, 10, 100 and 330 μM respectively. Similarly in the case of flufenamic acid, IC_{50} values of 0.8, 3, 30 and 48 μM were separately reported using substrate levels of 1, 10, 100 and 300 μM respectively. Such varied results illustrate the shift in IC_{50} values expected for a competitive inhibition for these agents (see Table 1). A more detailed kinetic analysis of mefenamic [69] gave a value of 1 μM

TABLE 2

Reported IC_{50} values for anti-inflammatory agents

The values in this table represent the values (in μM) for the IC_{50} and the arachidonate concentration used in the assay; the letter designates the reference indicated below. Thus, '204/330/d' indicates that an IC_{50} value of 204 μM was obtained when 330 μM archidonate were used as cited by Taylor and Salata [72]. Abbreviations indicate tissues for which the archidonate concentration was not specified: BSV, bovine seminal vesicles; HRS, human rheumatoid synovium; cell, MC5-5 cell line.

Phenylbutazone	7.2/33/a, 12.0/cell/b, 150/10/c, 204/330/d, 420/330/e, 875/100/f, 1400/100/g
Ibuprofen	3.8/cell/b, 6/1/h, 34.9/30/i, 1200/330/e, 2000/100/g
Naproxen	6.8/cell/b, 32/330/d, 100/330/j, 220/330/e, 370/100/g
Tolmetin	5.4/cell/b, 11.7/330/d
Ketoprofen	0.9/cell/b, 9.0/30/i
Niflumic acid	0.11/33/a, 0.3/1/h, 18/100/k
Flufenamic	0.8/1/h, 3/10/c, 6/330/d, 8.5/100/K, 30/100/f, 48/330/e
Mefenamic	0.7/1/h, 0.75/33/a, 2/10/c, 4/330/d, 6.3/100/k, 15/330/e
Meclofenamic	0.1/33/a, 0.6/1/h, 10/100/g
Flubiprofen	0.017/BSV/1, 0.136/150/m, 0.17/HRS/1, 1.4/cell/b
Indomethacin	0.36/HRS/1, 0.6/cell/1, b, h, 0.88/3.3/n, 1.4/330/a, 1.7/150/m, 2/330/e, c, 2.8/100/f, 7.0/330/j, 10/330/d, 17/33/a, 40/100/g, 43.3/30/i
Aspirin	2.3/330/d, 37/33/a, 60/330/o, 93/HRS/1, 110/cell/b, 120/3.3/n, 476/BSV/1, 600/10/c, 820/330/e, 1,100/1/h, 1,600/100/f, 4,400/30/i, 9,000/100/g, 15,000/330/j

a-Flower et al. [96]; b-Carty et al. [97]; c-Ziel and Krupp [98]; d-Taylor and Salata [72]; e-Takeguchi and Sih [99]; f-Horodniak et al. [100]; g-Flower et al. [101]; h-Cushman and Chueng [102]; i-Tachizawa et al. [103]; j-Tomlinson et al. [104]; k-Egan et al. [105]; 1-Crook et al. [106]; m-Nozu [107]; n-Gafni et al. [108]; o-Horodniak et al. [109].

for the competitive inhibition constant, K_I. This single value is consistent with the various IC_{50} values reported from other laboratories. The value of this K_I constant is independent of varying substrate concentration, and it corresponds, for example, to an IC_{50} value of 2 μM when the substrate concentration in the assay is the K_s value of 10 μM (see Table 1).

The relationship between reported IC_{50} values and substrate concentrations are not as easily interpreted for the agents known to cause a time-dependent, irreversible inactivation of the cyclooxygenase activity such as meclofenamic acid, flurbiprofen, indomethacin and aspirin [69]. The IC_{50} values for these agents also reflect the duration of exposure of enzyme to the inhibitor, and appreciable preincubation can produce very low IC_{50} values. Thus, the apparent "effectiveness" of these agents is a complex result of several factors that investigators may wish to avoid (for example, see ref. 72). Nevertheless, IC_{50} values can cause considerable confusion in comparisons between different systems with different substrate and cofactor levels. Also, neglect of irreversible inactivation in assessing inhibitors of cyclooxygenase activity can make subsequent interpretations somewhat compromised. An example is the report that IC_{50} values for fenaprofen varied from 1 to 100 μM with varied substrate levels from 1 to 82 μM, and relatively invariant IC_{50} values occurred for indomethacin [95]. The assays were initiated by adding enzyme to substrate and inhibitor, and products were isolated after 15 minutes of incubation. The competition of substrate and inhibitor for the cyclooxygenase active site during that time provides complex kinetics not easily summarized in a single value such as an IC_{50}.

4. Summary

The cyclooxygenase catalyzed formation of prostaglandin G_2 from arachidonic acid appears to be a hydroperoxide initiated free radical chain reaction. Physiologic suppression of this synthetic event is primarily achieved by suppressing the availability of both the nonesterified substrate acid and the hydroperoxide activator. Pharmacologic suppression of prostaglandin biosynthesis has been achieved: by limiting the availability of the nonesterified substrate acid with antiinflammatory steroids; by competitively interfering with hydrophobic analogs; by antagonizing the action of hydroperoxide activators with antioxidant radical trapping agents; by irreversibly inactivating the cyclooxygenase activity with specific acidic compounds. The complexity of the activator and inhibitor interactions has often provided paradoxical reports that require more complete consideration of the factors involved to fully evaluate the mechanism of action and relative effectiveness of an agent.

Acknowledgment

This review was supported in part by a grant (PCM-80-15638) from the National Science Foundation, and an award from the E.M. Bane Estate Trust, University of Illinois.

References

1 Samuelsson, B. (1965) J. Am. Chem. Soc. 87, 1011–1013.
2 Hemler, M.E., Smith, W.L. and Lands, W.E.M. (1976) J. Biol. Chem. 251, 5575–5579.
3 Miyamoto, T., Ogino, N., Yamamoto, S. and Hayaishi, O. (1976) J. Biol. Chem. 251, 2629–2636.
4 van Der Ouderaa, F.J., Buytenhek, M., Nugteren, D.H., and van Dorp, D.A. (1977) Biochim. Biophys. Acta 487, 315–331.
5 Vane, J.R. (1971) Nat. New Biol. 231, 232–235.
6 Hemler, M.E. and Lands, W.E.M. (1980) J. Biol. Chem. 255, 6253–6261.
7 van Der Ouderaa, F.J., Buytenek, M., Slikkerveer, F.J. and Van Dorp, D.A. (1979) Biochim. Biophys. Acta 572, 29–42.
8 Hemler, M.E. and Lands, W.E.M. (1977) Lipids 12, 591–595.
9 Smith, W.L. and Lands, W.E.M. (1971) J. Biol. Chem. 246, 6700–6704.
10 Lands, W.E.M., LeTellier, P.R., Rome, L.H. and Vanderhoek, J.Y. (1974) in Prostaglandin Synthetase Inhibitors (Robinson, H.J. and Vane, J.R., eds.) pp. 1–7, Raven Press, New York.
11 Hemler, M.E. and Lands, W.E.M. (1980) Arch. Biochem. Biophys. 201, 586–593.
12 Rollins, T.E. and Smith, W.L. (1980) J. Biol. Chem. 255, 4872–4875.
13 Ogino, N., Ohki, S., Yamamoto, S., Okuma, M. and Hayaishi, O. (1978) J. Biol. Chem. 252, 5871–5874.
14 Hemler, M.E., Graff, G. and Lands, W.E.M. (1978) Biochem. Biophys. Res. Commun. 85, 1325–1331.
15 Nugteren, D.H., Beerthius, R.K. and van Dorp, D.A. (1966) Recl. Trav. Chim. Pays-Bas Belg. 86, 1237–1245.
16 Takeguchi, C., Kohno, E. and Sih, C.J. (1971) Biochemistry 10, 2372–2376.
17 Yamazaki, I. (1974) in Molecular Mechanisms of Oxygen Activation (Hayaishi, O., ed.) pp. 535–554, Academic Press, New York.
18 Dewhirst, F. (1980) Prostaglandins 20, 209–222.
19 Smith, W.L. and Lands, W.E.M. (1972) J. Biol. Chem. 247, 1038–1047.
20 Smith, W.L. and Lands, W.E.M. (1972) Biochemistry 11, 3276–3285.
21 Cook, H.W. and Lands, W.E.M. (1976) Nature 276, 630–632.
22 Hemler, M.E., Cook, H.W. and Lands (1979) Arch. Biochem. Biophys. 193, 340–345.
23 Lands, W.E.M., Cook, H.W. and Rome, L.H. (1976) in Advances in Prostaglandin and Thromboxane Research Vol. 1 (Samuelsson, B. and Paoletti, R., eds.) pp. 7–17, Raven Press, New York.
24 Hemler, M.E., Graff, G. and Lands, W.E.M. (1978) Biochem. Biophys. Res. Commun. 85, 1325–1331.
25 Lands, W.E.M. and Brynes, M.J. (1982) Prog. Lipid Res. 20, 287–290.
26 Saeed, S.A., McDonald-Gibson, W.J., Cuthbert, J., Copas, J.L., Schneider, C., Gardiner, P.J., Butt, N.M. and Collier, H.O.J. (1977) Nature 270, 32–36.
27 Kawamura, M., Koshihara, Y., Senshu, T. and Murota, S. (1980) Prostaglandins 19, 659–669.
28 Koshihara, Y., Senshu, T., Kawamura, M. and Murota, S. (1980) Biochim. Biophys. Acta 617, 536–539.
29 Jaffe, E.A., and Weksler, B.B. (1979) J. Clin. Invest. 63, 532–535.
30 Di Rosa, M., Papadimitriou, J.M. and Willoughby, D.A. (1971) J. Pathol. 105, 239–256.
31 Flower, R. (1981) Trends Pharmacol. Sci. 2, 186–189.
32 Samuelsson, B., Borgeat, P., Hammarstrom, S. and Murphy, R.C. (1980) in Advances in Prostaglandin and Thromboxane Research, Vol. 6 (Samuelsson, B., Ramwell, P. and Paoletti, R., eds.) pp. 1–18, Raven Press, New York.
33 Samuelsson, B., Goldyne, M., Granstrom, E., Hamberg, S., Hammarstrom, S. and Malmsten, C. (1978) Annu. Rev. Biochem., 47, 997–1029.
34 Bang, H.O., Dyerberg, J. and Hjorne, N. (1975) Am. J. Clin. Nut. 28, 958–966.
35 Dyerberg, J., Bang, H.O., Stoffersen, E., Moncada, S. and Vane, J.R. (1978) Lancet i, 117–119.
36 Lands, W.E.M., LeTellier, P.R., Rome, L.H. and Vanderhoek, J.Y. (1973) Adv. Biosci. 9, 15–27.
37 Needleman, P., Raz, A., Minkes, M.S., Ferrendelli, J.A. and Sprecher, H. (1979) Proc. Natl. Acad. Sci. USA 76, 944–948.
38 Hamberg, M. (1980) Biochim. Biophys. Acta 618, 389–398.

39 Moncada, S. and Vane, J.R. (1979) Fed. Proc. 38, 66–71.
40 Culp, B.R., Titus, B.G. and Lands, W.E.M. (1979) Prostaglandins and Medicine 3, 269.
41 Ohki, S., Ogino, N., Yamamoto, S. and Hayaishi, O. (1979) J. Biol. Chem. 254, 829–836.
42 Lands, W.E.M., Sauter, J. and Stone, G.W. (1978) Prostaglandins and Medicine 1, 117–120.
43 Jobsis, F.F., (1964) in Handbook of Physiologic Respiration Section 3, Vol. 1, Chap. 2, pp. 63–84, Am. Physiol. Soc., Wash. D.C.
44 Stossel, T.P. (1974) N. Engl. J. Med. 290, 717–780.
45 Simon, L.S. and Mills, J.A. (1980) N. Engl. J. Med. 302, 1179–1185.
46 Pryor, W.A. (1973) Fed. Proc. 32, 1862–1869.
47 Nugteren, D.H. (1975) Biochim. Biophys. Acta 380, 299–307.
48 Badway, T.A. and Karnovsky, M.L. (1980) Annu. Rev. Biochem. 49, 625–726.
49 Chance, B., Sies, H. and Boveries, A. (1979) Physiol. Rev. 59, 527–613.
50 Cohen, G. (1975) in Progress in Clinical and Biological Research (ed. Brewer, G.) pp. 685–698, Liss, New York.
51 Fong, K.L., McCay, P.B., Poyer, J.L., Keele, B.B and Misra, H. (1973) J. Biol. Chem. 248. 7792–7797.
52 Anderson, S.M., Krinsky, N.I., Stone, M.J. and Clagett, D.C. (1974) Photochem. Photobiol. 20, 65–69.
53 Kellog, E.W. III and Fridovich, I. (1975) J. Biol. Chem. 250, 8812–8817.
54 Grossman, S., Shahin, I., and Sredni, B. (1979) Biochim. Biophys. Acta 572, 293–297.
55 Hamberg, M. and Samuelsson, B. (1974) Proc. Natl. Acad. Sci. USA 71, 3400–3404.
56 Borgeat, P., Hamberg, M. and Samuelsson, B. (1976) J. Biol. Chem. 251, 7816–7820.
57 Rapoport, S.M., Schewe, T., Wiesner, R., Halangk, W., Ludwig, P., Janicke-Hohne, M., Tannert, C., Hiebsch, C. and Klatt, D. (1979) Eur. J. Biochem. 96, 545–561.
58 Goetzl, E.J. and Sun, F.F. (1979) J. Exp. Med. 150, 406–411.
59 Murphy, R.C., Hammarstrom, S. and Samuelsson, B. (1979) Proc. Natl. Acad. Sci. USA 76, 4275–79.
60 Flohe, L., Gunzler, W.A. and Ladenstein, R. (1976) in Glutathione: Metabolism and Function (Arias, I.M. and Jakoby, B., eds.) pp. 115–138 Raven Press, New York.
61 Reddy, J.K. and Tappel, A.L. (1974) J. Nutr. 104, 1069–1078.
62 Pace-Asciak, C. and Wolfe, L.S. (1969) Biochim. Biophys. Acta 152, 784–787.
63 Nugteren, D.H. (1970) Biochim. Biophys. Acta 210, 171–176.
64 Lands, W.E.M., LeTellier, P., Rome, L. and Vanderhoek, J. (1972) Fed. Proc. 31, 476.
65 Ziboh, V.A., Vanderhoek, J.Y. and Lands, W.E.M. (1974) Prostaglandins 5, 233–240.
66 Black, K.L., Culp, B.R., Madison, D., Randall, O.S. and Lands, W.E.M. (1979) Prostaglandins and Medicine 3, 257–268.
67 Culp, B.R., Lands, W.E.M., Lucchesi, B.R., Pitt, B. and Romson, J. (1980) Prostaglandins 20, 1021–1031.
68 Bang, H.O. and Dyerberg, J. (1972) Acta Med. Scand. 192, 85–94.
69 Rome, L.H. and Lands, W.E.M. (1975) Proc. Natl. Acad. Sci. USA 72, 4863–4865.
70 Juby, P.F., Goodwin, W.R., Hudyma, T.W. and Partyka, R.A. (1972) J. Med. Chem. 15, 1297–1306.
71 Ku, E.C. and Wasvary, J.M. (1975) Biochim. Biophys. Acta 384, 360–368.
72 Taylor, R.J. and Salata, J.J. (1976) Biochem. Pharmacol. 25, 2479–2484.
73 Van Den Berg, G., Bultsma, T. and Nauta, W.T. (1975) Biochem. Pharmacol. 24, 1115–1119.
74 Procacinni, R.L., Smyth, R.D. and Reavey-Cantwell, N.H. (1977) Biochem. Pharmacol. 26, 1051–1057.
75 Shibata, Y. (1980) Arzneim-Forsch. 30, 1074–1076.
76 Shen, T.Y., Ham, E.A., Cirillo, V.J. and Zanetti, M. (1974) in Prostaglandin Synthetase Inhibitors, pp. 19–31, Raven Press, New York.
77 Gryglewski, R.J. (1974) in Prostaglandin Synthetase Inhibitors (1974) pp. 33–52, Raven Press, New York.
78 Shen, T.Y. (1967) Top. Med. Chem. 1, 29.
79 Gund, P. and Shen, T.Y. (1977) J. Med. Chem. 20, 1146–1152.
80 Appleton, R.A. and Brown, K. (1979) Prostaglandins 18, 29–34.

81 Vanderhoek, J. and Lands, W.E.M. (1973) Biochim. Biophys. Acta 296, 374–381.
82 Ahern, D.G. and Downing, D.T. (1970) Biochim. Biophys. Acta 210, 456–461.
83 Downing, D.T., Barve, J.A., Gunstone, F.D., Jacobsberg, F.R. and Lie Ken Jie, M. (1972) Biochim. Biophys. Acta 280, 343–347.
84 Vanderhoek, J.Y. and Lands, W.E.M. (1978) Prostaglandins and Medicine 1, 251–263.
85 Humes, J.L., Winter, C.A., Sadowski, S.J. and Kuehl, F.A. (1981) Proc. Natl. Acad. Sci. USA 78, 2053–2056.
86 Lands, W.E.M. and Rome, L.H. (1976) in Prostaglandins: Chemical and Biochemical Aspects (Karim, S., ed.) pp. 87–137, University Park Press.
87 Takeguchi, C. and Sih, C.J. (1972) Prostaglandins 2, 169–184.
88 Vanderhoek, J. and Lands, W.E.M. (1973) Biochim. Biophys. Acta 296, 382–385.
89 Lindgren, J.A., Claesson, H. and Hammarstrom, S. (1977) Prostaglandins 13, 1093–1102.
90 Kuehl, F.A., Humes, J.L., Egan, R.W., Ham, E.A., Beveridge, G.C. and Van Arman, C.G. (1977) Nature 265, 170–172.
91 Egan, R.W., Gale, P.H., Beveridge, G.C., Phillips, G.B. and Marnett, L.J. (1978) Prostaglandins 16, 861–869.
92 Lands, W.E.M. and Hemler, M.E. (1979) in Biochemical and Clinical Aspects of Oxygen (Caughey, W.S., ed.) pp. 213–223, Academic Press, New York.
93 Cook, H.W. and Lands, W.E.M. (1975) Can. J. Biochem. 53, 1220–1231.
94 Ohki, S., Ogino, N., Yamamoto, S. and Hayaishi, M. (1977) J. Biol. Chem. 144–148.
95 Ho, P.P.K. and Esterman, M.A. (1974) Prostaglandins 6, 107–111.
96 Flower, R., Gryglewski, R., Herbaczynska Cedro, K. and Vane, J.R. (1972) Nat. New Biol. 238, 104–106.
97 Carty, T.J., Eskra, J.D., Lombardino, J.G. and Hoffman, W.W. (1980) Prostaglandin 19, 51–59.
98 Ziel, R., Krupp, P. (1975) Int. J. Clin. Pharmacol. 12, 186–191.
99 Takeguchi, C. and Sih, C.J. (1972) Prostaglandins 2, 169–184.
100 Horodniak, J.W., Matz, E.D., Walz, D.T., Sutton, B.M., Berkoff, C.E., Zarembo, J.E. and Bender, A.D. (1975) Res. Commun. Chem. Path. Pharmacol. 11, 533–542.
101 Flower, R.J., Cheung, H.S., and Cushman, D.W. (1973) Prostaglandins 4, 325–341.
102 Cushman, D.W. and Cheung, H.S. (1976) Biochim. Biophys. Acta 424, 449–459.
103 Tachizawa, H., Tsukada, W., Saito, T. and Akomoto, T. (1977) Jpn J. Pharmacol. 27, 351–359.
104 Tomlinson, R.V., Ringold, H.J., Qureshi, M.C. and Forchielli, E. (1972) Biochem. Biophys. Res. Commun. 46, 552–558.
105 Egan, R.W., Humes, J.L. and Kuehl, F. (1977) Biochemistry 17, 2230–2233.
106 Crook, D., Collins, J. and Rose, A.J. (1976) J. Pharm. Pharmacol. 28, 535.
107 Nozu, K. (1978) Biochim. Biophys. Acta 529, 493–496.
108 Gafni, Y., Schwantzman, M. and Raz, A. (1978) Prostaglandins 15, 759–772.
109 Horodniak, J.W., Julius, M., Zarembo, J.E. and Bender, A.D. (1974) Biochem. Biophys. Res. Commun. 57, 539–545.

Subject index

Activation of prostaglandin biosynthesis
ferriprotoporphyrin 175, 206
heme requirement 174, 205
lag phase 206
lipid hydroperoxides 179, 206
manganoprotoporphyrin 175, 205
peroxide levels 209
Agonists of Thromboxane A
derivatives of $PGF_{2\alpha}$
16-fluorophenoxy (ICI 79939) 68
structural analogues to PGH_2
9,11-azo 67
9,11-etheno 67
9,11-dithio 67
9,11-epoxy (GBR 30728) 67
9,11-epoxy (SQ 26,536) 67
9,11-methanoepoxy (U 46619) 67
structural analogues to TXA_2
carbocyclic TXA_2 68
9,11-epithio-11,12-methylene TXA_2 68
9,11-methylene-11,12-epithio TXA_2 68
Antagonists of
leukotrienes
benzopyrones, 158
FPL 55712 158
rotenone 158
prostaglandin D_2
N-0164 109
Thromboxane A_2
other compounds
AH 19437 69
EP 045 70
7-oxabicyclo [2.2.1]heptane prostaglandins 70
phthalazinol (EG 626) 70
structural analogues to PGH_2
13-aza 69
9,11-azo 68
9,11-epoxy (SQ 26,536) 69
9,11-epoxyimino (EIP) 68
structural analogues to TXA_2
11α-carbathromboxane A_2 69
carbocyclic thromboxane A_2 (CTA_2) 69
15-deoxy-15,16-dihydro-11αcarbathromboxane A_2 69
9,11-epoxy-11α-carbathrombanoic acid 69
Assay of, 6-keto $PGF_{1\alpha}$
gas chromatography-mass spectrometry 108
levels in blood, urine, CSF and amniotic fluid 104–107
radioimmunoassay 108
Leukotrienes
aggregation of leukocytes 152
chemotaxis/chemokineses 152
gas chromatography-mass spectrometry 154
high performance liquid chromatography 152
smooth muscle strips 150
use of antagonists 150, 151
prostacyclin
cardiovascular effects 108
inhibition of platelet aggregation 107
smooth muscle strips 107
prostaglandins 23
11-deoxy-13,14-dihydro-15-keto-11β, 16ξ-cyclo PGE_2 24
15-keto-13,14-dihydro compounds 24
levels in blood and urine 24
measurement of capacity 23
methods
bioassay on superfusion cascade 25
gas chromatography 26
gas chromatography-mass spectrometry 25
high performance liquid chromatography 26
radioimmunoassay 25
urinary-type metabolites in blood 25
thromboxane A_2
antagonists 63
delay coil 63
lung parenchymal strip 63
methods
electron capture-gas chromatography 65
fluorescence-HPLC 65
gas chromatography-mass spectrometry 65

pitfalls in 66
radioimmunoassay 65
platelet aggregation 63
thromboxane metabolites
gas chromatography-mass spectrometry 67
radioimmunoassay 67
vascular preparations 62

Biological effects of, leukotrienes on
aggregation/adhesion 145
chemokinesis 142
chemotaxis 142
enzyme secretion 144
smooth muscle 148
superoxide production 145
vascular permeability 149
prostacyclin on
adenylate cyclase 110
blood pressure 112
blood vessels 112
collagen strips 110
gastric mucosa 109
microcirculation 113
platelet aggregates 110
platelets 109
pulmonary vascular bed 112
rabbit aortic strip 112
renin 109
template bleeding time 110
prostaglandins on
bone resorption 12
cyclic AMP 12
fever 12
gastric acid secretion 12, 15, 16
cytoprotection 15
enteropooling 16
gastrointestinal bleeding 15
kidney function 14
Bartter's syndrome 15
essential fatty acid deficiency 14
medullary flow 14
renal failure 14
renin release 15
sodium balance 14
tubular flow 14
lipolysis 12
nervous system 17, 18
alcoholism 19
cerebral blood vessels 18
fever 18
manodepressive psychoses 19
migraine 19
neuronal activity 18
schizophrenia 19
sedation 18
seizures 18
temperature regulation 18
pancreatic secretion 12
platelet aggregation 12, 15
reproductive system 13
artificial insemination 14
endogenous luteolytic hormone 14
labour induction 14
resorption of sodium and water 12
respiratory system 16
smooth muscle 11
vascular beds 12
vascular leakage 12
vascular system 16
blood pressure 12
microcirculation 16
Raynaud's disease 16
thromboxanes on
chemotaxis 52
gastric mucosa 50
polymorphonuclear leukocytes
adhesiveness 51
effect of TX synthase inhibitors 51
smooth muscle 50
Biosynthesis of, leukotrienes
A 129, 130
B 130
C 131
D 131
E 131
distribution 134, 135
prostaglandins
fatty acid cyclooxygenase 10, 171
catalytic properties 173
distribution 172
localisation 172
molecular properties 172
prostaglandin hydroperoxidase
association with cyclooxygenase 178
chemiluminescence 181
co-oxygenation of xenobiotics 180
hydrogen acceptors 179
hydrogen donors 179
lack of GSH peroxidase 178
PGA synthase 186
PGB synthase 186
PGC synthase 186
PGD synthase
occurrence 11, 184
PGE synthase

occurrence 11, 185
purification 185
requirement for glutathione 185
PGF synthase
occurrence 11, 185
PGI synthase, 6(9) oxycyclase
formation of HHD from PGH_1 101
localisation in endoplasmic reticulum 100
occurrence 99, 185
properties 101
purification 101, 185
thromboxanes
TXA synthase 52, 183
formation of TXA_3 55
HHD 55, 184
C21-TXA_2 55
MDA 184
localisation in dense tubular system 53
modulation 55
occurrence 52
properties 54
purification 53, 183
stimulation in sensitised lung 53, 71
stimulation in ureteral obstruction 52
stimulation with thrombin 54

Clinical trials with prostacyclin in
acute cerebral ischaemia 115
arteriosclerosis obliterans 114
cardiopulmonary bypass 116
central retinal vein occlusion 115
hemolytic uremic syndrome 116
ischaemic stroke 117
ischaemic ulceration 117
peripheral vascular disease 114
preeclamptic toxemia 116
pulmonary artery stenosis 116
pulmonary hypertension 115
Raynaud's syndrome 117
renal transplants 117
spontaneous angina 115
thrombotic thrombocytopenia purpura 116

Dietary influences on, prostaglandin production
dihomo-γ-linolenate-rich diet 32
effects on
arterial thrombosis 31
bleeding time 32
cardiovascular disease 31
platelet aggregation 31
salt-induced hypertension 31
fish oil feeding 32
linoleic acid-rich diet 31
thromboxane production
fish oil feeding
effects on bleeding time 59
effects on myocardial infarction 59, 209
formation of PGI_3 59
garlic 60
onion 60
Discovery of
essential fatty acids 1
HHT 46
12L-HPETE 46
6-keto $PGF_{1\alpha}$ 96
leukotrienes 127
6(9)oxy product 95
prostacyclin, PGX 96
prostaglandin endoperoxides – PGG, PGH 45
prostaglandins 1
SRS-A 131
thromboxanes 45

Inhibition of fatty acid cyclooxygenase by non-steroidal antiinflammatory drugs
aspirin 13, 177, 211, 212, 217, 220
ETYA 211
flubiprofen 217
flufenamic acid 217
ibuprofen 217
indomethacin 13, 177, 211, 212, 217, 220
ketoprofen 217
meclofenamic acid 217
mefenamic acid 217, 219, 220
naproxen 211
niflufenamic acid 217
phenylbutazone 217
tolmetin 217
other compounds
β-carotene 210
mannitol 210
tricresol 214
vitamin E 210
xylenols 214
leukotriene synthesis
AT-125 140
L-cysteine 141
δ-D-glutamyl-O-carboxy phenylhydrazine 140
some lipoxygenase inhibitors 157
3-mercaptopropionic acid 141
D-pencillamine 141

lipoxygenase
acetone phenylhydrazone 156
benoxaprofen 156
BW 755C 156
β-carotene 210
chlorpromazine 155
cyanide 155
EDTA 155
ETYA 155, 211
ETYA analogues 156
flavonoids 155
flurbiprofen 157
indomethacin 157
mannitol 210
NDGA 155
phenidone 156
toluene-3,4-dithiol 155
PGI synthase
9,11-diaza-PGH analogue 102
9,11-epoxyimino-PGH analogue 102
15-hydroperoxy arachidonic acid 101
nicotinic acid 108
tranylcypromine 102
vitamin E deficiency 102
TXA_2 synthetase
9,11-azo analogue 57
9,11-azo-15-deoxy analogue 57
9,11-azo-13-oxa analogue 57
benzydamine 55
burimamide 57
1-carboxyheptylimidazole 56
cimetidine 57
clotrimazole 56
diazoxide 57
dipyridamole 57
9,11-epoxymethano analogue 57
hydralazine 57
imidazole 56
9,11-iminoepoxy analogue 58
3-(1-imidazolylmethyl) indole 56
L-8027 56
metapyrone 56
9,11-methanoepoxy analogue (U46619) 57
metiamide 57
MPAA 111
N-0164 56
nicotinic acid 57
nonyl imidazole 56
OKY-046 111
OKY-1580 111
OKY-1581 57
SQ 80, 338 56
timnodonic acid (EPA) 59
TPCK 58
UK-34787 56
UK-37, 248 57

Metabolism of, arachidonic acid by
autoxidation 8, 139
cyclooxygenase 10
co-oxygenation of xenobiotics 11
PGG and PGH formation 11
13-pro S hydrogen elimination 10
monooxygenase system (cytochrome P-450)
epoxidation 27, 196
epoxide hydrolase 27, 196
lipogenases
5- 129, 134, 136, 193, 194, 195
8- 136
9- 136
11- 136, 139
12- 136, 138, 193, 194, 195
15- 136, 139, 194, 195, 196
soybean L-2 196
leukotrienes by
dipeptidase 141
γ-glutamyltranspeptidase 133, 141
glutathione-S-transferase 133
ω-oxidation 142
prostacyclin and 6-keto $PGF_{1\alpha}$
amniotic fluid levels 105, 106
cerebrospinal fluid levels 107
circulating metabolites 103
NADP-linked 15-PGDH 103
9-PGDH, 6-keto PGE_1 103
plasma levels 104, 106
urinary levels 105, 106
urinary metabolites 103, 106
prostaglandins and thromboxane by
15-hydroxyprostaglandin dehydrogenase,
inhibition by ethacrynic acid 189
furosemide 189
indomethacin 189
NAD (Type I) 19, 61, 187
NADP (Type II) 189
occurrence 187, 189
PGA-specific dehydrogenase 189
PGD-specific dehydrogenase 189
PGI-specific dehydrogenase 190
9-hydroxyprostaglandin dehydrogenase 190
9-keto prostaglandin reductase 191
11-keto prostaglandin reductase, 22
Δ13-prostaglandin reductase 61, 192

β-oxidation 60, 61, 192
ω-oxidation 192
11-dehydrogenation of thromboxanes 61
Metabolites, plasma
of 6-keto $PGF_{1\alpha}$ 102, 104, 106
of prostacyclin 102, 104, 106
of prostaglandins 20, 24
of thromboxanes 60, 66
urine
of 6-keto $PGF_{1\alpha}$ 102, 105, 106
of prostacyclin 102, 105, 106
of prostaglandins 21
of thromboxanes 61, 66

Nomenclature of
leukotrienes, 127, 128
prostacyclin and 6-keto $PGF_{1\alpha}$ 96
prostaglandins 2
thromboxanes 49

Protection from inhibition of fatty acid cyclox-ygenase by
arachidonic acid 212
diflunesal 213
docosa hexaenoic acid 212
O-phenanthroline 212
salicyclic acid 213

Release of, precursor fatty acids, by
inhibition by
glucocorticoids 8
macrocortin 8
lipomodulin 8
mechanism 7
phospholipase A_2 5, 208
phospholipase C 6
stimulation by
bradykinin 6
calcium 7
ischaemia 6
thrombin 6
leukotrienes 130, 131, 135
prostacyclin 99, 104–107
prostaglandins 17, 24
thromboxane from sensitised lungs
blocked by β-adrenergic receptor compounds 72
non steroidal antiinflammatory drugs, 72
TXA_2 blockers 72
FPL 55712 72
lack of effect by, α-adrenergic receptor agonists 72
reversal by, β-adrenergic blocking drugs 72
stimulated by histamine, 72
SRS-A 72

Side effects of prostacyclin administration
drowsiness 116
facial flush 116
headache 116
hypotension 116
restlessness 116
tachychardia 116
Stimulation of, fatty acid cyclooxygenase
epinephrine 175
hydroquinone 175
MK-447 214
phenol 175, 214
tryptophan 175
leukotriene synthesis
calcium ionophore 132
cyclooxygenase inhibitors 134
fMLP 142
prostaglandin hydroperoxidase
p-aminophenol 179
benzidine 179
epinephrine 179
guiaicol 179
hydroquinone 179
phenol 179
serotonin 179
tetrahydrofolic acid 179
tetramethylphenylenediamine 179
tryptophan 179
uric acid 179
TXA_2 synthetase
calcium ionophores A23187 58
X538A 58
estrogens 59
heparin 58
norepinephrine 59
vasopressin 59
Structure of
dihomoprostaglandins 4
6-keto $PGF_{1\alpha}$ 97
leukotrienes 128
mono-O-methyl thromboxanes 47
oxetane-oxane ring of thromboxanes 48
primary prostaglandins 4, 96
prostacyclin 97
prostaglandin endoperoxides, PGG, PGH 4
prostaglandin metabolites 4